Decolonizing Global Healt

A Critical Realist Perspecti

AF760595

This insightful work uses a critical realist perspective to unpack the colonially informed culture, structures, and mechanisms which exist across global health institutions, offering a vision for radical change through a process of decolonization.

Shedding light on the institutional structures that perpetuate and sustain long-standing power imbalances in global health research and practice, postcolonial critical realism provides a cogent, meta-theoretical basis for understanding colonialism and decolonization. It reveals these structures as social constructions rather than naturally occurring phenomena. In astutely examining a range of factors, from the language of global health to the principles and practice of research in this field, the book identifies not only the role that colonialism continues to play, but also the means by which it can be subverted.

Written by a prominent author in this important field of study, this book will be key reading for students and scholars from public health to medicine, as well as philosophy, anthropology, and development studies.

Ferdinand C. Mukumbang is an Assistant Professor at the Department of Global Health, University of Washington, US. He is a public health scientist specializing in health policy and systems research, with a specific focus on implementation sciences. He is particularly interested in the development and adoption of realist-informed research methods for evidence-based theorizing in health care and global health. He actively champions the decolonization of global health, striving to dismantle systemic inequities and promote equitable healthcare access worldwide.

"This is a long overdue book. It offers a much-needed philosophical synthesis of the broad range of demands and goals embedded in the growing quest to 'decolonize' global health."

Seye Abimbola, *University of Sydney, Australia*

"This unique, important contribution synthesizes Mukumbang's extensive international experience collaborating within the field of Global Health [...] Mukumbang lays a viable, sensitive, and assertive pathway for decolonizing Global Health."

Denise De Souza, *Torrens University Australia*

"In a highly polarized topic Mukumbang manages to keep his cool and dig deep into the underlying structures of coloniality and decolonization [...] A must-read for anyone with or without power in the global health domain."

Dimitri Renmans, *Université Libre de Bruxelles*

"This is an impressive book that traces the historical roots of colonialism, unpacks its persistence through coloniality and neo-colonialism, and outlines detailed steps for decolonizing global health."

Dr. Bipin Adhikari, *Senior Social Scientist, Mahidol-Oxford Tropical Medicine Research Unit, Bangkok*

Decolonizing Global Health

A Critical Realist Perspective

Ferdinand C. Mukumbang

Routledge
Taylor & Francis Group
LONDON AND NEW YORK

Designed cover image: Ferdinand C. Mukumbang and Sophie Lane

First published 2026
by Routledge
4 Park Square, Milton Park, Abingdon, Oxon OX14 4RN

and by Routledge
605 Third Avenue, New York, NY 10158

Routledge is an imprint of the Taylor & Francis Group, an informa business

© 2026 Ferdinand C. Mukumbang

The right of Ferdinand C. Mukumbang to be identified as author of this work has been asserted in accordance with sections 77 and 78 of the Copyright, Designs and Patents Act 1988.

All rights reserved. No part of this book may be reprinted or reproduced or utilised in any form or by any electronic, mechanical, or other means, now known or hereafter invented, including photocopying and recording, or in any information storage or retrieval system, without permission in writing from the publishers.

For Product Safety Concerns and Information please contact our EU representative GPSR@taylorandfrancis.com. Taylor & Francis Verlag GmbH, Kaufingerstraße 24, 80331 München, Germany.

Trademark notice: Product or corporate names may be trademarks or registered trademarks, and are used only for identification and explanation without intent to infringe.

British Library Cataloguing-in-Publication Data
A catalogue record for this book is available from the British Library

ISBN: 978-1-032-70092-2 (hbk)
ISBN: 978-1-032-70077-9 (pbk)
ISBN: 978-1-032-70078-6 (ebk)

DOI: 10.4324/9781032700786

Typeset in Times New Roman
by SPi Technologies India Pvt Ltd (Straive)

To my wife and children

Contents

Figures

Tables

Preface

Addressing colonization and advocating for the decolonization of global health has primarily been achieved in academia through the publication of commentaries based on the perspectives and experiences of global health specialists. However, decolonization agendas are often not informed by empirical evidence, and there is a lack of a philosophical foundation underpinning calls for decolonization in global health. This book addresses this gap by providing a robust philosophical foundation to support the calls for decolonizing global health. By establishing these philosophical foundations, the book also lays the groundwork for empirical inquiries that can inform evidence-based approaches to decolonization.

The notion that society and its institutions can be rationally transformed to improve human well-being and happiness is still debated. We have gained a clearer understanding of how individuals and cultures influence health outcomes, medical practices, and the implementation of health policies and programs. There is also a greater awareness of colonialism's impact on shifting power dynamics in social relationships, which has contributed to health disparities and inequities between countries and regions. Furthermore, we have developed insights into the ideas, emotions, and fantasies that drive the processes initiated by colonialism, as well as its ongoing effects on contemporary global health practices.

These insights have significant implications for certain groups, particularly those who suffered the most from colonialism and civil society shaped by the politics of memory. In global health, as in many other fields, a knowledge community is emerging that can meaningfully address geopolitical issues and contribute to understanding coexistence locally and globally. This community critically examines the role of colonialism and its enduring effects on contemporary global health practices. Discussions about colonialism's ongoing influence on today's world are often categorized as "postcolonialism," "postcolonial criticism," or a "postcolonial approach."

In this book, I will explore the concepts of colonialism, colonization, coloniality, decoloniality, and decolonization in conjunction with the critical realist philosophy of science and its application in global health research and practice.

The central thesis of this book, "Decolonizing Global Health: A Critical Realist Approach," is that we can decolonize global health research and practice by understanding society through critical realism and the decolonization agenda through the postcolonial critical realist lens. Engaging in this discourse requires (1) a clear understanding of colonialism, colonization, coloniality, decoloniality, and decolonization as both historical events and ideologies, (2) a comprehensive grasp of the field of global health, including the study of diseases, international relations, interdependence, and the formation of partnerships among institutions, organizations, and countries to tackle global health issues, (3) the political/structural origins/determination of inequity in health within and between countries, and (4) a solid foundation in critical realism, which aims to address inequity and promote human emancipation.

My goal is to guide the reader through the colonial origins and evolution of global health research and practice while amplifying the calls from others to dismantle these colonial foundations for a more effective global health system. In this book, I adopt a postcolonial approach. The term "post" in postcolonialism does not imply that colonialism's influence and impact have ended, but rather a mark placed on the period of political decolonization. It is important to note that the colonialism often referenced in postcolonial studies pertains to the nineteenth and twentieth centuries. This era of colonialism coincided with the rise of capitalism, as many colonies were established to supply raw materials that fueled Western imperialism. This work is postcolonial because it focuses on the current state of affairs reflecting Western colonialism's aftermath. Additionally, decolonization aims to address and reverse the lingering effects of colonialism.

In Europe, many perceive the postcolonial approach as a provocative challenge that seeks to impose ideas and theories developed outside traditional European thought. Terms like "postcolonialism," "postcolonial criticism," and "decolonization" often evoke strong reactions, ranging from enthusiasm and constructive acceptance to arrogant dismissal and even anger. I anticipate similar responses to the arguments in this book, which address both postcolonialism and the decolonization of global health.

Sustainable development has not matched the political independence and decolonization of formerly colonized nations in the Global South. Colonialism and imperialism (neo-colonialism) continue to impact global health through complex pathways often less appreciated or understood. While several postcolonial theories have been explored to explain how (neo)colonialism continues to influence almost every aspect of contemporary national and international engagements in different walks of life, the use of meta-philosophical positions to unpack the complexities around the continued influence of (neo)colonialism has been limited. To this end, I used critical realist tenets to explore the influence of colonialism on global health and to propose a plausible approach to decolonizing global health.

The countries/regions facing significant health challenges have critical political and socioeconomic dimensions that require political solutions at the domestic and international levels. Decolonizing global health has recently filled academic spaces on blogs and social media, activist circles, and even high school debate culture. It is arguably one of the buzzwords that have dominated the field of global health and academia since around 2020.

Arguments have been made that the major sociocultural structures must be decolonized for true decolonization of global health. The decolonizing of the global health movement will not succeed without decolonizing the world's political economy. Systemic reforms must be the main action to target the fundamental forces shaping global health. Such systemic reforms involve removing the underpinning social-economic inequities exacerbated by colonization, which have never been undone since.

The proposed approaches are often practical but lack philosophical foundations. In particular, critical realism has not fully explored its potential as a philosophical framework for understanding the social processes of colonization and decolonization within global health. This book aims to fill this gap by employing postcolonial critical realism as a philosophical foundation to scaffold my engagement with (de)colonization. To this end, I drew heavily from Bhaskar's critical realist philosophy of science (Bhaskar, 2014), dialectical critical realism based on the MELD model (Bhaskar, 2020), Archer's Morphogenetic approach (M. Archer, 1995), Gilbert and Sliep's inter-relational reflexivity (Gilbert & Sliep, 2009), Erik Olin Wright's definition and classification of utopias (Wright, 2010), and Elder-Vass's notion of responsible critique (Elder-Vass, 2019).

Chapter 1 starts by outlining the historical events and forces or structures that perpetuated the ideology of colonialism and colonization. It also outlines the forces behind the political decolonization of formerly colonized nations and how and why countries fought for their decolonization. This chapter also establishes a working definition of global health and its colonial foundation.

Chapter 2 provides historical background on the development of global health, elucidates the role of coloniality in colonizing global health, and thematically conceptualizes the nature of current global health practice. I identified health inequities and disparities, dependency syndrome, global health agenda monopoly, knowledge hegemony and epistemic injustice, and pervasive inequitable global health partnerships as the expression of a colonized global health. The goal of unpacking the nature and historical background of global health and the role of coloniality forms the foundation for exploring the possibilities of decolonizing global health from a critical realist perspective.

Chapter 3 provides historical background on the development of global health, elucidating the role of coloniality in colonizing global health, and thematically conceptualizes the nature of current global health practice. I identified health inequities and disparities, dependency syndrome, global health agenda monopoly, knowledge hegemony and epistemic injustice, and pervasive inequitable global health partnerships as the expression of a colonized global health. The goal of unpacking the nature and historical background of global health and the role of coloniality forms the foundation for exploring the possibilities of decolonizing global health from a critical realist perspective.

Chapter 3 proposes postcolonial critical realism as a robust postcolonial ontology for understanding global health colonization's social processes (coloniality) and the possibilities (decoloniality) of decolonizing global health. The chapter focuses on integrating the relevant basic critical realist tenets of the existence of a mind-independent reality, concept-dependence of the social world, (in)transitive entities, generative causation, stratified reality, emergence, open systems, and retroductive theorizing with colonial reflections. To this end, I focused on establishing postcolonial critical realism as an ontological position that can allow me and other scholars to engage with the literature on (de) colonialism.

Chapter 4 focuses on five mindsets and ideologies with causal tendencies that underpin coloniality and orchestrate the colonial practice of global health. The mindsets and ideologies of hegemony, (internalized) racism, religious paternalism, white supremacy, and white saviorism are operationalized as generative mechanisms of health inequities and (social and epistemic) injustices experienced and observed in global health. The interactions and connections between these mindsets and ideologies form the colonial matrix of power in global health. The chapter also conceptualizes coloniality as the plurality of these causal mechanisms operating in the postcolonial era. Using Sayer's conceptualization of causality (introduced in Chapter 3), the chapter explores how relevant structures sustaining colonial practices globally within which the bundles of causal mechanisms operate to cause health inequity, epistemic injustice, global health agenda monopoly, and inequitable collaborations, experienced in the Global South. Sayer's conceptualization provides a robust framework for understanding and conceptualizing decoloniality and the decolonization of global health.

Decoloniality in global health practice entails challenging the colonial matrix of power that underpins global health practice—research and curricula, partnerships, and the attitude that ignores the capacity, knowledge, and contributions of the Global South. To decolonize global health, Chapter 5 proposes a change of mindset or epistemic orientation, which entails decolonizing the mind, combating colonial amnesia, going beyond traditional mastery (global health expertise), establishing meaningful global health collaborations, valorizing local knowledge and having a self-reliant mindset—decoloniality. This chapter argues that these mindsets and their corresponding activities and relevant context conditions are the bedrock to reducing health inequities and ushering in social justice in global health practice and research in the Global South.

In Chapter 6, Bhaskar's Dialectic of freedom, a transformative approach operationalized through his MELD Schema, was adopted as a framework within postcolonial critical realism to envisage a process for decolonizing global health. Using the MELD Schema, where 1M explores "what is and what is not," the chapter discusses how global health is inequitable and unjust to the Global South underpinned by coloniality—the instrumentalization of colonial powers. At 2E, I explored the nature of global health: rid of coloniality in global health research and practice. At 3L, the chapter explores what global health should be: equitable and just, representing the interest of all the parties involved, including the disenfranchised. In alignment with 4D, the chapter calls for equitable participation of Global South experts in governance structures and advisory bodies on improving health outcomes in the Global South to illustrate how global health can be. The chapter also shows that dialectical critical realism provides the rationale and an opportunity to decolonize global health beyond current propositions and practices.

Chapter 7 focuses on illuminating the intricate interactions among structure (an organized set of social institutions and patterns of institutionalized relationships), agency (the thoughts and actions of individuals), and culture (the dynamic interplay between cultural systems and sociocultural interactions) that perpetuate the entrenched power imbalances in global health established by colonialism. These dynamic interactions contribute to social processes that reproduce or transform individuals and society over time—called social morphogenesis. To this end, social morphogenesis is proposed as a robust theoretical framework, informed by critical realism, to elucidate how decolonization can be achieved in global health. I use Margaret Archer's structure–agency–culture framework to analyze the eras of colonization, neo-colonization, and decolonization in this context. A philosophical understanding of these complexities can inform practical interventions to advance decolonization in Global Health.

Chapter 8 reviews three existing approaches (the instrumentalist, democratic, and associative views) proposed by Stilz (2015) to achieve political decolonization. The chapter further explored the potential application of these three views to decolonization to achieve decoloniality in global health. Finally, the chapter proposes a decolonial reflexivity underpinned by a postcolonial critical realist approach informed by Archer's morphogenetic approach and Bhaskar's MELD planar model. The proposed decolonial reflexivity approach has four interlinked steps:

1. Develop a responsible critique, which entails making arguments and providing justifications for the decolonization of global health.
2. Formulate concrete utopias or decolonization goals. Formulate realistic decolonization goals with strategic mobilization of resources.
3. Establishing commitment requiring all global health interest holders to be committed to the decolonization project.
4. Action, which requires converting the set goals into practical actions with measurable outcomes.

The decolonial reflexivity approach focuses on undoing the colonial matrix of power—mindsets of hegemony, racism, religious paternalism, white supremacy, and white saviorism by decolonizing the mind, combating colonial amnesia, redefining global health expertise, establishing meaningful global health collaborations, valorizing local knowledge and having a self-reliant mindset. Decolonial reflexivity offers a concrete approach to achieving equity and justice in global health.

Reflexive statement

After reviewing a book chapter, one of my collaborators, Denise De Souza, wrote, "It would be good for you to explain why critical realism is suitable for decolonizing global health. Does critical realism align with more indigenous (Asian, African, etc.), perspectives or at least allow these perspectives to be considered within the critical realism and dialectical critical realist frameworks?"

I realized I needed to justify using a philosophical approach considered to be a Western philosophy to support my work while advocating for an indigenous knowledge base as part of decolonial reflexivity. While I do not consider critical realism to be a Western philosophy based on Bhaskar's background and focus on human freedom and emancipation, this conundrum led me to engage in deeper reflexivity. Addressing global health's coloniality and exploring its potential for decolonization requires alignment with postcolonial and decolonial agendas. These agendas seek to analyze colonialism's power dynamics and effects on colonized societies by amplifying their voices, reclaiming marginalized narratives, and revealing how colonial power structures continue to shape contemporary society—particularly through language, culture, and politics. The goal is to shift away from the colonizer's perspective and empower marginalized voices.

Postcolonial literature is primarily created by individuals from formerly colonized states, particularly those who are natives of these colonies and now live and work in the diaspora. These authors explore the structures of pre-colonialism, the narratives and events of colonialism, and its lasting effects. As someone from a country that both France and England have colonized, and currently residing in the Global North while writing about the impact of colonialism on global health—a field in which I am active—I identify as a postcolonial diasporic author. Postcolonial and decolonial authors pursue the postcolonial and decolonial agenda, which aligns with my goals of writing this book. However, I was reluctant to abandon the strong ontological foundation of critical realism, which offers valuable insights into society and social events, particularly regarding human emancipation and freedom—principles that resonate with the postcolonial agenda of decoloniality. Therefore, I chose to retain critical realism as a framework for my work due to its explanatory potential and emancipatory framework while incorporating the perspectives of decolonial scholars and postcolonial discourses.

To this end, I found Tinsley's (2021) initial work on postcolonial critical realism most appealing as she attempted to integrate the core elements of these philosophical positions to formulate a cogent meta-theory suitable for engaging the decolonization agenda of global health. The postcolonial critical realist theoretical foundation allowed me to bring a nuanced explanation to (de)colonialism and how equitable and just global health practices can be achieved. While there is value in underpinning this work in a cogent theoretical framework, there is greater value in grounding the discussion and suggestions in practicality. The practicality of the recommendations offered in this book based on the philosophical reflections of coloniality and decoloniality is informed by my growing up in Cameroon, a country which to date typifies a country soaked in coloniality. Therefore, I aim to understand how colonialism continues to impact the public and global health practice in Cameroon, Africa, and the Global South, with Africa being the predominant geographical focus of the book, and provide practical recommendations that could be useful to various global health actors and institutions.

Writing this book while teaching, doing research, writing grants, mentoring students, serving in departmental committees, and publishing articles simultaneously was an arduous endeavor. I found it strange that my department does not consider book writing an important scholarly contribution; thus, it does not contribute during annual evaluations. Therefore, this lack of consideration meant that writing this book was only secondary to all the activities I had to do to meet my annual milestones. This book is, therefore, born of sheer passion and dedication to the agenda and cause to achieve equity and justice in global health research and practice. It consumed my thoughts and reflections for the best part of two years, and I am thankful for not giving up. I thank myself for not giving up.

References

Archer, M. (1995). *Realist social theory: the morphogenetic approach*. Cambridge University Press.

Bhaskar, R. (2014). *The possibility of naturalism: A philosophical critique of the contemporary human sciences*. Routledge.

Bhaskar, R. (2020). Critical realism and the ontology of persons. *Journal of Critical Realism*, 19(2), 113–120. https://doi.org/10.1080/14767430.2020.1734736

Elder-Vass, D. (2019). Realism, values and critique. *Journal of Critical Realism*, 18(3), 314–318. https://doi.org/10.1080/14767430.2019.1614744

Gilbert, A., & Sliep, Y. (2009). Reflexivity in the practice of social action: From self-to inter-relational reflexivity. *South African Journal of Psychology*, 39(4), 468–479. https://doi.org/10.1177/008124630903900408

Stilz, A. (2015). Decolonization and self-determination. *Social Philosophy and Policy*, 32(1), 1–24. https://doi.org/10.1017/S0265052515000059

Tinsley, M. (2021). Towards a postcolonial critical realism. *Critical Sociology*, 48(2). https://doi.org/10.1177/08969205211003962

Wright, E. O. (2010). *Envisioning real utopias*. Verso.

Acknowledgements

I extend my deepest gratitude to Glendy Mukumbang for her unwavering love, support, and patience, which made this project possible.

I want to thank my editor, George Russell, and editorial assistant, Amy Thompson, and the team at Routledge for their invaluable expertise, which shaped this work in ways I could not have achieved alone. My heartfelt appreciation also goes to my beta readers, Denise De Souza, Dimitri Renmans, Bipin Adhikari, and Seye Abimbola, for their time and constructive feedback on the resubmitted version of the book.

I am indebted to Brian Van Wyk for introducing me to realist evaluation, which sparked my curiosity in critical realism as a philosophy of science. I am also grateful to Bruno Marchal, who guided me through my early days of realist-informed work, enhancing my understanding of the foundational principles of critical realism. I want to thank my friends and colleagues Brynne Gilmore, James Pfeiffer, Steve Gloyd, Sara van Belle, Catherine Hastings, Priscilla Anderson, and Dave Elder-Vass for their rigorous feedback and encouragement during moments of doubt and for reviewing various book chapters. I am especially thankful to my brother, Anthony Ambe, for his support in writing the first chapter. His historical insights and presentation of ideas significantly shaped my understanding of colonization and political decolonization.

I appreciate my colleagues, Megan Coe (University of Washington) and Nancy Clark (University of Victoria), along with the International Association of Critical Realism, for inviting me to lecture to their students and present on materials from the book. Their support helped me refine my thoughts and presentation skills. I am also grateful to other colleagues who published thought-provoking pieces addressing various aspects that enriched my conceptualization of decolonizing global health, including Alison Wiyeh, Bipin Adhikari, and Shiva Raj Mishra.

Additionally, I am thankful for my creative collaborators, Patrick Lane, his daughter, Sophie Lane, and Alberto Reyes, who helped translate some of my ideas into artwork to represent some key concepts and ideas better.

This book is built upon the foundations laid by critical realist thinkers such as Roy Bhaskar, Margaret Archer, and Dave Elder-Vass. In decolonizing global health, I drew inspiration from the outstanding work of Seye Abimbola and Mahdukar Pai, whose ideas fueled my curiosity.

Any errors in this work are solely my own.

Finally, I thank the readers for allowing these pages to resonate with meaning and inspiration in your hands.

1 Colonial Foundations of Global Health

Introduction

Colonial settlement conditions or the colonizer's identity continue to shape medicine, health, and healthcare delivery globally. Colonialism of the nineteenth century was the most important in magnitude and the most fraught with consequences. Its legacy persists today, manifesting in systemic inequalities and ongoing conflicts. The imposition of foreign rule often dismantled local institutions, leading to exploitation and cultural erasure. While some argue colonialism spurred development, the overwhelming consensus is of its destructive impact on colonized societies. The repercussions of colonialism continue to affect contemporary relationships between nations, highlighting the need for critical reflection on its historical and ongoing effects. Understanding this complex legacy is essential for addressing global disparities and fostering equitable relationships. This chapter will focus on colonialism and its continued influence on modernity, especially contemporary global health practice.

The extant literature is rife with references to colonialism, colonization, coloniality, decolonial, and their respective antonyms of decolonization and decoloniality (decolonial reflections). Unsurprisingly, the literature's conceptualization of colonialism and its cognates and how they apply and relate to global health remains fragmented and sometimes confusing. One of my goals in this chapter, and indeed this book, is to clarify and operationalize these terms to ground our understanding of the structure and function of the current-day practice of global health through a postcolonial critical realist lens. I briefly conceptualize colonialism as a construct and an ideology to achieve this goal. Then, I provide a brief historical narrative of colonization. Most importantly, I relate colonialism and colonization to global health's inception, development, and evolution as a research and practice field.

I relate most of my arguments and illustrations to the colonization of Africa because the African form of colonialism is considered the most recent in historical timelines as it emerged from the early nineteenth to mid-twentieth centuries; consequently, its consequences have continued into the present. Also, as an area of intellectual discourse, I am more familiar with the global health landscape of Africa as I was born and educated in Africa, and my global health

DOI: 10.4324/9781032700786-1

work focuses predominantly on the African continent. My familiarity with the goings-on on the continent makes me draw most of my illustrations from the continent. Nevertheless, because this book is meant to serve as an intellectual discourse and possibly as a practical guideline to decolonizing global health, I will draw lessons from other parts of the world and the writings of other scholars.

Talking about relying on the writings of other scholars both from the historical perspective or from a social scientific perspective, I organized this chapter in a way that introduces the reader to the history of colonization to the development of global health as a field and navigate through the different terminologies and variants of colonialism. To this end, I will start by unpacking what colonialism entails. This chapter will provide a brief historical picture of colonization, focusing on the three phases of European colonization. The ideas and processes of political decolonization and independence naturally follow from that. To link the (de)colonization to global health, I will provide a synopsis of global health and the key issues related to global health. I conclude the chapter by providing a historical development of the field of global health and how it was born from the need to address the mortality and morbidity that the colonizers and the colonized experienced while working to achieve the goals of the colonizers.

Colonialism

Western Europe's capitalist agendas and imperial ideologies strongly influenced the modern international system. The term colonialism is used to describe the process of European settlement, violent dispossession, and political domination over much of the world, including the Americas, Australia, and parts of Africa and Asia (Kohn, 2008). Colonialism is defined as a domination practice involving subjugating one person to another. According to Manning (1974), colonialism (especially in Africa) was driven by three European agendas: (1) European economic and cultural penetration, (2) European political control, and (3) the primacy of European economic interests over the interests of the colonized. Modern colonialism began 400 years ago, fundamentally altering the world's economic landscape. It allowed Europe to amass considerable wealth through trade, and during this era, the foundations of what we now recognize as free-market capitalism were established to facilitate that trade. There is an ongoing debate among historians about whether colonialism's importance lies solely in its economic consequences, while others contend that cultural factors, such as missionary Christianity and a sense of racial superiority, also played a crucial role.

In this book, I use "colonialism" as an ideology driven by a core set of comprehensive arguments and principles that modern European thinkers present to persuade a broader audience of the advantages of imperial processes and colonization (Arneil, 2023). As an ideology, colonialism includes both action and advocacy, and it is through advocacy that most individuals become associated with the phenomenon (Wright, 1967). Closely linked to the ideology of colonialism is imperialism, which many modern scholars have argued that it is hard to distinguish from colonialism (Pitts, 2010). This conflation stems from the fact that imperialism[1] is also an ideology promoting a form of international hierarchy where one political community effectively governs or controls another, often characterized by the domination of one political society over another through establishing and maintaining an empire. Thus, imperialism is an ideology that extends a country's power and influence through military force or other means. It involves controlling or dominating other territories, often through establishing colonies or imposing economic and political control over other regions (Veltmeyer, 2020). Imperialism can manifest in various forms, including direct territorial acquisition, economic exploitation, and cultural influence. Historically, it has been driven by various factors, such as the desire for resources, strategic military positions, and the spread of a nation's culture or ideology.

Colonial advocacy served as a primary mechanism through which individuals engage with colonialism—whether by perpetuating its logic like neoliberal policy advocacy (Willmott & Skillings, 2021), resisting its legacies (e.g., reparations campaigns), or navigating its cultural aftermath (e.g., mental health decolonization). Western colonial powers historically used advocacy (e.g., "civilizing missions") to legitimize exploitation and domination, a legacy critiqued as a "historical original sin." For example, The Colonial Advocate newspaper in Upper Canada (1824–1834) demonstrates how nineteenth-century reformers used advocacy to critique and operate within colonial power structures, making colonial governance a central focus for its readers (Karsgaard et al., 2024). Historical and modern advocacy for colonialism, such as Bruce Gilley's argument for a "new colonialism" dependent on local leaders promoting colonial agendas, directly ties individuals to colonial ideologies. Clinical legal practices in settler-colonial contexts often perpetuate coloniality by sustaining structural violence against indigenous communities despite claims of neutrality (Getgen et al., 2023).

It has been argued that imperialism was the necessary and inevitable result of capitalism[2] (Veltmeyer, 2020) and so was colonialism. It is also now established that the wellspring of colonialism and imperialism is the power-seeking behavior of men leading to intergroup domination. Because colonialism and imperialism were two forms of conquest expected to benefit Europe economically and strategically, it is conceptually challenging to distinguish between them (Kohn & Reddy, 2024). Indeed, while attempting to define colonialism, Horvath (1972) suggested that the conceptual distinction between the two constructs is subtle. Arneil (2023) argues that the conflation of colonialism and imperialism occurred after World War II when colonialism and imperialism converged through the UN decolonization process, as the "saltwater thesis" defines colonialism as foreign racialized domination, making it synonymous with imperialism. To distinguish between the two concepts or ideologies, Kohn and Reddy (2024) argue that colonialism is mostly associated with settlements in places controlled by a large population, while imperialism is associated with administratively controlling another territory occupied by another population. Nevertheless, because settlement has been found in both instances, Horvath (1972) suggested that the difference lies in the levels of settlement, with greater number of permanent settlers observed in colonialism as seen in the colonization of Latin America, North America, Australia, New Zealand, and South Africa. Based on this distinction,[3] Horvath (1972) argues that most of Africa and Asia, was imperialized—dominated but not settled—and the countries involved are noticeably different today (worst off), in part, because of the nature of the domination process. Whichever style of domination was adopted, colonialism and imperialism led to indigenous people becoming a minority or subjugated in their land and being limited to menial jobs and limited opportunities, while the ruling class benefits from the land's natural resources. Branch (2011) argues that many of the foundational ideas and practices of modern statehood were formed in the interactions of Europeans with the unknown, resulting in colonial reflection. To this end, Arneil (2023) insists that the distinction between colonialism and imperialism should be maintained as it shows how colonialism's characteristic form of colonial power manifests in its negative effects on those subjected to it in colonial institutions and processes.

I have defined colonialism as an ideology with two clear components: advocacy and action (not that they are practically distinguishable). Up to this point, I have focused on the advocacy aspect of the colonial ideology. Regarding the action, the European colonial rule in Africa, Asia, and the Americas employed various modes of exploitation, including slavery, feudal dependence on landowners, usury from merchants and moneylenders, and capitalist exploitation, which extracts surplus labor from nominally free wage earners (Bagchi, 2021). However, in colonial countries, pre-capitalist modes of exploitation were the most prevalent. The prevalence of pre-capitalist modes of exploitation in colonial territories corresponds broadly to the period from 1492 to the late nineteenth/early twentieth century, with regional variations. Because different exploitation approaches were adopted, different institutions and actors were also involved. In addition to having different actors involved in the colonization apparatus, they collaborated to achieve the colonial project (Figure 1.1). The idea of collaboration as a key character of imperial expansion and maintenance is well established.

This imperialist agenda and, indeed, the connection between the advocacy and action components of colonialism is succinctly described by Simmons (2020, p. 191) in the following excerpt:

> European colonial projects included much more than military and administrative dominance; they were more thorough and aimed to change how the colonized viewed and operated in the world. Colonizing powers sought to change their colonial worlds, reshaping indigenous religious beliefs and practices while altering the related and intertwining social, political, and cosmological structures by which they were upheld.

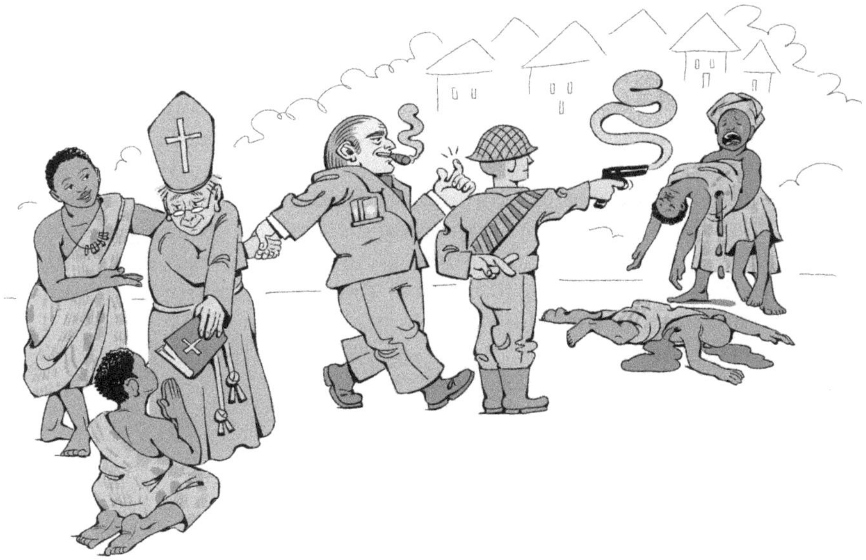

Figure 1.1 Approaches to colonialism.

Figure 1.1 illustrates the involvement of three key institutions represented by different actors. The Priest represents the role of religion, particularly Christianity, the capitalist represents the economic interests of colonialism, and the soldier represents the political involvement in colonialism. The Priest and the colonizer had their arms on each other's shoulders, and at the side of the colonizer, who was armed, was a soldier with another type of weapon as they invaded the natives, a sign of strong collaboration and alliance. The purposes of colonialism included economic exploitation of the colony's people and natural resources, creating new markets for the colonizer, and extending the colonizer's way of life to populations beyond its national borders. On the other hand, missionaries believed it was their duty to spread Christianity, and the Church leaders believed colonization was necessary to save souls. To this end, the different actors found the need to work together to achieve their different objectives in the colonized nations.

While the literature often links religious organizations to colonialism, their presence within European empires did not always support colonial rule (McKay, 2007). As noted above, they had precise mandates to spread their religious values and save souls. These mandates warranted missionaries to occasionally challenge imperial racial divides and were often the most vocal opponents of racist officials and legislation. Most of these missionaries came from Scandinavia or other nations that were generally unsympathetic to colonialism. Consequently, in some instances, imperial officials restricted missionaries from entering peripheral regions like Bhutan and Tibet, arguing that their presence could disrupt local communal relations.

Owing to the challenges in distinguishing between colonialism and imperialism, in this book, I will consider colonialism as a broad concept that refers to the project of European social, economic, and political domination that began in the early sixteenth century. I conceptualized colonialism as a systematic process of exercising military, political, economic, cultural, and religious control and domination over the land, resources, and native populations. These acts of political, physical, cultural, spiritual, economic, and intellectual occupation of space through mostly forceful displacement of indigenous populations gave rise to colonialism, settler colonialism, neo-colonial relations, and coloniality. In the next section, I will discuss how European countries colonized other countries politically, physically, culturally, spiritually, economically, and intellectually.

Colonization

The history of humankind is replete with instances of one society conquering another's territory and expanding its control by settling its people there. Colonization is the action component of colonialism. The colonial activities warranted the movement of large populations to distant lands across oceans (Kohn & Reddy, 2024). The activity of conquering and ruling another territory for expansion and control marked the beginning of what is now referred to as the European colonial project—colonization. During this time (the fifteenth and sixteenth centuries), several European countries engaged in "European settlement, violent dispossession, and political domination over the rest of the world, including the Americas, Australia, parts of Asia, and Africa" (Kohn & Reddy, 2024). It was in this context that the term colonialism gained significant emphasis.

My thinking resonates with those of Arneil (2023), who also believes there is a clear distinction between colonialism and colonization. She argued that while colonization is the historical process through which people were colonized, colonialism is the underlying ideology that was used to justify such entities and processes. Colonization has a lengthy history that begins in the sixth century with the Phoenicians, Greeks, and Romans, and extends to modern times with nations such as Portugal, Spain, the Netherlands, China, Japan, Denmark, Germany, England, France, Russia, Belgium, and the USA. These nations established colonies throughout various periods. The Western historical tradition links the colonial phenomenon to the era of the Great Discovery (Ferro, 1997). This perspective suggests that significant colonial endeavors began with the fifteenth-century explorers, particularly those from Portugal, Spain, and England. These explorers set out to "discover" distant lands in the West Indies and subsequently established trading posts along routes in Africa, India, and Asia (Ferro, 1997). As a result, terms like "colonist" and "colonization" largely disappear from historical accounts from the times of the Phoenicians, Greeks, and Romans until the rise of the Portuguese, Spanish, and English in the fifteenth century (Ferro, 1997).

Cooper (2006) challenges the notion that the empires of the nineteenth and twentieth centuries were more colonial than those that came before them. He argues that little has fundamentally changed, as colonialism endures in "the post-Enlightenment penchant for classification and hence invidious distinction based not on the give and take of relations between the unequal but on the systemic ranking of people" (Cooper, 2006, p. 28). In the context of European colonization of Africa, "the colonizing country arrogated to itself a civilizing mission while Africa was projected as the very paradigm of the non-civilized world" (Césaire & Kelley, 2007). In addition to the civilization mission of Africa, there was also the agenda of expanding Christianity and commercial goals.

European colonial history is commonly categorized into three distinct waves. The initial wave commenced with the Portuguese conquest of Ceuta in 1415, marking the beginning of the exploration and conquest of various African territories, a period frequently referred to as the "Age of Discovery." This invasion was followed by the colonization of the Americas by the Spanish and Portuguese, later joined by the British, French, and Dutch. The second wave, starting in the 1870s, was instigated by the British expansion in Asia through the British East India Company, during which France, Portugal, and the Netherlands were active participants. The Scramble for Africa (1880s–1914) is widely regarded as the third major phase of colonialism, often termed the "New Imperialism" period. This phase was marked by rapid partition, during which European powers (e.g., Britain, France, and Germany) competed to colonize nearly 90% of Africa within decades.

Political Decolonization and Independence

The resolutions made after World War I aimed to prevent future conflicts but often led to more tensions, contributing to the outbreak of World War II. Key factors included the Treaty of Versailles, the Great Depression, appeasement policies, militarism in Germany and Japan, and the League of Nations' failures. Colonies in Asia, Africa, and the Caribbean played crucial roles in World War II, providing soldiers and resources to the Allies. India, for example, contributed over half a million soldiers, while African and Caribbean colonies offered military support and labor.

The United Nations was established in 1945 to prevent future conflicts, with the UN Charter emphasizing international peace, economic and social issues, and human rights. The principle of self-determination in the Charter encouraged colonized peoples to seek independence. After World War II, decolonization became a significant movement, with the UN Charter providing a framework for anticolonial movements. Decolonization varied across Asia and Africa, with some countries achieving independence peacefully and others through conflict.

In Asia, nationalist movements emerged after Japan's occupation during World War II, leading to independence struggles. Southeast Asian countries like Malaya and Vietnam faced prolonged conflicts. The Philippines' journey to independence was marked by centuries of resistance against Spanish and American colonialism. By the late 1940s and early 1950s, many colonies gained independence, with Southeast Asian nations leading the way. India, Burma, and Ceylon also achieved independence, with India's movement characterized by nonviolent resistance under Mahatma Gandhi.

In Latin America, most colonies gained independence between 1808 and 1826, driven by rising tensions and global events. The Spanish Bourbons' reforms in the eighteenth century led to instability, and Enlightenment ideas challenged monarchial authority. Despite the end of formal colonial administrations, colonial dominance persists in global relations, as argued by Quijano (2007) through a "colonization of the imagination."

Grosfoguel (2007) describes the belief that removing colonial administrations equated to decolonization as a powerful myth. He points out that while formal colonialism ended, global coloniality continues, with colonized individuals still facing similar oppressions and exploitations. Ndlovu-Gatsheni (2013) uses the phrase "postcolonial neo-colonized world" to explain current forms of Colonialism in Africa, noting that the neocolonial influences have undermined the liberation struggle. Ndlovu-Gatsheni (2013) also argues that this situation affects Africa, revealing invisible matrices of power that maintain inequality and prevent true decolonization. His analysis suggests a need to interrogate these subtle forms of coloniality that remain influential in the present.

The current decolonization movement is aimed at undoing the continued negative influence of colonialism even after the legal-political decolonization. Following this line of thinking, Táíwò (2022) distinguishes between two forms of decolonization:[4] Decolonization$_1$, which achieved political independence and sovereignty, and Decolonization$_2$, a post-independence ideological project seeking to purge all colonial influences. I will use Táíwò's (2022) distinction of decolonization throughout the book, as it clarifies the distinction between colonization, decolonization, and their cognates.

The "Benefits" of Colonialism

Providing an overview of colonialism and its cognates is not comprehensive without mentioning its perceived "benefits." Unsurprisingly, discussions on the cost and benefits of colonialism dominated the second half of the twentieth century, when most colonized nations gained their independence. The prevailing argument was whether colonialism improved or worsened the conditions of the colonized nations (Manning, 1974). A cursory engagement with the extant literature reveals an inclination to colonialism being more detrimental to the colonized nations and beneficial to the colonizers. Emerson (1969) argued that if people did not praise or dismiss colonialism as a "normal part of history," critics would not blame the entire system. Instead, they would focus on calling out its specific harms or unfair practices.

While several authors looked at colonialism from a beneficial perspective in the second half of the twentieth century, I will focus mostly on recent arguments for colonialism. For example, Bruce Gilley (2023), who authored "The Case for Colonialism," argues that colonialism benefited colonized peoples through improved governance, economic development, and infrastructure while criticizing anticolonial narratives as oversimplified. Adam Smith is also cited by Williams (2023) for framing colonialism as ultimately "beneficial for humanity." Nigel Biggar (2023), a theologian and ethicist whose book "Colonialism: A Moral Reckoning" engages in a moral defense of colonialism, emphasizes alleged positive legacies while acknowledging critiques. He sees denigrating colonialism as an "important way of corroding faith in the West" (p. 276). These authors represent contemporary academic efforts to re-examine colonialism through frameworks emphasizing purported "benefits" or moral complexity.

Contrary to the understanding that colonialism in all its manifestations is an evil that should speedily be ended, in recent times, there are claims that colonial rule introduced efficient governance, state-building, and technocratic administration that laid the foundations for modernization and progress (Gilley, 2023). Specifically, it is argued that colonialism spurred infrastructure (e.g., railways, institutions), trade integration, and economic growth beneficial to colonized societies (Williams, 2023). It is also highlighted that colonial governments and missionary organizations also invested in education in the colonized nations, which resulted in educational advances for the colonized (Manning, 1974). Colonial powers also trained local elites in governance, law, and bureaucracy to prepare colonies for eventual independence. Manning (1974) explained that European firms and governments invested in enterprises like railroads and ports in their colonies, and these investments brought wages to workers, and better transport brought better prices to producers and consumers. It has also been argued that the adoption of the language spoken by the colonial masters played a crucial role in fostering unity in the African nations that have multilingual tribal languages (Manning, 1974).

Despite the cited arguments for the "benefits" of colonialism, Emerson (1969) reported that "Colonial and ex-colonial peoples have from time to time found it tempting to assume that if they had remained free, all kinds of good things would have fallen to their lot, enabling them to advance on the path to modernity, prosperity, strength, and national unity far more rapidly than proved possible under alien control." (p. 7). This alternative approach is, of course, globalization. It has been argued that Globalization achieves economic integration and wealth generation comparable to colonialism's "benefits" for dominant powers but through market-driven, non-coercive frameworks. However, persistent inequality and power imbalances suggest it risks replicating colonial patterns in subtler forms. To this end, many authors have argued that globalization is simply a new form of imperialism (Chilcote, 2002; Vilas, 2002; Went, 2002). The challenge, therefore, lies in creating inclusive systems that avoid (historical) abuses.

Global Health and Colonialism

Abimbola (2024), in his book *The Foreign Gaze: Essays on Global Health*, suggested that any book on global health must start by engaging with what global health means or should mean. A logical explanation for this request would be that there are diverse perspectives on what global health constitutes. According to Koplan et al. (2009), in addition to variability in the definition of global health, these definitions are often linked to common definitions of public health or a politically correct updating of international health. The evolution from "international health" to "global health" represents a politically correct update that aligns with contemporary inclusivity, equity, and collaboration values. This shift acknowledges the limitations of traditional approaches, which often neglected underlying determinants of health and reinforced colonial power dynamics. However, while the updated terminology and frameworks are steps forward, true progress depends on translating these ideals into concrete actions that address structural inequities and empower marginalized communities.

The change in terminology from public and international health to global health was intended to shift from the narrow view of global health as the problems of the world's poorest societies, to global health as the health of an interdependent global population (Frenk et al., 2014). Nevertheless, of course, the change in terminology is not simply attributable to expanding our views on health; there are logical arguments backing this expansive perspective, such as the notions of interconnection and interdependence. Interconnection refers to the nature of health threats and their effects, while interdependence pertains to the distribution of power, responsibility, and capacity to respond to health threats (Frenk et al., 2014). While the World Health Organization did not conceptualize "global health," it played a pivotal role in the transition of International Health to Global through coordinating, strategic planning, and leadership of "global health" initiatives, which must be acknowledged (Brown et al., 2006).

Linking global health to public and international health makes sense because, as we will see while reviewing the history of global health, what we know today as global health has metamorphosed through various stages, from colonial medicine to tropical medicine and international health (Chen et al., 2020). For instance, "tropical medicine," which focused on diseases prevalent in colonized regions like malaria, was a key development during colonialism and was a foundation for early global health research. Indeed, MacFarlane et al. (2008) argue that the accelerated development of programs in global health, particularly in North American academic institutions, is informed by earlier programs in tropical medicine and international health that originated predominantly in Europe. The metamorphosis of global health from its colonial larva form changes its current definition and, in most cases, is linked to its colonial larva forms. The implication is that whatever form global health has today results from its differentiation from its colonial larva form during its transformative phases. To this end, the adult form of global health shares the same DNA as its larva. For instance, Gichane et al. (2022) define global health as "a distinct public health discipline."

Responding to the suggestion Abimbola (2024) made that "Any book on global health must first get one thing out of the way: what global health means, or should mean" (p. 8), I found it befitting to have a section of the introductory chapter dedicated to outlining how I have defined and operationalized global health in this book since the book is about decolonizing global health. Identifying that consensus around a precise definition remains elusive, Salm et al. (2021) conducted a systematic review with qualitative synthesis to identify common themes highlighted in the literature associated with global health. The following four themes were distilled from the extant literature revealed that global health is:

> (1) a multiplex approach to worldwide health improvement taught and pursued at research institutions; (2) an ethically oriented initiative that is guided by justice principles; (3) a mode of governance that yields influence through problem identification, political decision-making, as well as the allocation and exchange of resources across borders and (4) a vague yet versatile concept with multiple meanings, historical antecedents and an emergent future.
>
> (Salm et al., 2021)

While global health was designed to focus on only medical and health issues that were transnational with global impact (Chen et al., 2020), an observation made by MacFarlane et al. (2008), which is still relevant today, is that global health predominantly focuses on the health needs of the Global South. According to Chen et al. (2020), "Global" is key to defining global health. I will start by offering a simplified version of global health: the study, research, and practice of improving health and equity for people worldwide. Global health adopts a multidisciplinary approach to fulfill its goals, considering social, cultural, economic, and environmental factors.

The World Health Organization played a key role in the evolution of global health. Through the formulation of the World Health Organization in 1948, global health governance was established in its current form. The governance ecosystem of bilateral donors, philanthropic organizations, non-government organizations, and multilateral organizations is rooted in political and historical relationships formed during colonial times—the 1885 Berlin Conference still influences twenty-first-century donor relationships and research partnerships between European universities and African institutions in former colonies (Erondu et al., 2025). In the 1950s and 1960s, changes in biology, economics, and global politics affected foreign relations and public health. The World Health Organization moved from focusing solely on malaria to developing health services and working on smallpox eradication. In the 1970s and 1980s, it introduced primary health care but later supported selective primary health care due to changing dynamics (Brown et al., 2006). In the 1990s, the World Health Organization tried to lead in global health as a strategy for survival but did not create its agenda.

The Colonial Foundation of Global Health

Besides the economic, social, and political impact of colonialism, an area in which colonialism also manifested strongly over time is healthcare. The manifestations of colonialism in medicine and healthcare have metamorphosed over the years, taking different forms, from colonial medicine to tropical medicine and international health. The role of colonialism in shaping global health's advent, evolution, ethos, education, and practices is rife in the literature (Abimbola & Pai, 2021; Bhakuni & Abimbola, 2021; Bump, 2025; Eichbaum et al., 2021; Hussain et al., 2023; Kwete et al., 2022; McCoy et al., 2024). My goal, therefore, is to provide a synopsis of how global health has evolved over the years (Figure 1.2), focusing on colonialism's role in how and why it is practiced the way it is today.

Like many other fields, global health has evolved over the years (centuries), including influences from the colonial era. The evolution of global health can be tracked through its different appellations, from "colonial medicine," which later became "tropical medicine," and then "international health," to "global health" (Holst, 2020; Hussain et al., 2023). Colonial medicine is the term used to describe the idea of taking medical practice across borders informed by colonial ideologies. The concept of colonial medicine captures colonial processes and actions, which orchestrated the formulation of the transferability of knowledge and resources for the prevention and treatment of diseases across international lines. Colonial medicine is, therefore, medicine practiced in the colonies, connected to the colonizing power through imperial/global processes and policies, but unique to each locale due to climate, indigenous beliefs and practices, regional geopolitics, and other complex factors (McCleery, 2015, p. 152). Colonial powers prioritized the advancement of medical knowledge and resources for their people when diseases arose and only extended such efforts to local populations in the colonies if it served their interests, such as when the colonial state wished to win their loyalty, protect a colonized labor force or prevent anticolonial revolution (Amster, 2022; Hussain et al., 2023). The non-medical component of public health also followed this pattern.

Around the turn of the nineteenth century, "missionary medicine" became the public-facing arm of colonial medicine, masking exploitation with altruism. This duality persists in global health, where faith-based organizations deliver 40% of Sub-Saharan Africa's healthcare today, often entangled with proselytization agendas. It is theorized that it was in missionary medicine that imperialists/capitalists collaborated with religious organizations to achieve colonial goals. This approach aimed to manage populations for both physical and moral health. As the name suggests, it involved physicians from colonizing the nation's leading medical missions, with an implicit goal of social and moral

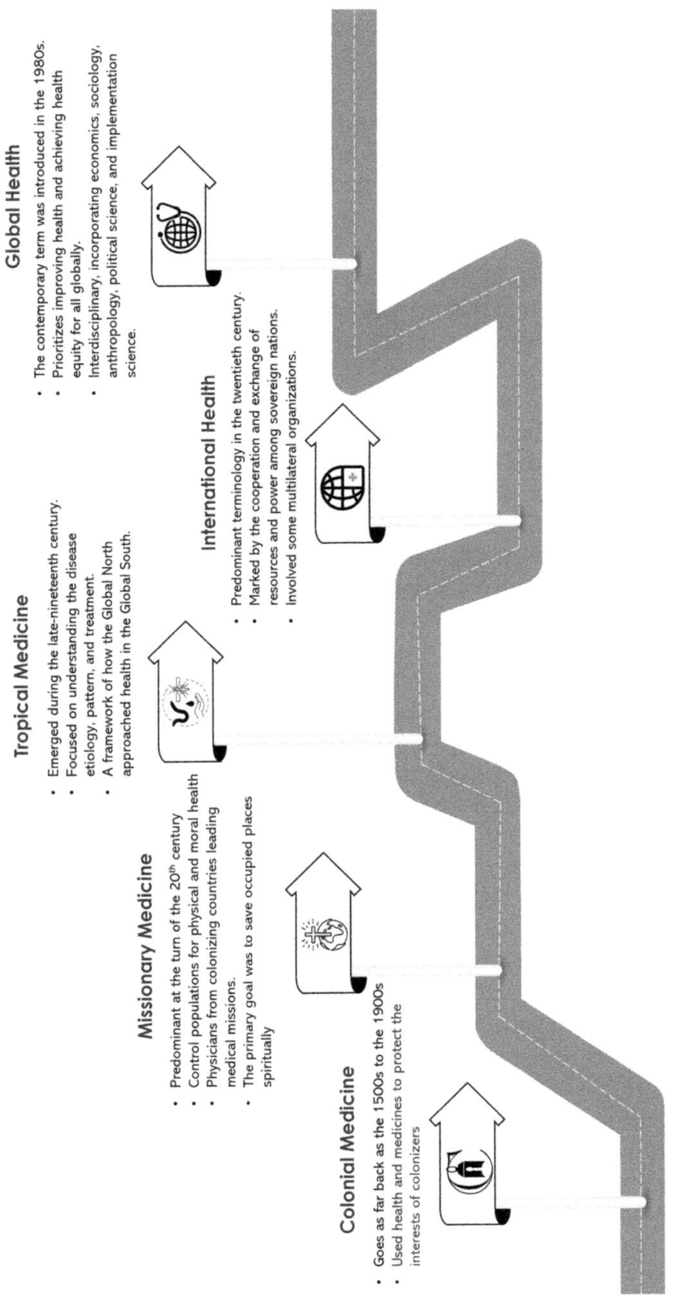

Figure 1.2 A synopsis of the historical evolution of global health.

engineering to "save" the occupied territories (Castor & Borrell, 2022). While pursuing their dual mission of soul conversion and pastoral service provision, missionaries embedded themselves within marginalized colonial communities often overlooked by imperial systems. They learned the local languages, studied the religions and cultures, and often dedicated their adult lives to these communities. While many missionaries were skilled at forming relationships with local leaders and the elite, others intentionally chose to serve the poorest of the poor. As a result, they documented the experiences of "subalterns" who are often overlooked in historical accounts (McKay, 2007).

The weaponization of medical discoveries allowed the colonial powers to establish themselves in colonies with tropical conditions and diseases. For instance, quinine extracted from cinchona bark (Andes) became a malaria preventive by the 1850s. British colonial troops in India saw malaria deaths drop from 76% (1823–1827) to 5% post-1850s. This discovery allowed sustained military presence in malarial zones like West Africa during the "scramble for Africa." Tropical medicine, which emerged in the late nineteenth century, aimed to understand the disease etiology, patterns, and treatments affecting indigenous populations in the Southern Hemisphere (Castor & Borrell, 2022). This discipline signifies a shift in how the Global North approached health issues in the Global South. Malaria was one of such problems that colonizers needed to address to achieve their successful colonization of Africa. In the practice of colonial medicine, racial superiority or inferiority was used as a rationale to impose restrictions on the movement of indigenous people in the name of infection control while exploiting local remedies and pursuing medical progress through unethical research practices. Through these colonial practices, it is fair to say that many medical advancements associated with the Global North and its scientists relied on exploiting vulnerable populations (Hussain et al., 2023). The history of "exotic syphilis" or "Arab syphilis" demonstrates how medicine upheld racist notions across various aspects, including pathology, research, conferences, journals, institutions, grants, and medical careers (Amster, 2022).

White settlers' permanent colonization of tropical regions became possible only when, at the end of the nineteenth century, more effective prevention measures reduced the newcomers' high mortality rates. While colonizers considered colonial medicine a tool to enable their settlement in the colonies, tropical medicine was seen as a method of carrying out the imperial project (McCleery, 2015). Tropical medicine[5] was deemed appropriate because doctors during the colonial era had to deal with tropical diseases such as malaria, dysentery, hookworm, and tuberculosis. Using malaria as a trace condition to establish the transition from colonial medicine to tropical medicine, Bump and Aniebo (2022) recounted how malaria, which was a colonial problem, rose to prominence as a colonial activity and how interest in malaria was harnessed to create the first schools of tropical medicine. The creation of academic tropical medicine, which combines laboratory science, medicine, hygiene, and public health, was primarily driven by the need to combat malaria and other tropical diseases affecting the labor force of the different plantations.

Because it was initially formed within colonial governments, tropical medicine became a specialization and independent academic profession with colonial features. Tropical medical research also held a political advantage regarding national and international prestige due to its distinctive nature of competition and exchange among European states (Bruchhausen, 2020). At the end of the nineteenth century, a new wave of imperialism led to the establishment of geographical societies and institutes of tropical medicine across Europe (Affun-Adegbulu et al., 2023) to preserve the health of European colonial rulers and protect them from the health hazards of tropical diseases (Holst, 2020). For example, the Institute of Tropical Medicine established in Belgium was mandated to extend Belgium's scientific enterprise to the Belgian colony to tackle colonial diseases and contribute to scientific progress in tropical medicine (Affun-Adegbulu et al., 2023). In this way, the institute was deeply involved in and had a central role in the colonial project and Belgium's oppressive and exploitative rule in Congo. Even today, the "neglected tropical disease" research ecosystem mirrors the colonial structure.

The profound influences of macroeconomic forces and financial power on defining global health priorities remain evident in academic and private sector engagement. This dynamic emerged directly out of colonialism by European nations and similar imperial activities by the United States, which created the demand for specialized knowledge about "tropical" diseases and other health obstacles to conquest (Bump, 2025). To this end, key global health funders continue to fund research led by tropical medicine institutes in the United Kingdom, Europe, and North America. Bhaumik (2024) argued that organizations in these non-endemic nations, where neglected tropical diseases are mostly non-existent, were recipients of 75% (47,997 million USD out of a total of 63,537 million USD) of direct research funding on neglected tropical diseases and 70% (40,940 million USD out of a total of 58,223 million USD) of indirect research funding on neglected tropical diseases between 2007 and 2022. These funds enable the institutes to continue to build on and modernize their research infrastructure, thus keeping the colonial essence of tropical medicine alive (Bhaumik, 2024).

During the second half of the twentieth century, particularly throughout the postcolonial period, the concept of international health gained recognition as a logical progression of traditional tropical medicine. The transition from tropical medicine to international health was not smooth, meaning these terms were used interchangeably during the second half of the twentieth century. While the colonial foundation of global health in the forms of colonial and tropical medicine was propelled by trade through imperialism, international health was mostly underpinned by geopolitics—grand strategies of nations that play out through competition for territory, energy, natural resources, and other forms of power (Bump, 2025). This understanding explains why the United Nations

Universal Declaration of Human Rights (Article 25) in 1948 and the Constitution of the World Health Organization played a significant role in addressing epidemics (Bruchhausen, 2020). These documents acknowledged that combatting epidemics should no longer be driven solely by political and economic interests but rather recognize the importance of healthcare as a fundamental human right. International Health was primarily focused on addressing health issues and obstacles in the Global South, strongly emphasizing preventing and treating infectious diseases, improving hygiene and water provision, and promoting the health of children and mothers (Holst, 2020). According to Castor and Borrell (2022), international health was also defined by cooperation and exchange of resources and power among sovereign nations based on their respective needs and the involvement of multilateral organizations.

Even today, numerous universities and scientific institutions employ this term, though its scope has broadened to encompass non-communicable diseases, injuries, and the reinforcement of health systems beyond tropical ailments. The era of international health also saw the commitment of the Global North and the international organizations to address the health issues of the Global South (Birn, 2009). This commitment includes helping the Global South address health-related issues, including development aid, which preceded overseas development aid and current international cooperation. Another important component of international health is the addition of public health concepts that evolved from social hygiene or social epidemiology. In this way, internation health also focused on addressing the social factors that influence health and illness, as well as the disparities in health resulting from an unequal distribution of social, political, and economic opportunities (Birn, 2009). It was practiced with a colonial mentality.

The goal from the late colonial period and early decolonization phase to make health care available to everyone was not taken up again until the détente policy of the 1970s and the announcement of primary health care (PHC) in Alma Ata in 1978 (Bruchhausen, 2020). In the last three decades, the terms "planetary health" and "global health" have replaced the concept of international health, with "global health" gaining more prominence in recent times. Some authors have argued that global health has become prominent because, in the twenty-first century, the world has become more globalized. In a broader sense, "global" includes all health challenges and transnational factors, such as the global eradication of diseases like polio, antibiotic resistance, food security, urbanization, migration, and climate change. Consequently, global health focuses primarily on addressing health issues that have a worldwide impact on humanity based on the eight elements of PHC, which are based on measures already implemented during the colonial period: health education, improved water supply, and nutrition (Bruchhausen, 2020).

What constitutes global health, or the nature of global health, remains controversial because there are disagreements among different authors and other stakeholders (Koplan et al., 2009). Despite the controversial nature of global health, the field has become interdisciplinary, incorporating economics, sociology, anthropology, political science, implementation science, and other fields within its practice (Rowson et al., 2012). For researchers and as a field of study, global health is a branch of health sciences and a specialized discipline within broader public health and medicine, which provides the guiding principles for achieving health for all (Koplan et al., 2009).

Braveman et al. (2011) argued that global health issues, such as health inequities and disparities, should be considered within the broader context of ethics and human rights to address its colonial legacy. They argue that achieving "health for all" requires the instrumentalist approach to disease prevention and treatment and ensuring equity and justice in the distribution of resources, which entails addressing broader political, economic, and social determinants of health because of colonialism. The "Healthy People" agenda also captures this dualistic goal of eliminating colonialism-related health disparities to achieve health equity (Braveman et al., 2011). However, Rowson et al. (2012) argue that "equity, a key element of many definitions of global health, is a value-laden concept and carries significant ideological baggage" (p. 1). While I agree that the notions of equity and justice are linked to different epistemological positions, they are at the heart of the ethos of global health: addressing inequities and injustice in the distribution of health resources and the creation and use of knowledge. Therefore, global health should consider addressing health disparities and equity concerns, which, for the most part, are enshrined in colonialism and are deeply ingrained in social values and human rights principles.

Conclusion

The inequity and injustice associated with the practice of global health also stem from the colonial foundation of global health, and the practice of global health will not be complete without considering the need to address the remnants of colonialism plaguing the ethos of global health. The central argument here is that the inequities and injustices introduced by colonial practices did not end abruptly with the political decolonization of formerly colonized nations but continue to influence international engagements, including global health practice. Consequently, global health's definition and practice have evolved to include language on autonomy, power, and health equity. In Chapter 2, I will illustrate how, by preserving certain power structures (coloniality), colonial ideologies and mindsets continue to influence global health practice.

Notes

1 There is also no commonly accepted definition of imperialism. The basic tenet that applies to it is that there is an international hierarchy, which is the basis for the political domination of one society over the other. Wright (1967) identified the following tenets across the different definitions of imperialism: (1) some political or social unit (such as state, nation or people), which is being imperialistic; (2) some unit which is the object of imperialism; (3) the nature of the relationship between the two; (4) the means of establishing this relationship; (5) the degree of realization of the relationship; (6) the reason and motive for establishing the relationships.

2 Imperialism is understood in its connection to capitalism as the projection of state power aimed at securing the conditions needed for capital accumulation.
3 Colonialism is that form of intergroup domination in which settlers in significant number migrate permanently to the colony from the colonizing power, while Imperialism is a form of intergroup domination in which few, if any, permanent settlers from the imperial homeland migrate to the colony.
4 Decolonization with the subscripts relates to political decolonization for Decolonization$_1$ and the proposed undoing of the remnants of colonialism for Decolonization$_2$. Decolonization$_2$ speaks to the systematic dismantling of colonial power structures and aiming to reclaim indigenous epistemologies and cultural identities. Decolonization without the subscript alludes to the ideology of self-governance, political autonomy, essentializing cultures or enabling authoritarian nationalism whether the one that has occurred (Decolonization$_1$) or the one that is being advocated for (Decolonization$_2$).
5 Although not all countries that were colonized are in tropical regions, this name was given based on the notion that tropical disease became problematic for the colonizers in those areas. Thus, the focus on tackling these tropical diseases led to the branch of medicine termed "tropical medicine." Today, topical medicine is a specialty that focuses on diagnosing and treating diseases and conditions that are more common, difficult to control, or unique to tropical and subtropical regions, which is a component of global health.

References

Abimbola, S. (2024). *The foreign gaze: Essays on global health*. IRD.

Abimbola, S., & Pai, M. (2021). Undoing supremacy in global health will require more than decolonisation—Authors' reply. *The Lancet*, 397(10279), 1058–1059. https://doi.org/10.1016/S0140-6736(21)00373-1

Affun-Adegbulu, C., Cosaert, T., Meudec, M., Michielsen, J., Van De Pas, R., Van Belle, S., Van De Put, W., Soors, W., Robertson, F., & Ddungu, C. (2023). Decolonisation initiatives at the Institute of Tropical Medicine, Antwerp, Belgium: ready for change? *BMJ Global Health*, 8(5), e011748. https://doi.org/10.1136/BMJGH-2023-011748

Amster, E. J. (2022). The past, present and future of race and colonialism in medicine. CMAJ: *Canadian Medical Association Journal*, 194(20), E708. https://doi.org/10.1503/CMAJ.212103

Arneil, B. (2023). Colonialism versus Imperialism. *Political Theory*, 52(1), 146. https://doi.org/10.1177/00905917231193107

Bagchi, A. (2021). On capitalist colonialism and imperialism. *Social Scientist*, 49(9), 19–28.

Bhakuni, H., & Abimbola, S. (2021). Epistemic injustice in academic global health. *The Lancet Global Health*, 9(10), e1465–e1470. https://doi.org/10.1016/S2214-109X(21)00301-6

Bhaumik, S. (2024). On the nature and structure of epistemic injustice in the neglected tropical disease knowledge ecosystem. *PLOS Neglected Tropical Diseases*, 18(12), e0012781. https://doi.org/10.1371/JOURNAL.PNTD.0012781

Biggar, N. (2023). *Colonialism: A moral reckoning*. HarperCollins Publishers.

Birn, A. E. (2009). The stages of international (global) health: Histories of success or successes of history? *Global Public Health*, 4(1), 50–68. https://doi.org/10.1080/17441690802017797

Branch, J. (2011). "Colonial reflection" and territoriality: The peripheral origins of sovereign statehood. *European Journal of International Relations*, 18(2), 277–297. https://doi.org/10.1177/1354066110383997

Braveman, P. A., Kumanyika, S., Fielding, J., LaVeist, T., Borrell, L. N., Manderscheid, R., & Troutman, A. (2011). Health disparities and health equity: The issue is justice. *American Journal of Public Health*, 101(Suppl 1), S149. https://doi.org/10.2105/AJPH.2010.300062

Brown, T. M., Cueto, M., & Fee, E. (2006). The World Health Organization and the transition from international to global public health. *American Journal of Public Health*. 96(1), 62–72. https://doi.org/10.2105/AJPH.2004.050831

Bruchhausen, W. (2020). Global health in the colonial era: The expansion of European medicine. In Europe History Online (Mainz). Leibniz Institute of European History (IEG). www.ieg-ego.eu/en/threads/theories-and-methods/knowledge-transfer/walter-bruchhausen-global-health-in-the-colonial-era-the-expansion-of-european-medicine

Bump, J. B. (2025). Global health and its limitations: An historical perspective. *Health Systems & Reform*, 11(2), 2478681. https://doi.org/10.1080/23288604.2025.2478681

Bump, J. B., & Aniebo, I. (2022). Colonialism, malaria, and the decolonization of global health. *PLOS Global Public Health*, 2(9), e0000936. https://doi.org/10.1371/JOURNAL.PGPH.0000936

Castor, D., & Borrell, L. N. (2022). The cognitive dissonance discourse of evolving terminology from colonial medicine to global health and inaction towards equity. *Preventive Medicine*, 163, 107227. https://doi.org/10.1016/J.YPMED.2022.107227

Césaire, A., & Kelley, R. (2007). *Discourse on colonialism* (J. Pinkham, Trans.). Monthly Review Press.

Chen, X., Li, H., Lucero-Prisno, D. E., Abdullah, A. S., Huang, J., Laurence, C., Liang, X., Ma, Z., Mao, Z., Ren, R., Wu, S., Wang, N., Wang, P., Wang, T., Yan, H., & Zou, Y. (2020). What is global health? Key concepts and clarification of misperceptions: Report of the 2019 GHRP editorial meeting. *Global Health Research and Policy*, 5(1), 14. https://doi.org/10.1186/S41256-020-00142-7

Chilcote, R. H. (2002). Globalization or imperialism? *Latin American Perspectives*, 29(6), 80–84. https://doi.org/10.1177/009458202237779

Cooper, Frederick. (2006). *Colonialism in question: Theory, knowledge, history* (1st ed.). University of California Press.

Eichbaum, Q. G., Adams, L. V., Evert, J., Ho, M.-J., Semali, I. A., & Van Schalkwyk, S. C. (2021). Decolonizing global health education: Rethinking institutional partnerships and approaches. *Academic Medicine*, 96(3), 329–335. https://doi.org/10.1097/ACM.0000000000003473

Emerson, R. (1969). Colonialism. *Journal of Contemporary History*, 4(1). https://about.jstor.org/terms

Erondu, N. A., Dhar Sharma, V., Mulumba, M., & na Haki, A. (2025). Decolonial framings in global health law: Redressing colonial legacies for a just and equitable future. *Journal of Law, Medicine & Ethics*, 1–3. https://doi.org/10.1017/JME.2025.25

Ferro, Marc. (1997). *Colonization: A global history*. Routledge.

Frenk, J., Gómez-Dantés, O., & Moon, S. (2014). From sovereignty to solidarity: A renewed concept of global health for an era of complex interdependence. *The Lancet*, 383(9911), 94–97. https://doi.org/10.1016/S0140-6736(13)62561-1

Getgen, J., Caroline, K., & Laporte, B. (2023). Unsettling human rights clinical pedagogy and practice in settler colonial contexts. *Journal of Gender, Social Policy & the Law*, 31(3). https://digitalcommons.wcl.american.edu/jgspl/vol31/iss3/4

Gichane, M. W., Wallace, D. D., & Wall, S. (2022). Dismantling and reimagining global health education. *Global Health Action*, 15. https://doi.org/10.1080/16549716.2022.2131967

Gilley, B. (2023). *The case for colonialism*. New English Review Press.

Grosfoguel, R. (2007). The epistemic decolonial turn: Beyond political-economy paradigms. *Cultural Studies*, 21(2–3), 211–223. https://doi.org/10.1080/09502380601162514

Holst, J. (2020). Global eealth—Emergence, hegemonic trends and biomedical reductionism. *Globalization and Health*, 16(1). https://doi.org/10.1186/S12992-020-00573-4

Horvath, R. J. (1972). A definition of colonialism. *Anthropology*, 13(1), 45–57. https://about.jstor.org/terms
Hussain, M., Sadigh, M., Sadigh, M., Rastegar, A., & Sewankambo, N. (2023). Colonization and decolonization of global health: which way forward? *Global Health Action*, 16(1). https://doi.org/10.1080/16549716.2023.2186575
Karsgaard, C., Pillay, T., & Shultz, L. (2024). Facing colonial Canada through pedagogies of equity for First Nations: An advocacy education project. *Journal of Curriculum and Pedagogy*. https://doi.org/10.1080/15505170.2022.2134948
Kohn, M. (2008). Colonialism. https://philpapers.org/rec/KOHC
Kohn, M., & Reddy, K. (2024). Colonialism. *Stanford Encyclopedia of Philosophy*. https://plato.stanford.edu/cgi-bin/encyclopedia/archinfo.cgi?entry=colonialism
Koplan, J. P., Bond, T. C., Merson, M. H., Reddy, K. S., Rodriguez, M. H., Sewankambo, N. K., & Wasserheit, J. N. (2009). Towards a common definition of global health. *The Lancet*, 373(9679), 1993–1995. https://doi.org/10.1016/S0140-6736(09)60332-9
Kwete, X., Tang, K., Chen, L., Ren, R., Chen, Q., Wu, Z., Cai, Y., & Li, H. (2022). Decolonizing global health: what should be the target of this movement and where does it lead us? *Global Health Research and Policy*, 7(1). https://doi.org/10.1186/s41256-022-00237-3
MacFarlane, S. B., Jacobs, M., & Kaaya, E. E. (2008). In the name of global health: Trends in academic institutions. *Journal of Public Health Policy*, 29(4), 383–401. https://doi.org/10.1057/JPHP.2008.25
Manning, P. (1974). Analyzing the costs and benefits of colonialism. *African Economic History Review*, 1(2), 15–22. www.jstor.org/stable/3601097
McCleery, I. (2015). What is "colonial" about medieval colonial medicine? Iberian health in global context. *Journal of Medieval Iberian Studies*, 7(2), 151. https://doi.org/10.1080/17546559.2015.1077390
McCoy, D., Kapilashrami, A., Kumar, R., Rhule, E., & Khosla, R. (2024). Developing an agenda for the decolonization of global health. *Bulletin of the World Health Organization*, 102(2), 130–136. https://doi.org/10.2471/BLT.23.289949
McKay, A. (2007). Towards a history of medical missions. *Medical History*, 51(4), 547. https://pmc.ncbi.nlm.nih.gov/articles/PMC2002588/
Ndlovu-Gatsheni, S. J. (2013). The entrapment of Africa within the global colonial matrices of power. *Journal of Developing Societies*, 29(4), 331–353. https://doi.org/10.1177/0169796X13503195
Pitts, J. (2010). Political theory of empire and imperialism. *Annual Review of Political Science*, 13, 211–235. https://doi.org/10.1146/annurev.polisci.051508.214538
Quijano, A. (2007). Coloniality and modernity/rationality. *Cultural Studies*, 21(2–3), 168–178. https://doi.org/10.1080/09502380601164353
Rowson, M., Willott, C., Hughes, R., Maini, A., Martin, S., Miranda, J. J., Pollit, V., Smith, A., Wake, R., & Yudkin, J. S. (2012). Conceptualising global health: Theoretical issues and their relevance for teaching. *Globalization and Health*, 8(1), 1–8.
Salm, M., Ali, M., Minihane, M., & Conrad, P. (2021). Defining global health: findings from a systematic review and thematic analysis of the literature. *BMJ Global Health*, 6(6), e005292. https://doi.org/10.1136/BMJGH-2021-005292
Simmons, C. (2020). Subtle subversions: resisting colonialism through religion. *Religion*, 50(2), 191–195. https://doi.org/10.1080/0048721X.2020.1713510
Táíwò, O. (2022). *Against decolonisation: Taking African agency seriously* (1st ed.). Hurst & Company.
Veltmeyer, H. (2020). Capitalism, development, imperialism, globalization: a tale of four concepts. *Globalizations*, 17(8), 1335–1349. https://doi.org/10.1080/14747731.2019.1699706
Vilas, C. M. (2002). Globalization as imperialism. *Latin American Perspectives*, 29(6), 70–79. https://doi.org/10.1177/009458202237778

Went, R. (2002). Globalization in the perspective of imperialism. In *Science & Society*, 66(4).
Williams, D. (2023). Adam Smith, colonialism, and liberal imperialism. *National Institute Economic Review*, 265, 39–50. https://doi.org/10.1017/NIE.2023.26
Willmott, K., & Skillings, A. (2021). Anti-Indigenous policy formation: Settler colonialism and neoliberal political advocacy. *Canadian Review of Sociology = Revue Canadienne de Sociologie*, 58(4), 513–530. https://doi.org/10.1111/CARS.12357
Wright, H. M. (1967). "Imperialism": The word and its meaning. *Social Research*, 34(4), 660–674.

2 Expressions of Coloniality in Global Health

Introduction

Some countries and regions persistently experience higher burdens of diseases, including epidemics and syndemics. These regions characteristically lack well-organized and functional health systems and inadequate human, financial, and material resources to address these disease burdens. Factors such as weak socioeconomic and political power, poor technological advancements, and inadequate resources (financial, material, and human) have been attributed to the higher burden of diseases and the poorer health outcomes experienced in these countries and regions. This inequitable wealth, resources, and health distribution is not serendipitous. The global and international health literature suggests that other systemic factors account for the inequities and disparities in the distribution of disease burdens and the availability of resources. These systemic factors have been linked to international relations between countries and regions worldwide.

Appellations such as "low- and middle-income countries," "developing countries," "underdeveloped nations," and "third-world countries" have been used to describe these countries with low socioeconomic status experiencing high population-level disease burdens characterized by weak health systems (including technological advancements). While these descriptions are not "natural," they distinguish these countries from well-resourced countries (wealthy nations), ascribed corresponding antonyms like high-income, developed, and first-world countries. Such classifications of the world, especially in global health, have been found to originate from oppressive structures like racism and colonialism (Khan et al., 2022). For instance, the term "sub-Saharan Africa," which is frequently used in global health research to distinguish countries in the North of Africa from the rest, is more racist than on a geographical basis. Going on the geographical argument, one would observe that the Sahara Desert extends to many other countries beyond the seven North African countries (Algeria, Egypt, Libya, Morocco, Sudan, Tunisia, Western Sahara) to accommodate countries like Chad, Niger, and Mali. What differentiates these seven North African countries from the other 47 African countries is that most of their populations are black. This observation supports the notion that the

DOI: 10.4324/9781032700786-2

pervasive use of "sub-Saharan Africa" to mark the African continent for global health practice is more racial than otherwise.

Countries predominantly described as underdeveloped (including the economic classification of low- and middle-income countries) are geographically concentrated in the Southern region of the globe, and their counterparts are found predominantly in the North. The term "Global South" has been used increasingly in the social sciences and has become a "common ground" concept for International Cooperation, Economics, and International Law and Inequality Studies (Lira, 2021). Consequently, the focus on addressing inequalities and inequities in the decolonization discourse popularizes the classification of "Global South"[1] and "Global North" in the global health literature. The "Global North" and "Global South" divide describes a grouping of countries along socioeconomic and political characteristics. The Global South broadly comprises countries in Africa, Latin America and the Caribbean, Asia (Israel, Japan, and South Korea), and Oceania (Australia and New Zealand). A keen observation reveals that the geographical classification of countries into "Global South" and "Global North" does not precisely align with the cardinal directions of north and south, as many of the Global South countries are geographically located in the Northern Hemisphere (Figure 2.1).

The temptation to categorize and dichotomize countries may appear helpful—for example, economic classifications by the International Monetary Fund and the World Bank for lending purposes and the analytical advancement of the social sciences. While this classification may have theoretical and analytical benefits, it is worth exploring whether such conceptualization promotes fair and positive change in international relations (Lira, 2021). For instance, it has been argued that the different appellations that have been used to classify nations based on different criteria create a *false* hierarchy among nations, as higher values are ascribed to wealthier nations, with the consequence that these nations have the power to exploit and subjugate less economically viable countries (Khan et al., 2022). As such, power asymmetries between countries and regions continue to engender a long heritage of unequal and unfair relationships, notably colonialism, imperialism, post-World War II governance structures, and patriarchal norms and practices. This imbalanced relationship manifests in unequal trade relations, appropriation of mind and capital, exploitative practices by transnational corporations, and technological dependencies.

Although Global North is commonly used in global health to describe resource-rich nations that are superior to those considered as Global South, the term "global" in global health is usually employed to refer to a world outside rich nations focusing on a world that needs development or assistance to address the different challenges that they are facing. According to Khan et al. (2022), the idea that countries are inherently different, ordered, or ranked along a hierarchy is a racist, colonialist construct originating from European and North American institutions and structures. The Global North and

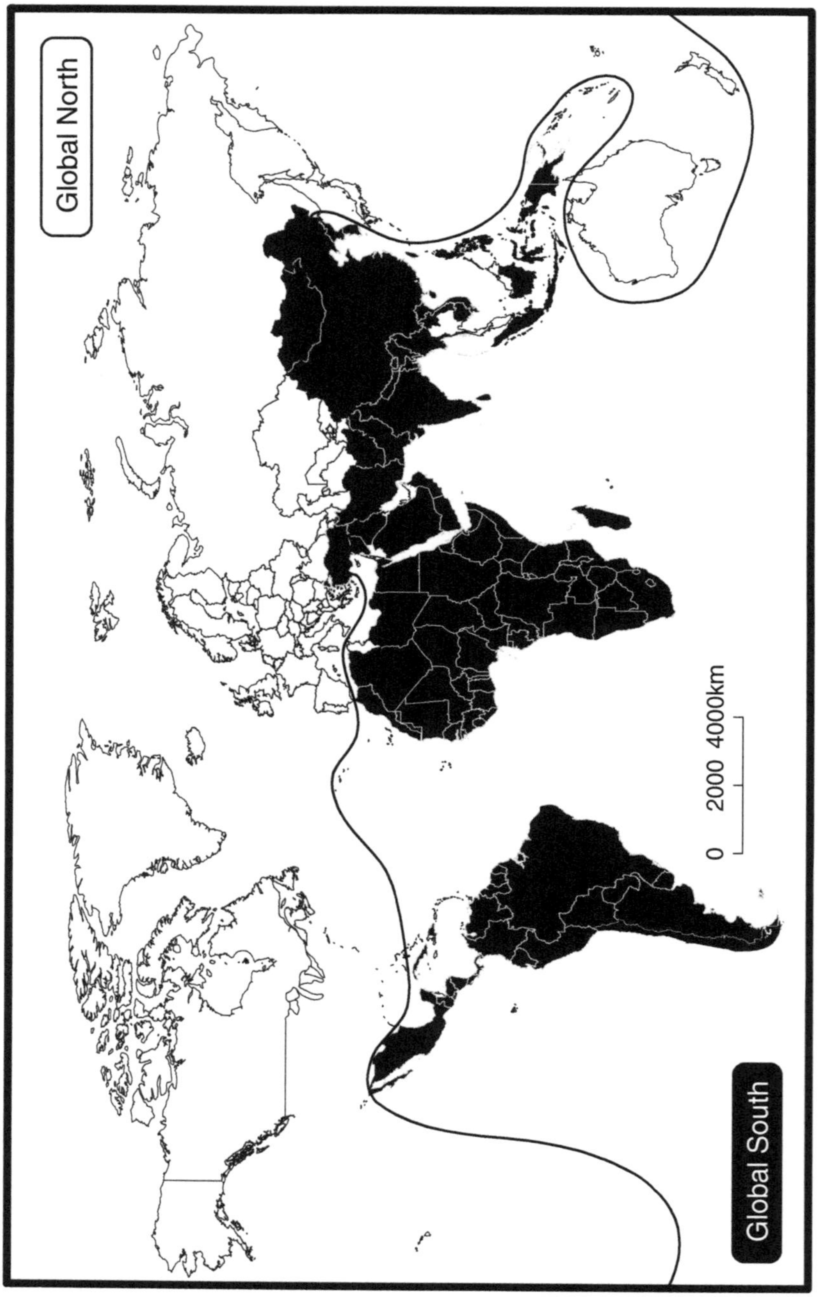

Figure 2.1 Global South and Global South regional divide.

Global South categorization is a "language that reinforces the hegemony of Europe and North America over the rest of the world" (Opara, 2021). Indeed, there are historical underpinnings of such power asymmetries between countries and regions of the North and those of the South, leading to a long heritage of unequal and unfair relationships.

Carl Oglesby, an American political activist, is credited for coining the term "Global South" in 1969 in Commonweal to describe a set of countries beset by the "dominance" of the "Global North" through political and economic exploitation (Oglesby, 1969). Therefore, when discussing the "Global South," it is necessary to consider the historical dispute between empires (center) and colonies (periphery). Consequently, ontologically, the terms "Global North" and "Global South" operationalize colonization. As it relates to global health, this classification implicitly describes the foundation of global health and the source of diverse health disparities, thus triggering reflection on inequities and injustice in health. Epistemically, these classifications sensitize readers to the "location" of knowledge production and encourage the development of critical consciousness, which is valuable to contesting colonial legacies, decolonizing knowledge systems, and promoting epistemic justice (Sims, 2023). One challenge with this epistemic conceptualization of the "Global South" is that it assumes that the regions of Africa, Asia, Latin America, and the Middle East are homogenous—immutably poor and disease-ridden (Daffé et al., 2021). Homogenizing countries from this region conceals their diversity and differences and how this may shape and inform their various expectations, positions, and ambitions (Cranston, 2025). While acknowledging the challenges and the consequences of using the terms "Global North" and "Global South" in this book, I adopted this categorization (albeit with reservations) because it "connote[s] the division of [countries] along the lines of power, [the most recent] colonial history, and associated wealth" (Wispelwey et al., 2023, p. e1469). This categorization supports my ontological and epistemological arguments toward building my postcolonial critical realist theory and contributions to decolonizing global health by acknowledging and addressing the contribution of these structures.

To understand the lines of power and colonial influences associated with the current practice of global health, I set out to capture the key stages associated with the advent and development of the field of global health as we know it today. The historical snapshot of the evolution of global health could be beneficial to researchers, policymakers, global health students, global health program managers, and others to get a sense of why global health is the way it is and critical structures that influenced and framed to inform how it could be better practiced (Packard, 2016). Nevertheless, the goal of providing narratives on the history of global health in this book is to help us better understand the role of colonialism in shaping the distinction between the "Global North" and "Global South" and, consequently, the nature of global health as practiced today.

For those working in global health, it is unsurprising that our understanding of disease patterns and distributions, the strengthening of resources for health and health systems, and global health research are rife with comparisons between what is happening in the Global North and Global South. This arbitrary division of the world as Global South and Global North is one of the most significant signs of the colonized situation of global health. We often find, conspicuously, that nations located in the Global North outperform their Global South counterparts in most health matrices and are closest to meeting the WHO sustainable development goals. As outlined in Chapter 1, the colonization of the Global South by nations of the Global North is one of the most striking reasons offered to explain the nature of the health systems and health status observed between nations of the Global North and those in the Global South.

In Chapter 1, I focused on establishing the colonial birth and foundations of global health. In this chapter, the focus will be on the colonial influences in contemporary global health. Accordingly, this chapter examines how colonial-era social architectures endure and analyzes the contested roles of key actors in perpetuating versus challenging those power frameworks. Particularly, this chapter will focus on unearthing the effects of these social structures and their influence on global health practice and research. The notion of coloniality is at the heart of the effect of colonial structures and relationships in global health. To this end, the chapter starts with the notion of coloniality.

Coloniality

Colonialism, in its various forms, established its authority to accumulate wealth through military conquest and subsequent political dictatorship. Nevertheless, its most insidious form of control extended to the mental world of the colonized. Through cultural influence (imperialism), colonial powers dictated how individuals perceived themselves and their place in the world. The diverse and intricate global structures erected during colonialism to amass wealth did not automatically, magically, or wishfully vanish after Decolonization$_1$ (Grosfoguel, 2007). The prevailing argument is that these global structures were not dismantled in Decolonization$_1$. Richardson (2019) contends that after Decolonization$_1$ colonial structure continues to exist under the same "colonial power matrix" as it did in the colonial era. He argues further that Decolonization$_1$ began a shift from "global colonialism" to the current era of "global coloniality." That is why when Gilley (2018) argues that "Western and non-Western countries should reclaim the colonial toolkit and language as part of their commitment to effective governance and international order" (p. 168), I wonder what he is talking about. My argument is that Decolonization$_1$ was largely theoretical as practically, there is an ongoing relevance of colonial structures in the postcolonial era, and it drives the colonial practices in global health.

Táíwò (2022), in his book *Against Decolonisation: Taking African Agency Seriously*, argues that decolonization in post-independence Africa must be abandoned since political decolonization (Decolonization$_1$) has already been achieved. He stated that advocating for Decolonization$_2$ denotes "forcing an ex-colony to forswear, on pain of being forever under the yoke of colonization, any and every cultural, political, intellectual, social and linguistic artifact, idea, process, institution and practice that retains even the slightest whiff of the colonial past" (p. 3). Basing his argument on Africa, Táíwò argued further:

> [T]o turn colonialism into the most important or even the only element in explaining social phenomena in Africa cannot be plausible, adequate, or correct. This is, for me, probably the most vexing aspect of the decolonisation trope. Because colonialism is adopted as the single or dominant axis on which to plot the continent's history and events post-colonisation—and no serious attention is paid to the fractures, cleavages, and different historicities as colonialism evolved—the many divergences that characterize it are glossed over in most analyses.
>
> (Táíwò, 2022, p. 148)

Táíwò's text suggests that coloniality may be overused in the African context, potentially undermining the recognition of African agency. However, these concerns serve as cautions against misusing the concept of coloniality rather than arguments for abandoning it altogether. Meagher (2023), engaging with Táíwò's work, argued that a meaningful sense of decolonization that emphasizes eradicating what has an enduring colonial function but not simply a colonial "tinge" should be made. To this end, my engagement with coloniality in this chapter is to capture those enduring colonial influences in global health practices and research.

Under colonialism, the interests of the colonialists were prioritized above all else, with the needs of the colonized addressed only when they aligned with those interests. The abuses of colonialism were intentional, as was the resulting resentment among the formerly colonized. Today, most formerly colonized economies, particularly in Africa, remain deeply connected to a Euro-American-dominated global system, but the terms of these connections typically disadvantage the formerly colonized. In this way, colonialism has evolved into neo-colonialism (Nkrumah, 1965). Following Decolonization$_1$, the colonizers intended to maintain a power hierarchy and control over their formal colonies and other nations under similar conditions. Whether for profit, prestige, political advantage, or from a sense of tasks left unaccomplished, the ex-colonial powers understandably sought to maintain a greater or lesser degree of contact with their former colonies (Emerson, 1969). Thus, based on this premise, there are calls for a second decolonization (Decolonization$_2$).

Understanding Decolonization$_2$ requires examining the continuing dynamics of internalized and systemic oppression of colonized countries, resulting in the reproduction of the colonial logic of commodifying human beings, labor, space, culture, and knowledge (Opara, 2021). The interlocking systems of principles and practices perpetuating inquiry-driven expansion and coercive control over existential, perceptual, embodied, cognitive, affective, and behavioral realms constitute a foundational pillar of modernity—a phenomenon rigorously scrutinized through postcolonial theoretical discourses. The structure of these often clandestine principles and practices established during and after colonialism is known as coloniality. Figure 2.2 is an illustration of how, in the eyes of the world, the colonizers left their colonies, represented by the soldiers leaving through the front and receiving farewells from the colonized while the capitalist and the priest are seeking to return through the backdoor through the different treaties and agreements that they signed with the colonized.

Colonialism results from power asymmetry, where one group dominates and subjugates another group(s) to exploit and extract from them. Formal colonialism was achieved through conquest, by force, trickery, or "agreement," but sometimes by combining these methods with an edifice of ideas, beliefs, and narratives that justify exploitation, extraction, and misappropriation. As a conceptual framework, "coloniality" seeks to describe the hierarchical systems of race, politics, economics, society, knowledge, language, and gender that were established through European colonization. These systems have persisted even after the juridical-political "decolonization" (Decolonization$_1$) and still perpetuate oppression to serve the interests of pan-capital (economic and cultural/symbolic) accumulation.

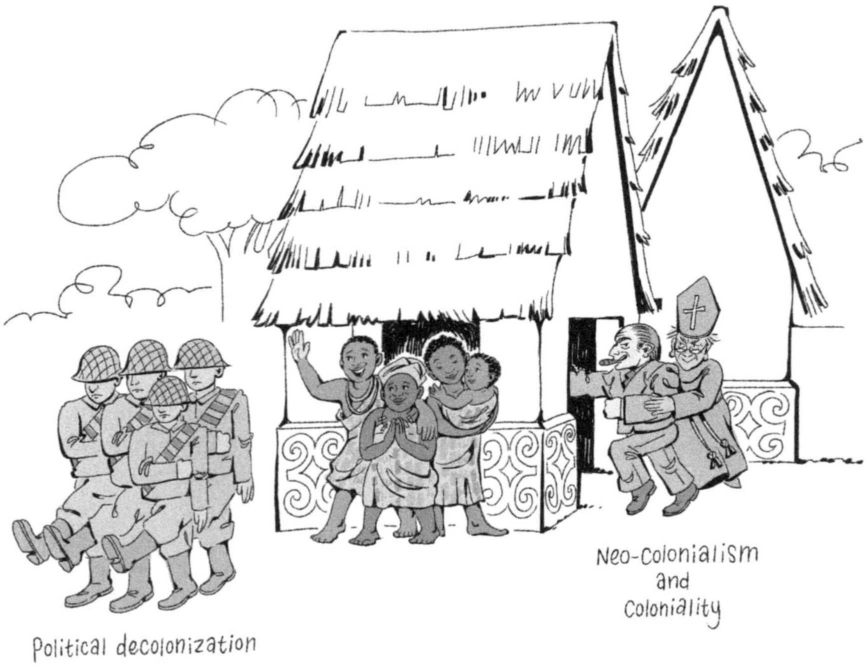

Figure 2.2 An illustration of the establishment of coloniality.

Coloniality, thus, goes beyond the historical reality of colonialism and transcends into an integral part of the logic of a wider range of international relations shaping modernity, including, of course, global health practice. Coloniality is. Therefore, the modus operandi perpetuates the inequities and injustices introduced by colonialism, even in the absence of evident colonizers. Coloniality is connected to the power structures established during colonization, which continue to exist even after the political decolonization (Tarusarira, 2020). As a result, it encompasses long-standing patterns of power that emerged because of colonialism, which were driven by capitalism and imperialism. According to Quijano (2007), colonialism was more associated with the power imbalance between the colonized and the colonizer than with an imposition from the colonizer.

Coloniality was predominantly achieved through the national middle class, which assumed power after the colonial regime, serving as the agents of the former colonial powers, which can be likened to feudalism (Ganshof, 1952). Keshri and Bhaumik (2022) argued that feudal structures helped imperial forces sustain political colonization. Through institutionalized relationships, the colonizers granted the elites proprietary rights to land, resources, and people, and implicitly, they gained the right to exploit these assets. Keshri and Bhaumik (2022) shared an example of this colonial feudal structure: the "*zamindari*" (landholder) system in British India. Under this system, *zamindars*—the economic and social elites—were given the authority to collect rent from peasants in exchange for an annual fee paid to the "Crown." It makes sense that feudalism was used to instill coloniality, as many historians consider it a crucial historical precursor to capitalism (Katz, 1993; Moore, 2003; Sen, 1984), which is at the heart of colonial agendas. By establishing feudal structures, former colonizers continued to exert control over their postcolonial states with less coercion than direct colonialism. Therefore, Fanon (1963) concluded that the goal of the immediate postcolonial government "has nothing to do with transforming the nation; it consists, prosaically, of being the transmission line between the nation and a capitalism, rampant though camouflaged, which today puts on the mask of neocolonialism" (p. 152). Imperialism and capitalism, thus, continue to shape culture, labor, intersubjectivity relations, and knowledge production, extending beyond the formal boundaries of colonial administrations (Maldonado-Torres, 2007).

Coloniality was sustained by making capitalism seductive and transformed into an aspiration for the colonized. For example, The Commonwealth of Nations, a voluntary political association of countries, was established in 1949 to maintain ties between former British colonies. The Commonwealth claims that these 56 member states, most of whom are in the Global South, are of equal status (even with those of the Global North like The United Kingdom, Australia, and New Zealand). Power (2009) used Mozambique as a case study to illustrate the neocolonial paternalism and sense of trusteeship that the Commonwealth has articulated to "foster its vision of African development which seems to rather lock the continent into a permanent stage of tutelage and to repetitively reduce Africa to a set of core deficiencies for which externally generated 'solutions' must be devised" (p. 14). Such structures were used to maintain the colonial ties that existed during the colonial days and maintain agendas of colonialism under the guise of promoting international understanding and world peace and influencing international society to the benefit of all. In this case, the colonial powers worked on shaping the perceptions and manipulating the wishes of the colonized to the extent that the colonized became persuaded to accept and even desire the entrapment policies they presented that were harmful to them.

The colonized were enticed to reach the same material benefits and the same power as the colonizers to become "developed." In this way, colonizers (developed countries) became the reference for colonized societies concerning civilization and development, engendering a power system strengthened by capitalism (Beghin, 2022). Therefore, coloniality was partly sustained by a pursuit of isomorphism (Dimaggio & Powell, 1983). The authors argue that organizations/Institutions within a field or industry become increasingly similar over time! The perception of global health institutions in the Global North as the "gold standard" has created a dynamic where institutions worldwide emulate their structures and practices to gain legitimacy in the eyes of funders. This drive for alignment with dominant ideologies can have profound implications. It reinforces a cycle where institutions in the Global South prioritize conformity to Northern models, often at the expense of innovation and locally driven solutions. It also skews collaborative efforts, favoring North–South partnerships over potentially impactful South–South collaborations.

Through imperialism and capitalism, the goals of the colonized nations now mirrored those of the ethos and praxis of the former colonizers. For example, according to Beghin (2022), after the end of colonialism, the governments of Latin American nations adopted economic, political, social, and cultural agendas like those of their formal colonizers that were of little benefit to most of their population. The culture of the colonized was made seductive and transformed into an aspiration for the colonized. The colonized became enticed to reach the same material benefits and the same power as the colonizers to become "developed." In this way, the colonizers (developed countries) became the reference for the colonized societies regarding civilization and development, engendering a power system strengthened by capitalism (Beghin, 2022). Quijano (2007) contends that capitalism formed the basis of exploitation and social domination that continues to determine the distribution of power and resources. For example, the International Monetary Fund (IMF) charges higher interest rates and compels countries of the Global South to cut government spending compared to countries from the Global North, like the USA, who are charged lower interest rates (Allen & Giovannetti, 2011). Therefore, coloniality is a structure of domination or a pattern of power sustained through established structures.

The premise of coloniality is that colonialism was cruel and that its deleterious effects did not leave the societies and people that were colonized. While the political liberation of colonized nations was largely achieved to maintain the power and control that the colonial nations had on the colonized nations, bilateral aid agencies were born, allowing the colonial colonies to manage the colonial assets of their regime. These bilateral aid agencies established social hierarchies, systems, and ideologies that centralized the interests of the formal colonial nations while denigrating those of the formal colonies.

Coloniality is not solely a product of a specific colonial relationship but rather arises within a specific socio-historical context. Therefore, coloniality encompasses the ongoing presence of power structures and relationships created through colonialism practices (Tarusarira, 2020). The power structures that emerged from the alliance of colonialism and imperialism have shaped the political landscape and became the driving force for other social relations between the colonized. Following the end of political colonialism, relations between former colonizers and the colonized were maintained through cooperation and agreements. These established relations undermined the culture, knowledge, and way of life of the colonized. At the same time, the former colonizers continued to impose a mystified image of their patterns of producing knowledge, meaning, and visions (Quijano, 2007).

Coloniality provides a framework for analyzing various power dynamics, which extends beyond just the relationships between former colonies and colonial powers. For example, during the colonial era, many medical advancements were made by exploiting colonized nations. History shows that colonial powers prioritized medical research and advancements when diseases impacted their populations. However, they only extended such efforts to local communities in the colonies when it served their interests, such as the need for a local workforce. A prime example of this can be seen in the case of malaria control during the construction of the Panama Canal. Most of the Tropical Medicine Institutes in the Global North were created to conduct medical research to serve colonizers during their colonial expeditions by focusing on addressing tropical diseases. Based on their agendas, these institutes continue to exist today and carry out research focused on tropical diseases, typically found in the Global South. The establishment of tropical medicine and hygiene schools during that period ensured that knowledge produced in colonial settings was integrated into international health and naturalized as global health science (Daffé et al., 2021). Although these institutes have transformed their agendas today to conduct research and implement programs and interventions to address health problems around the world, colonialism is the backbone of their existence, scaffolding their operations even to the present date.

The Expression of Coloniality in Global Health

Although global health is centered on ensuring equity, eliminating barriers, and addressing disparities in health throughout the world (Bain et al., 2024), global health practice itself is being accused of being inequitable and unjust (Affun-Adegbulu et al., 2023). The colonial practice of medicine laid the foundation for health inequity, systematic differences in the opportunity for different groups of people to achieve optimal health, leading to unfair and avoidable health outcomes (Tangcharoensathien et al., 2023). For example, in the early twentieth century, French colonial governments undertook extensive medical campaigns in sub-Saharan Africa to manage tropical diseases. The French colonial government organized campaigns against diseases such as sleeping sickness, leprosy, yaws, syphilis, and malaria. This medical exercise aimed to guarantee the health of the colonial masters occupying the colonized territories. Over several decades, millions of inhabitants in the sub-Saharan region were subjected to medical examinations and forced to receive injections of medications with unestablished efficacy and side effects, including blindness, gangrene, and death (Lowes, 2020). This practice led to mistrust in medicine, negatively affecting current health seeker behavior and meaningful health outcomes, such as vaccination rates, leading to underusing health care and health inequity (Lowes, 2020).

Table 2.1 illustrates the possible manifestation of coloniality in global health, indicating the influence of the Global North over health policies, research agendas, funding priorities, publications, and interventions in the Global South while disregarding Global South knowledge systems and community priorities.

Health Inequities and Disparities

Most of the world's population resides in the Global South, which also bears the brunt of diseases, described as health inequality. Health inequities, the differences in health status or the distribution of health resources between different population groups, are the most conspicuous picture of contemporary global health. Monitoring the trends of health inequities in countries indicates a conspicuous disparity between countries in the Global North and those in the Global South. For example, according to the World Health Organization (WHO), children are 14 times more likely to die before the age of five in sub-Saharan Africa than in the rest of the world (Alkema et al., 2014; UNICEF, 2024).

The lack of COVID-19 vaccines in Africa during the COVID-19 pandemic outbreak due to vaccine hoarding in the Global North typifies health resource inequities as a characteristic of global health. Mendelson et al. (2024) also demonstrated the huge disparities in resource availability for managing the global antimicrobial resistance pandemic between the Global North and the Global South. They argued that the disparities in resource availabilities, needs, and priorities of the Global North and the Global South regarding the actions required to mitigate the antimicrobial resistance pandemic directly threaten to successfully address the problem of antimicrobial resistance globally (Mendelson et al., 2024).

Although global healthcare access and quality have improved since 1990, inequalities between the best and worst-performing countries have grown. It has been argued that having a robust economy does not automatically ensure

Table 2.1 Manifestation of coloniality in global health

Effects of global health coloniality	*Global health coloniality*	*Characteristic colonial global health practices*
Health inequities and disparities	• Narratives obscuring relationships that favor and sustain the progress and wealth of the Global North and the under-development and poverty of the Global South. • Funding processes, practices, policies, and partnerships that replicate colonial dynamics of extraction and exploitation.	• Patent rights and the overall intellectual property framework underlying life sciences development and innovation are retained in the Global North with less willingness to share with countries in the Global South.
Dependency syndrome	• The white savior industrial complex is the trademark of colonization in global health. • Discourse that ignores the role of (neo)colonizer economic and national security decisions and policies that suppress indigenous independence.	• Advanced methodological training or high-tech techniques are required and are always offered in the partner Global North country, with little consideration for it being offered in the partner Global South in-country. • Global health research funding primarily comes from the Global North. When HIC donors give grants, they predominantly fund institutions, contractors, and principal investigators in their countries.
Agenda monopoly	• Limited participation of experts and community representatives from the Global South in governance structures and advisory bodies of organizations that focus on improving health in the Global South. • Limited considerations of the expertise and knowledge base of the researcher from the Global South.	• Global health practitioners often develop their hypotheses, goals, work plans, research strategies, and timelines before deciding whom to collaborate with in the Global South. • Global North researchers generally avoid brainstorming with anyone with overlapping or complementary expertise.

(*Continued*)

Table 2.1 (Continued)

Effects of global health coloniality	*Global health coloniality*	*Characteristic colonial global health practices*
Knowledge hegemony and epistemic injustice	• Maintenance of a global health hegemonic power hierarchy in global health. • Curricula and practice that remarginalize, deprioritize, and minimize indigenous communities' lived experiences, expertise, and epistemologies.	• Global North researchers often adopt methods they have perfected themselves or in their institutions. • Global health practitioners do not often invite individuals working in the Global South to share their experiences and lessons learned on working in the local settings. • Global health researchers strive to make their protocols different from any existing consensus guidelines for working in resource-limited settings so that they are credited for originality and innovation.
Normalized unequal partnerships	• Using language that reinforces the hegemony of the Global North over the Global South by defining nations by economic status set to Euro-American indices of prosperity and development. • Maintenance of a global health hegemonic power hierarchy in global health.	• Presentations on the work done in the Global South are often done by partners and trainees in the Global North because it is difficult for researchers from the Global South to secure visas for international conferences. • Global South partners are less often invited to lead the writing of manuscripts and papers published from collaborative work. • Global South partners are rarely included in the authorship list and are rarely given meaningful positions when included.

access to quality healthcare (Kruk et al., 2018). Also, a robust economy alone does not guarantee equitable access to quality healthcare, as evidenced by disparities in high-income nations. For example, Saudi Arabia has a high gross development product but struggles with uneven rural healthcare quality despite free universal care (Alfaqeeh et al., 2017). Similarly, advanced medical technology does not guarantee superior healthcare outcomes. This perspective is evident when individuals do not receive care. Advanced technology is a tool, not a solution. Superior outcomes require equitable systems that address access, education, and holistic care. They should be for ailments with established treatment options due to poor access to health services. For example, Cuba achieves better outcomes than the United States with minimal advanced technology by prioritizing universal primary care and social determinants of health. Other authors have argued that larger systemic issues are at play, perpetuating health inequities rather than relying on a strong economy (Spiegel & Yassi, 2004).

Health inequity is "the presence of unfair, avoidable, or remediable differences in achieving optimal health and well-being among people" (Tangcharoensathien et al., 2024, p.86). This definition suggests that the underlying forces orchestrate or drive continuous disease prevalence and health outcomes inequities. Tangcharoensathien et al. (2024) explained that "contemporary forms of colonialism, notably corporate and financialized colonialism through globalized systems of wealth extraction and profiteering, lead to inequitable global health systems" (p. 86). Mukherjee (2017) argues further that the impoverishment of countries by colonial powers and other systemic forces and international relations causes global health inequities. Colonialism established centuries of the monopoly of global capital and advanced technology by countries of the Global North. The Global South thus depends on international financial institutions and other multilateral agencies (Aginam, 2000).

Colonialism played a significant role in worsening the spread and impact of diseases. Packard's research unveiled the devastating effects of colonial practices like large-scale agriculture, forced labor, and forced migration on the prevalence of malaria (Anon, 2018). Additionally, colonialism contributed to health disparities by introducing new diseases, uprooting populations, and creating poor working conditions and famine. European powers brought infectious diseases to Africa during their voyages to colonize new lands and establish trade routes (Okuonzi, 2009). These diseases affected people who had no immunity, leading to widespread infection.

Furthermore, colonialism compelled people to relocate to new regions, such as mosquito-infested lowlands, making them more vulnerable to diseases (Bump & Aniebo, 2022). For instance, the Swazi people were forced to move to the lowlands after being displaced from their homelands by colonists, exposing them to higher risks of malaria. The colonial pursuit of export economies often exposed workers to diseases without adequate occupational protections. Workers in mining areas of Southern Africa and the Belgian Congo, for instance, experienced higher rates of tuberculosis. At the same time, those in plantation agriculture became more susceptible to water-borne, mosquito-borne, and worm diseases (Bruchhausen, 2020).

Moreover, colonialism could lead to famine conditions that heightened susceptibility to diseases. For example, the imposition of taxes on the Swazi people, coupled with drought conditions and the exportation of their crops, resulted in famines that left them vulnerable to malaria. When people sought food and work during these famines, they lost their acquired immunity, making them susceptible to infection upon their return.

Dependency Syndrome

The Global South is said to suffer from a dependency syndrome. The dependency theory is a seminal concept developed in the late 1950s by Raul Prebisch, the director of the United Nations Economic Commission for Latin America. Dependency theory is based on the Marxian notion of exploitation and backwardness (Edelstein, 1981). Prebisch and colleagues found that economic growth in advanced industrialized countries did not always result in progress in poorer nations but often led to significant economic challenges in poorer countries (Edelstein, 1981). This finding challenged the neoclassical and modernization theories, which assume that economic growth universally benefits all, albeit sometimes unevenly (Brand-Correa et al., 2022).

Prebisch's initial explanation for this phenomenon was that poorer countries exported raw materials to richer countries, which manufactured products using those materials and sold them back to the poorer countries (Ferraro et al., 1996). The cost of manufacturing a usable product was always higher than the cost of the raw materials used. According to this theory, Global South countries are locked in a state of dependency because they primarily export raw resources to wealthy countries of the Global North, which then export value-added manufactured goods back to the Global South. In this way, the Global North nations control the terms of trade, perpetuating this dependence as the Global South countries inevitably confront higher import prices and lower export earnings, leading to rising debt and shrinking ability to finance the debt.

Rising debt and diminishing ability to repay national debts and loans have implications for money that a country allocates for the smooth running of the country annually, including the amount allocated for health. Kalipso Chalkidou, the director of the World Health Organization's Department on Health Financing and Economics in a 2024 report, shared that in 42 countries found in the Global South, mainly in Africa and South Asia, domestic public spending per capita on health remains below $30 per person per year. Experts have explained that these countries are dealing with high debts that they must pay to maintain their credibility and borrow more money. The World Health Organization report also showed that while public health expenditure remained stagnant over the years, donor aid rose, and out-of-pocket spending grew faster in these Global South countries. These countries depend on donor aid to complement the insignificant amounts allocated for public health spending in this climate. The outcome of this dynamic is that very few effective programs will be conceived, designed, and implemented for disease prevention and health promotion, leading to inequities in health outcomes compared to countries in the Global North. African nations receiving the US President's Emergency Plan for AIDS Relief (PEPFAR) account for 49% (27 out of 55) of all PEPFAR-supported countries globally (Bendavid, 2016). The level of dependency of most Global South countries on donor aid was typified when millions of lives were at stake when President Donald Trump put a pause on all PEPFAR funds at the start of his second term in office.

Related to the type of dependency proposed by Raul Prebisch is path dependency. Path dependency is a concept that shows how past decisions and long-lasting institutional practices limit future policy choices (Dimaggio & Powell, 1983). Early decisions significantly influence later progress, creating systems and norms that make change difficult. Path dependency, therefore, refers to the tendency to rely on past practices, decisions, and actions for the outcome rather than current conditions (Figure 2.3). Thus, those who repeat the same strategies will almost certainly get the same results. This phenomenon is marked by increasing returns, institutional lock-in, and high costs of changing paths. When a country or institution starts on a certain trajectory, the resulting policies and investments create benefits that make it harder to stray from that path (Mahoney, 2000). Politically, existing power structures encourage policymakers to keep the current model, as altering it could harm established interests. Socially, professional standards and public beliefs support current methods, making alternatives seem extreme, even if they could lead to better results (Peters et al., 2005). Therefore, despite their advantages, different policy options face strong challenges like economic limits, political pushback, and resistance to change.

The stagnation of African healthcare systems originated from two pivotal fractures. First, the 1980s structural adjustment programs imposed by the International Monetary Fund and World Bank as loan prerequisites fundamentally redefined health governance. These neoliberal reforms mandated austerity measures—slashing public expenditure, privatizing services, and

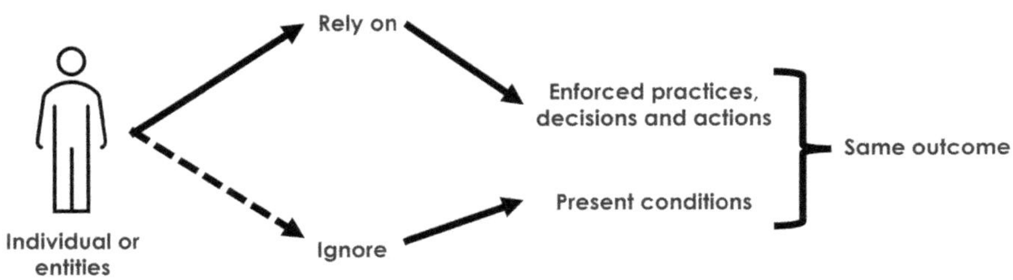

Figure 2.3 A conceptual representation of path dependency.

prioritizing debt reduction—effectively dismantled state capacity to finance social services, including health care (Guleid, 2025). African governments, for example, constrained by spending cuts, saw public health collapse: citizen expenditures on medical care surged by 63% in structural adjustment program-adherent nations between 1980-1995, while maternal mortality ratios worsened by 15% across sub-Saharan Africa.

Second, the vacuum created by structural adjustment programs enabled donor-driven neo-patrimonialism in healthcare, in which the ruler governs based on personal loyalties. International aid agencies responded to the crisis not by rebuilding national health systems but by establishing 87 parallel disease-specific initiatives (e.g., PEPFAR, Global Fund) between 1995 and 2010 (Kruk et al., 2010). These vertically structured programs—each with discrete budgets, personnel, and reporting protocols—diverted 68% of sub-Saharan Africa's health funding to external priorities by 2005. Consequently, health ministries became administrative appendages to donor agendas, with 73% of Mozambique's health budget in 2008 tied to externally dictated HIV/AIDS programming rather than national epidemiological needs (Guleid, 2025).

A recent publication by Wiyeh et al. (2025) demonstrated how the PEPFAR funding mechanism instilled path dependency in most Global South recipient countries (Figure 2.4). First, PEPFAR's disease-specific focus has inadvertently distorted health workforce distribution through its compensation

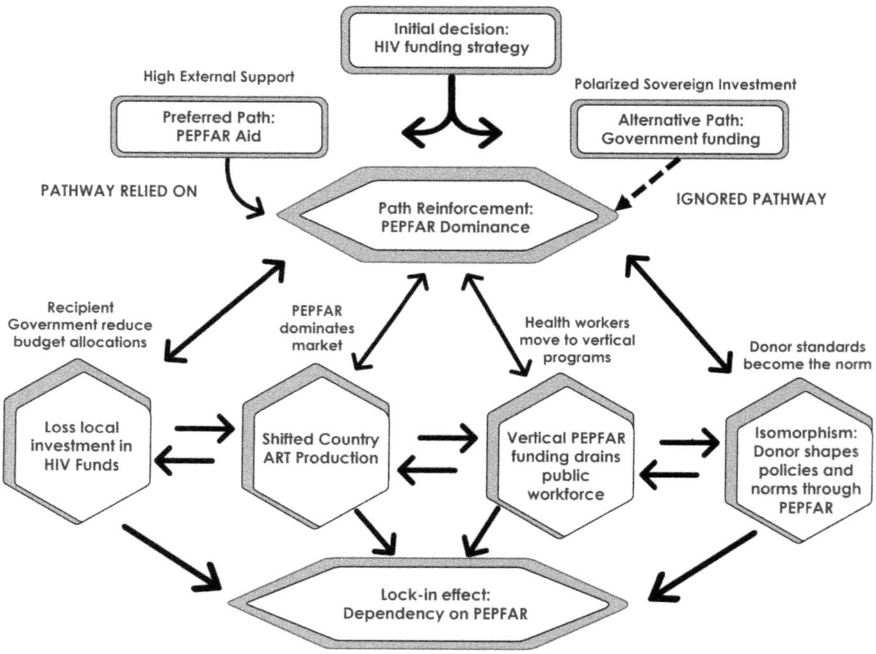

Figure 2.4 A conceptual representation of PEPFAR path dependency.

structures, which prioritize HIV/AIDS specialists over general practitioners. This remuneration disparity has precipitated a brain drain from essential health sectors—including maternal care and chronic disease management—thereby undermining primary healthcare infrastructure and systemic resilience (Kavanagh, 2014). Concurrently, the program's vertically integrated procurement mechanisms for antiretroviral therapies (ARTs) have stifled the development of autonomous pharmaceutical supply chains in recipient nations. As evidenced by the predominant reliance on imported ARVs, while PEPFAR's bulk purchasing expanded treatment coverage, it simultaneously perpetuated dependence on foreign manufacturers, constraining local production capacity. This dynamic exemplifies what Dambisa Moyo terms the "micro-macro paradox," wherein targeted aid achieves narrow programmatic success while failing to catalyze sustainable economic development (Moyo, 2009). As countries transition from PEPFAR-controlled procurement, many face acute cost escalations and supply chain disruptions, jeopardizing long-term medication accessibility (Kavanagh, 2014). Furthermore, the initiative has engendered a crowding-out effect on domestic health financing: by subsidizing HIV/AIDS care costs, PEPFAR inadvertently compressed national health budgets, as governments reallocated domestic resources away from HIV care, thereby institutionalizing fiscal dependency (Zakumumpa et al., 2024). This bifurcated governance architecture entrenched systemic fragmentation, prioritizing donor-mandated performance metrics over sustainable capacity building.

Additionally, countries in the Global South frequently adopt health policies based on high-income countries, driven by external legitimacy and donor preferences rather than local needs. This approach mimics "successful" models that may not fit their realities. Network effects also favor established organizations, restricting local policymakers' ability to influence their national health policies (Hacker, 2004). Consequently, countries in the Global South are stuck in a system of external dependency, limiting their ability to develop strong public health and economic structures.

Global Health Agenda Monopoly

Beaglehole and Bonita (2010) define global health as "collaborative transnational research and action for promoting health for all." Considering this definition, we notice that in the practice of global health, global health partnerships are characterized by unequal and inequitable partnerships between the actors from the Global North and those from the Global South. These "collaborations," therefore, often mirror colonial relationships, with countries from the Global North dictating the direction of proceedings and, consequently, the agenda and standards of practice to the rest of the world.

Büyüm et al. (2020) argued that colonization and the predatory nature of capitalism underpin the design of global and public health systems, resulting in structural, racial, and ethnic inequities within black, indigenous, and people of color (BIPOC) communities worldwide. He argued that colonial patterns were also used through the Euro-Western knowledge system to shape language and response to the recent COVID-19 pandemic (Büyüm et al., 2020). To this end, many Global North and South scholars have been questioning the nature and practice of Global Health in contemporary times. The argument is that contemporary global health practice still carries the legacy of Colonial Medicine to a more significant extent. To a greater extent, global health practice takes the form of (white) saviorism, an idea in which a (white) person, or (white) culture, "rescues" people of color from their situation. Weekes-Richemond (2022) shared that coloniality is rife among donors, who are usually from the Global North, and they are increasingly exerting their influence and dangling checkbooks in the face of cash-strapped global health governments.

In 2020, an estimated 85% of global health organizations had headquarters in Europe and North America. The predominant existence of Global Health organizations in the Global North feeds the imbalance of power that maintains the colonial status quo. Consequently, working and training younger generations on global health occurs predominantly based on visions, agendas, and a culture of saviorism in institutions in the North. According to Banerjee et al. (2023), irrespective of where the individual is originally from, those who work in global health in the Global North (me included) benefit from an imbalance of power perpetuated by this culture of saviorism that maintains inequity and consequently an entrenched divide in global health. Therefore, nonwhites can also perpetuate white saviorism by their proximity to whiteness, power, or privilege because it relies on these structures to maintain inequality. Similarly, not only do countries found in the Global North have colonial mindsets and systems that perpetuate power imbalances, but there are organizations in the Global South that also perpetuate power imbalances through these systems (Khan et al., 2021). In a PLoS Blog entitled "Why I left my career in global health," Weekes-Richemond (2022) shared the following experiences being in global health practice and research for 14 years:

> I left the sector because it is racist and has a White savior complex. I have sat in too many boardrooms where well-meaning White middle-class individuals draw up projects that White donors have deemed to be global health priorities and then dictate how Low- and Middle-Income Countries (LMICs) should execute the project with little regard for cultural sensitivities. The racist assumption that black and brown people do not have the solutions to their problems has resulted in White individuals from the Global North at the seat of power, making decisions and speaking on behalf of black and brown people.

Learning institutions in the Global North promote a predominately white, Eurocentric curriculum, conveying that Western civilizations are far superior (better) than others. Banerjee et al. (2023) contend that with global health organizations situated predominantly in the Global North, global health education remains underpinned by harmful colonial worldviews and saviorism. These institutions are purported to teach based on curricula that remarginalize, deprioritize, and minimize indigenous communities' lived experiences, expertise, and epistemology (Opara, 2021). Because white saviorism dominates how global health institutes practice global health, the question is whether global health students are being trained to be saviors to less privileged countries in the Global South. The issue with the saviorism trope is that it foments a narrative that those being saved cannot address their problems and are victims. In the case of global health, only nations in the Global North can address the challenges of most countries in the Global South. A clear example was during the COVID-19 pandemic when many countries in the Global South could not purchase the COVID-19 vaccine unless they received help from countries and organizations in the Global North.

Knowledge Hegemony and Epistemic Injustice

"Knowledge is power" is a cardinal principle that guides the practice of global health, giving credence to the guardians of knowledge, the recognized "knowers," the knowledge community, who are thus powerful (Eichbaum et al., 2021). The current approach to global health is Eurocentric, rooted in a hierarchical perspective of humanity. This approach validates the notion that the Western way of life, knowledge, and practices are universally applicable and represent the goal of progress and modernity (Affun-Adegbulu et al., 2023; Affun-Adegbulu & Adegbulu, 2020). Also, in global health, greater value is attached to the skill sets of Global North partners, and little value is attached to the skill sets of Global South partners unless educated in the Global North. White supremacy takes both overt and subtle forms. However, they both perpetuate the privilege that white individuals consciously or subconsciously enjoy, often at the expense of those with nonwhite skin color. Global health partnerships that aim to "help," like philanthropic healthcare services, often replicate colonial relationships with a white supremacist mindset. Members from the Global North are often given more opportunities in the Global South, such as mentorship, employment, leadership positions, and compensation (Binagwaho et al., 2022). However, what reciprocity should be involved regarding benefits for the Global South is still unclear.

In perpetuating the legacy of white supremacy, partners from the Global North tend to share knowledge without demonstrating a willingness to learn from their counterparts in the Global South (Binagwaho et al., 2022; Galtung, 1967). Galtung (1967) adopted the term "Knowledge colonialism" to describe the asymmetric research and knowledge-sharing patterns adopted during colonialism, which is prevalent today, especially in global health. There is a long history of systematic data collection by donors, which is one way of maintaining the primacy of Northern institutions in debates about the global South (Bump & Aniebo, 2022). After the end of formal colonialism, "knowledge colonialism" metamorphosized into the "coloniality of knowledge," describing the structure of control whereby knowledge and ways of knowing are ascribed exclusively to colonial powers—which appears in global health norms and perceptions surrounding expertise (Daffé et al., 2021, p. 558). By knowingly or unwittingly devaluing the expertise of local collaborators and indigenous populations—their lived experience or other ways of knowing, we reproduce colonial practices and miss critical opportunities for impact.

Discrediting, devaluing, or undervaluing knowledge from local scientists and indigenous populations in the Global South has led to the perception of "epistemic indebtedness." Mishra et al. (2022) define epistemic indebtedness as a state of owing debt and gratitude to the global knowledge reserve (aka knowledge pool) that subsequently engenders a moral obligation to contribute (p. 1). For instance, very little is known about the contributions of Asian and African traditional medicine, its practice, and its impact on the epistemic pool of disease prevention, treatment, and management. In contrast, these traditional medicines and practitioners are part of the deeper cultural practices of these communities. It must be highlighted, too, that the minimalist appearance of this localized knowledge cannot be completely attributed to it being less considered by the global North but also that there might be a tradition to maintain this knowledge and practices amongst a specific hierarchy and circle (Mishra et al., 2022). Whatever perspective holds, or whether it is a combination of these two schools of thought, the observation is that there is epistemic indebtedness from the Global South.

Knowledge hegemony and epistemic injustice entail prioritizing knowledge generated by researchers from the Global North over that generated by Global South researchers with little collaboration with researchers from the Global North. Consequently, Global South researchers have succumbed to both enacted and perceived inferiority in how they could contribute to global epistemic reserve (Mishra et al., 2022). The term epistemic imposition has been used to describe this phenomenon, whereby hierarchical preference is afforded to knowledge generated by Global North researchers (with or without collaborations with Global South researchers). In this way, the knowledge of the locals or scientists from the Global South is considered less valuable than that from the Global North—prioritizing outsiders' perspectives over local wisdom and needs. This phenomenon is known as epistemic injustice—pervasive wrongs concerning knowledge production, use, and circulation in global health (Bhakuni & Abimbola, 2021). Epistemic injustice through the lens of white supremacy suggests that the Global North is recognized as a credible knowledge producer whose interpretive tools are used to make sense of existing or new knowledge (Bhakuni & Abimbola, 2021). The premise of epistemic injustice is that Scholars from the Global North often know more about other nations than these nations know about themselves (Galtung, 1967). The effects of such asymmetry can be seen in aspects like discrimination against underrepresented groups in academic publishing in global health, research partnerships, authorship practices, and academic writing (Bhakuni & Abimbola, 2021), evidenced by lower citation rates, fewer editorial board positions, and longer manuscript review periods (Heidt, 2023; Manan et al., 2023).

Publication equity is a potent tool for combating the issue of parachute research and its associated inequities in global health. The Global Public

Health journal is committed to ensuring that papers submitted by global health authors conducting primary research in the Global South must include the author(s) from the research setting (Robinsonid et al., 2023). This approach promotes a more inclusive and equitable research environment. While authorship equity is a practical and commendable approach to combating the practice of parachute research, it is unlikely to engender meaningful transformation to achieve epistemic decolonization. Parachute research is complex and requires multiple perspectives and approaches to address effectively. Therefore, it is our collective responsibility to champion the cause of publication equity and authorship diversity, as these are crucial steps toward achieving epistemic decolonization in global health.

The application of the dependency theory to helicopter research and, consequently, the fueling of systemic injustice in global health would suggest that the epistemic exploitation of the Global South hails from the colonial period. Colonial masters established a system of collecting data indiscriminately and unethically from countries of the Global South, a practice described by Galtung (1967) as "scientific colonialism." Galtung (1967) describes scientific colonialism as claiming unlimited access to data from other countries, predominantly from the Global South. These data are subsequently exported (representing raw material) to be processed in the Global North as published books and peer-reviewed articles (manufactured goods).

In their article "The Problem of 'Trickle-down Science' from the Global North to the Global South," Reidpath and Allotey (2019) argued that countries in the Global South continue to struggle to train and retain good researchers and practitioners to address local, regional, and global health challenges and consequently depend on knowledge generated from the Global North to inform health care practice in the Global South. They pointed out that the result of the Global South depending on the Global North for epistemic global health practice is that the knowledge obtained from the Global North is "(1) often not fit for purpose; (2) designed to accrue the greatest intellectual benefit to the North and (3) not supportive of subaltern science in the Global South (Reidpath & Allotey, 2019, p. 2). While global health institutions, researchers, and priorities are predominantly in the Global North, the bulk of Global Health activities (research work and intervention programs) are implemented in the Global South (Mogaka et al., 2021). It is also common knowledge that those involved in research, data collection, and research assistance in studies conducted in the Global South are hardly recognized for their contributions when the findings obtained from such studies are published. The practice of obtaining data from the Global South to analyze and publish in the Global North is described in the global health literature as parachute or parasite research.

Parachute or parasite research, a pervasive form of epistemic injustice, continues to shape global health discourse (Smith, 2018). The term "parachute researcher" refers to someone who enters a country (usually in the Global South), utilizes local resources, personnel, and research participants, and then returns home (in the Global North) to write an academic paper or book, without establishing long-term partnerships or contributing to the local research infrastructure. In this way, the Global South continues to depend on the Global North for evidence-based global health practices. I found the dependency theory helpful in understanding how the global South depends on the Global North for global health practice knowledge.

Scientific colonialism has transfigured into the "coloniality of knowledge" (Daffé et al., 2021), describing the structure of control whereby knowledge and ways of knowing are ascribed and accessible exclusively to the Global North. Articles and books published based on the data obtained from the Global South are usually monetized through paywall models, making them inaccessible to researchers and other stakeholders in the Global South, thus constituting a barrier to global health policymaking (Yamey & Feachem, 2011). When Global South researchers collect data from the Global South, they struggle to publish in high-impact (Global North) journals (Naidu et al., 2024). Consequently, Global South researchers must depend on collaborations with Global North researchers to publish in these journals and afford the exorbitant article processing charges.

The Global South's dependence on the Global North is perpetuated through global health research funding opportunities, funding systems, and funding organizations. Most organizations funding global health research, such as the US and European governments, and philanthropies like the Bill & Melinda Gates Foundation and the World Bank and Global Fund, come from the Global North (Head et al., 2020). Consequently, they favor global health research institutions and principal investigators in their own countries, even for the research proposed to be conducted in the Global South. For instance, Flint et al. (2022) uncovered asymmetries in how research is funded and assessed in the United Kingdom, suggesting that the UK–Global South partnerships prioritize the agendas of UK funding bodies and institutions. For instance, 70% of Fogarty grants are awarded to recipients in the US and other high-income countries. Similarly, 73% of Wellcome Trust grants support activities based in the UK, 80% of USAID contracts are awarded to firms based in the US, and it is estimated that 88% of grants provided by the Bill & Melinda Gates Foundation are held by institutions in the Global North (Charani et al., 2022). With minimal global health research opportunities and support for global health research emanating from the Global South (Abouzeid et al., 2022), the Global South tends to rely on the funding and support that the global health research institutions and principal investigators from the Global North obtain. This situation creates inequities and a situation where the Global South researchers rely on the Global North researchers and funders to conduct research in the South.

Pervasive Inequitable Global Health Partnerships

Equitable partnerships are fundamental to global health practice and research (Zaman et al., 2020). The "global" nature of global health relies on robust partnerships between the Global North and Global South (North–South partnerships) to achieve its goals of equitable access to healthcare services for all. Unfortunately, inequitable partnerships and collaborations are pervasive in global health. Nevertheless, North–South partnerships are often dynamic and often portrayed as complex and characterized by asymmetries in power and resources (Plamondon et al., 2021). Two hypotheses have been put forth to account for these inequitable partnerships in global health. The first thesis relates to the fact that global health is dominated by researchers from the Global North, thus leading to an imbalance stemming from entrenched power asymmetries (often linked to resource availability) that can undermine the contributions and knowledge of local experts (Zaman et al., 2020). The second thesis relates to the fact that global health partnerships are predominantly formed between researchers from the Global South who were previously colonized and the Global North representing the colonizers (Eichbaum et al., 2021). Owing to the historical inequitable and unjust nature of the relationship between these two halves of the globe, one of the goals of global health practice is to address the inequitable nature of these relationships.

North–South partnerships aim to achieve Sustainable Development Goals by mutually supporting research, offering technical assistance and service support, engaging in advocacy, and providing financing. Working on achieving Sustainable Development Goals indicates that involvement is distributed unevenly and upholds the North–South divide regarding countries' resources, such as access to data and scientific capabilities (Blicharska et al., 2021). Collaborative co-creation, communication, commitment, and continuous review support equitable partnerships. These pillars are underpinned by values of fairness, respect, care, and honesty, as described in the Global Code of Conduct for Research in Resource-Poor settings.

While global health strives to achieve epistemic justice and address inequities in access to healthcare services globally through an equitable positioning and engagement of the Global North and Global South actors, inequity remains ubiquitous in most global health partnerships (Bain et al., 2024). Plamondon et al. (2021) conducted a study in which they analyzed 30 peer-reviewed articles focusing on power dynamics, inequities, and contradictions or challenges present in North–South partnerships. They observed that global health partnerships are often depicted as inherently advantageous for Southern partners while neglecting to acknowledge power dynamics and inequities. Indeed, authorship inequity in global health research is representative of the unequal partnerships in global health, as research shows that Global South authors are under-represented in publications from global collaborative research North–South partnerships (Kaufman et al., 2023). Publication inequity highlights a specific aspect of power imbalances in global health collaborations or partnerships and reveals much about whose narratives are represented in academia.

Global health inequality affects scientific partnerships and other aspects of global health, such as humanitarian aid and medical practice. Global health partnerships occur in complex political and economic relationships and involve partners (e.g., government agencies, non-governmental organizations, corporations, universities, professional associations, philanthropic organizations, and communities) with different needs and interests (Plamondon et al., 2021). The inequitable nature of Global North–South partnerships is undergirded by inequities in power, privilege, and finances between partners involved in the formulated partnerships. Some structures underpinning the inequitable nature of Global North–South partnerships include disparities in access to good quality training, funding opportunities (fellowships, travel grants to attend international conferences, etc.), and publishing opportunities (Gautier et al., 2018).

Unearthing the historical events of the relationships between the Global North and the Global South helps unpack the inequitable nature of Global North–South partnerships in global health research and practice (Bump, 2025). Molosi-France and Makoni (2020) argue that relational power is at the heart of global North–South partnerships, and these partnerships are influenced by the contemporary remnants of established power patterns between the former colonizer and colonized. Gautier et al. (2018) cited as an example the creation of a scientific hub of working relationships based on material differences in the 1980s as an apparatus for tensions in Global North–South partnerships. Flint et al. (2022) concluded that differences in access to resources mean that global health practice asymmetries in Global North–South partnerships will continue unless more is done to ensure "equitable" engagements.

Discussion

There is overwhelming advocacy for Decolonization$_2$ based on the oft-cited hegemonic nature of coloniality. Indeed, the postcolonial and decolonial discourse literature is dedicated to examining and bringing to the fore the consequences of coloniality in modernity, hence the advocacy for Decolonization$_2$. While there seems to be overwhelming support for decoloniality and decolonization, some authors have focused on highlighting the positive side of colonization. Táíwò (2022), as seen earlier, has argued for abandoning the Decolonization$_2$ project. He contends that Decolonization$_2$ stifles African intellectual and social progress by framing Africans as perpetual victims of colonial legacy, thereby denying their capacity to critically engage with global ideas—including those labeled "Western"—and to shape their futures. Táíwò (2022) rejects the romanticization of pre-colonial purity, emphasizing instead Africa's dynamic agency in selectively adapting to and transforming external influences, as exemplified by historical figures like Frantz Fanon and Amílcar Cabral, who leveraged Enlightenment ideals against colonial oppression.

Despite the arguments of Táíwò (2022), the historical debilitation of Africa through colonialism continues to affect the level and the degree to which they can engage in global efforts to literate their pollution. McCoy et al. (2024) argue that coloniality limits the agency of the Global South in global health practices owing to the dominance over the structures and systems of global health governance by actors from the Global North who are pushing ideas and narratives. They explained that this dominance can be traced back to how powerful actors challenged and undermined the anticolonial vision of the Alma Ata Declaration and then proposed the more conservative vision of selective primary health care. This understanding is what they described as the colonization of global health, which is characterized by richer nations and organizations from the Global North dictating the direction of global health research and practice. Ultimately, the book advocates for a pragmatic focus on political and economic sovereignty while embracing Africa's right to participate in universal philosophical and cultural discourses without ideological constraints.

Conclusions

My goal in this chapter was three-fold. (1) Outline the concepts that guide current global health practice. (2) Unpack the concept of coloniality as an influence on how global health is practiced. (3) Discuss the expression of coloniality in Global Health. It was important to ask whose actions were responsible for the colonized status of global health, through which interactions, when and where, and with what consequences? To this end, the historical origins and current global operations were required, thus the value and contributions of this chapter. I identified health inequities, dependency syndrome, global health agenda monopoly, knowledge hegemony, epistemic injustice, and pervasive inequitable global health partnerships. The historical foundation, the role of coloniality, and the expression of coloniality in global health form the basis for a critical realist perspective on the possibility of decolonizing global health.

Note

1 "Global North/South" is within quotation marks in this text when describing the development of the concept. Without the quotation marks is when the definition of the term has been established.

References

Abouzeid, M., Muthanna, A., Nuwayhid, I. et al. (2022). Barriers to sustainable health research leadership in the Global South: Time for a grand bargain on localization of research leadership?. *Health Research Policy and Systems*, 20(136). https://doi.org/10.1186/s12961-022-00910-6

Affun-Adegbulu, C., & Adegbulu, O. (2020). Decolonising global (public) health: from Western universalism to Global pluriversalities. *BMJ Global Health*, 5(8), e002947. https://doi.org/10.1136/BMJGH-2020-002947

Affun-Adegbulu, C., Cosaert, T., Meudec, M., Michielsen, J., Van De Pas, R., Van Belle, S., Van De Put, W., Soors, W., Robertson, F., & Ddungu, C. (2023). Decolonisation initiatives at the Institute of Tropical Medicine, Antwerp, Belgium: ready for change? *BMJ Global Health*, 8(5), e011748. https://doi.org/10.1136/BMJGH-2023-011748

Aginam, O. (2000). Global village, divided world: South–North gap and global health global village. *Indiana Journal of Global Legal Studies Studies*, 7(2), 10.

Alfaqeeh, G., Cook, E. J., Randhawa, G., & Ali, N. (2017). Access and utilisation of primary health care services comparing urban and rural areas of Riyadh Providence, Kingdom of Saudi Arabia. *BMC Health Services Research*, 17(1), 1–13.

Alkema, L., Chao, F., You, D., Pedersen, J., & Sawyer, C. C. (2014). National, regional, and global sex ratios of infant, child, and under-5 mortality and identification of countries with outlying ratios: A systematic assessment. *The Lancet Global Health*, 2(9), e521–e530. https://doi.org/10.1016/S2214-109X(14)70280-3

Anon. (2018). Randall Packard: learning to learn from global health history. *Bull World Health Organ*, 96(4), 231–232. doi:10.2471/BLT.18.030418

Allen, F., & Giovannetti, G. (2011). The effects of the financial crisis on Sub-Saharan Africa. *Review of Development Finance*, 1(1), 1–27. https://doi.org/10.1016/J.RDF.2010.10.002

Bain, L. E., Adeagbo, O. A., Avoka, C. K., Amu, H., Memiah, P., & Ebuenyi, I. D. (2024). Identifying the conundrums of "global health" in the Global North and Global South: a case for Sub-Saharan Africa. *Frontiers in Public Health*, 12, 1168505.

Banerjee, A. T., Bandara, S., Senga, J., González-Domínguez, N., & Pai, M. (2023). Are we training our students to be white saviours in global health? *The Lancet*, 402(10401), 520–521. https://doi.org/10.1016/S0140-6736(23)01629-X

Beaglehole, R., & Bonita, R. (2010). What is global health? *Global Health Action*, 3(1), 5142. https://doi.org/10.3402/GHA.V3I0.5142

Beghin, N. (2022). Decoloniality as the only pathway to the right to development in Latin America. *Development*, 65(2–4), 178. https://doi.org/10.1057/S41301-022-00349-W

Bendavid, E. (2016). Past and future performance: PEPFAR in the landscape of foreign aid for health. *Current HIV/AIDS Reports*, 13(5), 256. https://doi.org/10.1007/S11904-016-0326-8

Bhakuni, H., & Abimbola, S. (2021). Epistemic injustice in academic global health. *The Lancet Global Health*, 9(10), e1465–e1470. https://doi.org/10.1016/S2214-109X(21)00301-6

Binagwaho, A., Ngarambe, B., & Mathewos, K. (2022). Eliminating the white supremacy mindset from global health education. *Annals of Global Health*, 88(1). https://doi.org/10.5334/AOGH.3578

Blicharska, M., Teutschbein, C., & Smithers, R. J. (2021). SDG partnerships may perpetuate the global North–South divide. *Scientific Reports*, 11(1), 1–11. https://doi.org/10.1038/s41598-021-01534-6

Brand-Correa, L., Brook, A., Büchs, M., Meier, P., Naik, Y., & O'Neill, D. W. (2022). Economics for people and planet-moving beyond the neoclassical paradigm. *Lancet Planet Health*, 6, e371–e379. www.thelancet.com/

Bruchhausen, W. (2020). Global health in the colonial era: The expansion of European medicine. www.ieg-ego.eu/en/threads/theories-and-methods/knowledge-transfer/walter-bruchhausen-global-health-in-the-colonial-era-the-expansion-of-european-medicine.

Bump, J. B. (2025). Global health and its limitations: An historical perspective. *Health Systems & Reform*, 11(2), 2478681. https://doi.org/10.1080/23288604.2025.2478681

Bump, J. B., & Aniebo, I. (2022). Colonialism, malaria, and the decolonization of global health. *PLOS Global Public Health*, 2(9), e0000936. https://doi.org/10.1371/JOURNAL.PGPH.0000936

Büyüm, A. M., Kenney, C., Koris, A., Mkumba, L., & Raveendran, Y. (2020). Decolonising global health: if not now, when? *BMJ Global Health*, 5(8), e003394. https://doi.org/10.1136/BMJGH-2020-003394

Charani, E., Abimbola, S., Pai, M., Adeyi, O., Mendelson, M., Laxminarayan, R., & Rasheed, M. A. (2022). Funders: The missing link in equitable global health research?. *PLOS Global Public Health*, 2(6), e0000583. https://doi.org/10.1371/journal.pgph.0000583

Cranston, G. (2025). Understanding the expectations, positions and ambitions of LMICs during pandemic treaty negotiations, and the factors contributing to them. *PLOS Global Public Health*, 5(3), e0003851. https://doi.org/10.1371/JOURNAL.PGPH.0003851

Daffé, Z. N., Guillaume, Y., & Ivers, L. C. (2021). Anti-racism and anti-colonialism praxis in global health—reflection and action for practitioners in US academic medical centers. *American Journal of Tropical Medicine and Hygiene*, 105(3), 557–560. https://doi.org/10.4269/ajtmh.21-0187

Dimaggio, P. J., & Powell, W. W. (1983). The iron cage revisited: Institutional isomorphism and collective rationality in organizational fields. *American Sociological Review*, 48(2).

Edelstein, J. C. (1981). Dependency: A special theory within Marxian analysis. Latin American Perspectives, 8(3/4), 103–107. www.jstor.org/stable/2633472

Eichbaum, Q. G., Adams, L. V., Evert, J., Ho, M.-J., Semali, I. A., & Van Schalkwyk, S. C. (2021). Scholarly perspective decolonizing global health education: Rethinking institutional partnerships and approaches. *Academic Medicine*, 96(3), 329–335. https://doi.org/10.1097/ACM.0000000000003473

Emerson, R. (1969). Colonialism. *Journal of Contemporary History*, 4(1).

Fanon, F. (1963). The pitfalls of national consciousness. In F. Fanon (Ed.), *The wretched of the earth* (pp. 148–205). Grove Press.

Ferraro, V., College, H., & Hadley, S. (1996). *Dependency theory: An introduction*. Mount Holyoke College.

Flint, A., Howard, G., Baidya, M., Wondim, T., Poudel, M., Nijhawan, A., Mulugeta, Y., & Sharma, S. (2022). Equity in Global North–South research partnerships: Interrogating UK funding models. *Global Social Challenges Journal*, 1(1), 76–93. https://doi.org/10.1332/VQIL8302

Galtung, J. (1967). Scientific Colonialism. *Transition*, 30, 10–15. https://about.jstor.org/terms

Ganshof, F. L. (1952). *Feudalism*. Longmans.

Gautier, L., Sieleunou, I., & Kalolo, A. (2018). Deconstructing the notion of "global health research partnerships" across Northern and African contexts. *BMC Medical Ethics*, 19(Suppl 1). https://doi.org/10.1186/S12910-018-0280-7

Gilley, B. (2018). The case for colonialism. *Academic Questions*, 31(2), 167–185.

Grosfoguel, R. (2007). The epistemic decolonial turn: Beyond political-economy paradigms. *Cultural Studies*, 21(2–3), 211–223. https://doi.org/10.1080/09502380601162514

Guleid, F. (2025, March 28). Why African health systems cannot simply move on. *International Health Policies*. www.internationalhealthpolicies.org/featured-article/why-african-health-systems-cannot-simply-move-on/

Hacker, J. S. (2004). Dismantling the health care state? Political institutions, public policies and the comparative politics of health reform. *British Journal of Political Science*, 34(4), 693–724. https://doi.org/10.1017/S0007123404000250

Head, M. G., Brown, R. J., Newell, M. L., Scott, J. A. G., Batchelor, J., & Atun, R. (2020). The allocation of USdollar;105 billion in global funding from G20 countries for infectious disease research between 2000 and 2017: a content analysis of investments. *The Lancet Global Health*, 8(10), e1295–e1304. https://doi.org/10.1016/S2214-109X(20)30357-0

Heidt, A. (2023). Racial inequalities in journals highlighted in giant study. *Nature*. https://doi.org/10.1038/D41586-023-01457-4

Katz, C. J. (1993). Karl Marx on the transition from feudalism to capitalism. *Theory and Society*, 22(3), 363–389. www.jstor.org/stable/657738
Kaufman, R., Fair, E., Reid, M., & Mirzazadeh, A. (2023). Authorship equity in global health research: Who gets the credit at University of California, San Francisco? *BMJ Global Health*, 8(10), 13713. https://doi.org/10.1136/BMJGH-2023-013713
Kavanagh, M. M. (2014). The politics and epidemiology of transition: PEPFAR and AIDS in South Africa. *Journal of Acquired Immune Deficiency Syndromes*, 65(3), 247–250. https://doi.org/10.1097/QAI.0000000000000093
Keshri, V. R., & Bhaumik, S. (2022). The feudal structure of global health and its implications for decolonisation. *BMJ Global Health*, 7(9), e010603. https://doi.org/10.1136/bmjgh-2022-010603
Khan, M., Abimbola, S., Aloudat, T., Capobianco, E., Hawkes, S., & Rahman-Shepherd, A. (2021). Decolonising global health in 2021: a roadmap to move from rhetoric to reform. *BMJ Global Health*, 6(3), e005604. https://doi.org/10.1136/BMJGH-2021-005604
Khan, T., Abimbola, S., Kyobutungi, C., & Pai, M. (2022). How we classify countries and people—and why it matters. *BMJ Global Health*, 7(6), e009704. https://doi.org/10.1136/BMJGH-2022-009704
Kruk, M. E., Freedman, L. P., Anglin, G. A., & Waldman, R. J. (2010). Rebuilding health systems to improve health and promote statebuilding in post-conflict countries: A theoretical framework and research agenda. *Social Science & Medicine*, 70(1), 89–97. https://doi.org/10.1016/J.SOCSCIMED.2009.09.042
Kruk, M. E., et al. (2018). High-quality health systems in the Sustainable Development Goals era: time for a revolution. *The Lancet Global Health*, 6(11), e1196. https://doi.org/10.1016/S2214-109X(18)30386-3
Lira, F. (2021, June 10). The Global South—from conceptualization to action? Research Institute for Sustainability. www.rifs-potsdam.de/en/blog/2021/06/global-south-conceptualization-action
Lowes, S. (2020). The legacy of colonial medicine in Central Africa. *Research Briefs in Economic Policies*, 209. https://scholar.harvard.edu/files/slowes/files/lowes_
Mahoney, J. (2000). Path dependence in historical sociology. *Theory and Society*, 29(4). www.jstor.org/stable/3108585?seq=1&cid=pdf-
Maldonado-Torres, N. (2007). On the coloniality of being: Contributions to the development of a concept. *Cultural Studies*, 21(2–3), 240–270. https://doi.org/10.1080/09502380601162548
Manan, M. R., Nawaz, I., Rahman, S., Razzaq, A., Zafar, F., Qazi, A., & Liblik, K. (2023). Diversity, equity, and inclusion on editorial boards of global health journals. *Asian Bioethics Review*, 15(3), 209–239.
McCoy, D., Kapilashrami, A., Kumar, R., Rhule, E., & Khosla, R. (2024). Developing an agenda for the decolonization of global health. *Bulletin of the World Health Organization*, 102(2), 130–136. https://doi.org/10.2471/BLT.23.289949
Meagher, T. (2023, April 11). For modernity: A review of Olúfẹ́mi Táíwò's *Against Decolonisation. Black Issues in Philosophy*. https://blog.apaonline.org/2023/04/11/for-modernity-a-review-of-olufemi-taiwos-against-decolonisation/
Mendelson, M., Laxminarayan, R., Limmathurotsakul, D., Kariuki, S., Gyansa-Lutterodt, M., Charani, E., Singh, S., Walia, K., Gales, A. C., & Mpundu, M. (2024). Antimicrobial resistance and the great divide: inequity in priorities and agendas between the Global North and the Global South threatens global mitigation of antimicrobial resistance. *The Lancet Global Health*, 12(3), e516–e521. https://doi.org/10.1016/S2214-109X(23)00554-5
Mishra, S. R., Joshi, B., Poudyal, Y., & Adhikari, B. (2022). Epistemic indebtedness: Do we owe to epistemic enterprises? *Journal of Global Health Economics and Policy*, 2, e2022012. https://doi.org/10.52872/001C.36869

Molosi-France, K., & Makoni, S. (2020). A partnership of un-equals: Global South–North research collaborations in higher education institutions. *Modern Africa*, 8(2), 9–24. https://doi.org/10.26806/MODAFR.V8I2.343

Moore, J. W. (2003). Capitalism as world-ecology: Braudel and Marx on environmental history. *Organization & Environment*, 16(4), 514–517. https://doi.org/10.1177/1086026603259091

Moyo, D. (2009). *Dead aid: Why aid is not working and how there is a better way for Africa*. Farrar, Straus and Giroux.

Mukherjee, J. S. (2017). The roots of global health inequity. https://doi.org/10.1093/OSO/9780190662455.003.0001

Naidu, T., Gingell, G., & Zaidi Z. (2024). Decolonial framework for applying reflexivity and positionality in global health research. *Global Health Promotion*, 31(2), 52–58. doi:10.1177/17579759241238016

Nkrumah, K. (1965). *Neo-colonialism, the last stage of imperialism*. Thomas Nelson & Sons.

Oglesby, C. (1969). "After Vietnam, what?" *Commonweal*, 90(1) (March 21).

Okuonzi, S. (2009). Colonial masters brought infectious diseases to Africa. www.newvision.co.ug/new_vision/news/1239715/colonial-masters-brought-infectitious-diseases-africa

Opara, I. N. (2021). It's time to decolonize the decolonization movement. PLoS Blogs. https://speakingofmedicine.plos.org/2021/07/29/its-time-to-decolonize-the-decolonization-movement/

Packard, R. M. (2016). The good and the bad campaigns. In *A history of global health: interventions into the lives of other peoples*. Johns Hopkins University Press.

Peters, B. G., Pierre, J., & King, D. S. (2005). The politics of path dependency: Political conflict in historical institutionalism. *The Journal of Politics*, 67(4), 1275–1300. https://doi.org/10.1111/J.1468-2508.2005.00360.X

Plamondon, K. M., Brisbois, B., Dubent, L., & Larson, C. P. (2021). Assessing how global health partnerships function: an equity-informed critical interpretive synthesis. *Globalization and Health*, 17(1). https://doi.org/10.1186/S12992-021-00726-Z

Power, M. (2009). The Commonwealth, "development" and post-colonial responsibility. *Geoforum*, 40(1), 14–24. https://doi.org/10.1016/J.GEOFORUM.2008.04.008

Quijano, A. (2007). Coloniality and modernity/rationality. *Cultural Studies*, 21(2–3), 168–178. https://doi.org/10.1080/09502380601164353

Reidpath, D. D., & Allotey, P. (2019). The problem of "trickle-down science" from the Global North to the Global South. *BMJ Global Health*, 4(4), e001719. https://doi.org/10.1136/bmjgh-2019-001719

Richardson, E. T., (2019). On the coloniality of global public health. *Medicine Anthropology Theory*, 6(4), 101–118. https://doi.org/10.17157/mat.6.4.761

Robinsonid, J., Kyobutungi, C., Nyakoojoid, Z., & Paiid, M. (2023). Editors as allies: Our two-year experience at PLOS Global Public Health. *PLOS Global Public Health*, 3(11), e0002644. https://doi.org/10.1371/JOURNAL.PGPH.0002644

Sen, A. (1984). *The transition from feudalism to capitalism*. The Institute of Development Studies and Partner Organisations. https://hdl.handle.net/20.500.12413/3260

Sims, D. A. (2023). When I say … Global South and Global North. *Medical Education*. https://doi.org/10.1111/MEDU.15263

Smith, J. (2018). Parasitic and parachute research in global health. *The Lancet Global Health*, 6(8), e838. https://doi.org/10.1016/S2214-109X(18)30315-2

Spiegel, J. M., & Yassi, A. (2004). Lessons from the margins of globalization: Appreciating the Cuban health paradox. *Journal of Public Health Policy*, 25(1), 85–110. https://doi.org/10.1057/PALGRAVE.JPHP.3190007

Táíwò, O. (2022). *Against decolonisation: Taking African agency seriously*. Hurst & Company.

Tangcharoensathien, V., Cetthakrikul, N., Lekagu, A., Ontong, S., Suphanchaimat, R., & Patcharanarumol, W. (2023). Global health inequities: A call for papers. *Bulletin of the World Health Organization*, 101(4), 230. https://doi.org/10.2471/BLT.23.289906

Tangcharoensathien, V., Lekagul, A., & Teo, Y. Y. (2024). Global health inequities: more challenges, some solutions. *Bulletin of the World Health Organization*, 102(2), 86. https://doi.org/10.2471/BLT.24.291326

Tarusarira, J. (2020). Religion and coloniality in diplomacy. *The Review of Faith & International Affairs*, 18(3), 87–96. https://doi.org/10.1080/15570274.2020.1795442

UNICEF. (2024). Child mortality. https://data.unicef.org/topic/child-survival/under-five-mortality.

Weekes-Richemond, L. (2022, March 29). Why I left my career in global health. PLoS Blogs. https://speakingofmedicine.plos.org/2022/03/29/why-i-left-my-career-in-global-health/

Wispelwey, B., Osuagwu, C., Mills, D., Goronga, T., & Morse, M. (2023). Towards a bidirectional decoloniality in academic global health: insights from settler colonialism and racial capitalism. *The Lancet Global Health*, 11(9), e1469–e1474. https://doi.org/10.1016/S2214-109X(23)00307-8

Wiyeh, A., Komba, P., Ojong, S.A., Wiysonge, C.S., Moki-Suh, B., Sadate-Ngatchou, P., et al. (2025). A critical juncture in global health: Leveraging historical institutionalism to examine PEPFAR dependency and inform the development of self-reliant public health systems. *PLOS Glob Public Health* 5(4), e0004440. https://doi.org/10.1371/journal.pgph.0004440

Yamey, G., & Feachem, R. (2011). Evidence-based policymaking in global health—The payoffs and pitfalls. *Evidence-Based Medicine*, 16(4), 97–99. https://doi.org/10.1136/ebm.2011.100060

Zakumumpa, H., Paina, L., Ssegujja, E., Shroff, Z. C., Namakula, J., & Ssengooba, F. (2024). The impact of shifts in PEPFAR funding policy on HIV services in Eastern Uganda (2015–21). *Health Policy and Planning*, 39(Supplement_1), i21–i32. https://doi.org/10.1093/HEAPOL/CZAD096

Zaman, M., Afridi, G., Ohly, H., McArdle, H. J., & Lowe, N. M. (2020). Equitable partnerships in global health research. *Nature Food*, 1(12), 760–761. https://doi.org/10.1038/s43016-020-00201-9

3 Postcolonial Critical Realism

Introduction

According to Samuel-Mbaekwe (1986), colonialism, especially in Africa, encompasses three distinct aspects of social reality in regions that experienced European conquest and rule during the nineteenth and twentieth centuries. First, it refers to European colonizers' activities in conquering and ruling the conquered colonies—colonization. For example, Wolfe (2006) tackled the idea of genocide during settler colonialism, which focuses on the activities of the colonizers. Second, it denotes the reactions of those subjected to European conquest and rule and the reactions of those recently emancipated. However, these two interpretations are limited because they focus solely on the act of colonization and the responses of the colonized to the colonial activities. These are the predominant discourses adopted by most postcolonial theoretical approaches. A third approach has emerged to address this limitation. This perspective integrates the first two by conceptualizing colonialism as a complex web of relationships between the colonizer and the colonized and between elements of European culture and indigenous cultures (Samuel-Mbaekwe, 1986). In this book, I engage with (de)colonization of global health as a social activity, which is dependent on the thoughts and actions of actors whose actions are guided by structures, and at the same time, their actions strive to change those very structures which control their actions or the actions of others. To this end, I found Balandier's (2020) conceptualization of colonialism a useful starting place.

Balandier (2020) suggested that studies focusing on understanding the current realities of formerly colonized societies must conceptualize colonialism as a colonial situation. He describes the colonial situation as the conditions whereby, while establishing itself, colonialism imposed on the colonized a very special type of situation (Balandier, 2020). It not only conditioned the reactions of the colonized but is still responsible for certain reactions of people recently emancipated. Balandier (2020) thus sees "the colonial situation" as the proper sociological conception of colonialism, as it encompasses the activities and dispositions of both the colonizer and the colonized, especially in their

DOI: 10.4324/9781032700786-3

interaction. Adopting a sociological conceptualization helps to unpack the roles of different actors and the formulation of social structures—elaborated social models, which are compositions of distinguishable sociological elements called institutions (Samuel-Mbaekwe, 1986).

Making the argument against the simple historical approach to unpacking colonialism, Samuel-Mbaekwe (1986) argued that the colonial situation approach to understanding colonialism transcends the activities of individuals as it leans more towards structuralism. Nevertheless, this hypothesis becomes less persuasive when actors' roles are undermined. In critical realism, this duality recognizes that the activities of agents contribute to the (re)formulation of structures. Therefore, studying colonialism as a colonial situation should consider colonialism as the creation of the actions of individuals or groups of individuals and social formations. Thus, the colonial situation represents a congenial of events and consequences requiring a robust approach to unpack it comprehensively.

My conceptualization of the colonial situation should allow us to examine colonialism's effects on colonized societies' social structures, hierarchies, and cultural practices. It should also highlight the power dynamics between colonizers and the colonized, including the imposition of new social norms, racial classifications, and the disruption of traditional social systems. This perspective views colonialism as a system of domination that extends beyond political control and economic exploitation, profoundly influencing the social fabric of society. The social approach (colonial situation) thus offers a robust platform for unpacking colonialism and its lingering effects on global health, therefore allowing for a deeper ontological engagement that critical realism promises.

Postcolonial Critical Realism

The traditions of thought around postcolonialism and decoloniality are diverse and longstanding. Postcolonialism[1] and its different strands (postcolonial theory, postcolonial studies, postcolonial thought, decolonial thought, and neo-colonial theory) have gained prominence across the social sciences and beyond, including political science, international studies, anthropology, sociology, area studies, geography, history, philosophy, literature and art (Felsch, 2023). Postcolonialism as a theoretical framework focuses on colonialism's cultural, political, and social effects and their lingering effects on modernity—coloniality. Its main objective is to comprehend how the effects of colonialism persist and impact modern societies. One of its primary concerns is examining how previous colonial relationships shape present-day racial, economic, and cultural dynamics (Young, 2021). To this end, postcolonial theory aims to challenge the hegemony of Western narratives and amplify the perspectives and voices of formerly colonized people.

Postcolonialism emerged as an intellectual movement that extensively explored political and socioeconomic issues, with a noticeable focus on the cultural aspects of decolonization. This way, decolonial dialogues are closely linked to world-systems theory, scholarly research in development and underdevelopment theory, and the critical social theory traditions. While postcolonialism primarily focuses on the colonial activities of the nineteenth and twentieth centuries, decoloniality traces its roots back to the earlier European invasions of the Americas in the fifteenth century (Bhambra, 2014). The decolonial theory builds upon the postcolonial theory project, extending its temporal and spatial scope, highlighting the coloniality of institutions, and grounding itself in praxis (Tinsley, 2021). Today, postcolonial and decolonial dialogues have evolved into a theoretical discourse on colonialism and its cognates and have received so much attention that it has become institutionalized through the journal *Postcolonial Studies*. The effect of such institutionalization is that many articles and scholarly works have been published advocating for decolonization (of different fields and areas of life) and knowledge production processes.

Postcolonial theory and Marxism have been the most influential theoretical approaches to studying decolonization in the Global South (D'Souza, 2010). Over the recent decades, there has been increasing recognition that philosophy should engage more with (de)colonial discourse (Gordon, 2019; Maldonado-Torres et al., 2018). A quick Google search of the literature using the keywords "philosophy" and "decolonization" in various combinations and variants reveals an agenda more inclined to decolonize the field of philosophy than adopting a philosophical position to engage with the concept and practice of decolonization. Few scholarly writings were found to have adopted or considered a philosophical or metatheoretical position to examine decolonization or what the process entails. For example, Talabi (2021) applied critical analysis and historical approaches to investigate the meaning of decolonization within the African context. Tobi (2020) also developed a distinctly epistemic rationale for epistemic decolonization that provides arguments for decolonizing knowledge as an epistemic virtue. Lacertosa (2025) concludes that scaffolding colonial discourses within a philosophical position addresses not only what decolonization entails but also provides a platform on how to implement it methodologically, which are not objects of analysis but living epistemological realities.

Colonialism gave rise to colonial discourse. Colonial discourse denotes the collection of statements and depictions that have historically portrayed the colonized and the colonizer in binary, dualistic terms (Ochoa, 1996), and this discourse persists today. To grasp the concept of postcolonialism, one must delve into the ideas of (de)coloniality and acknowledge the intricate and sometimes conflicting relationships between the colonizers and the colonized. This theoretical framework allows us to examine how historical colonial structures continue to influence present-day economic and cultural realms while offering avenues for resistance and reassessing global power dynamics (Young, 2021).

Postcolonial and decolonial dialogues have (to a certain extent) successfully challenged the insular nature of historical narratives and historiographical traditions originating from Europe. The effects of these dialogues are especially evident in their critique of arguments that attribute the origins of modernity solely to Europe and their exploratory activities over the last two centuries. The dialogues also advocate for understanding the emergence of the modern world within the comprehensive lens of colonialism, the building of empires and their operations, and enslavement (Bhambra, 2014).

The philosophical foundations of postcolonial discourse are attributed to critical theory, which includes Marxism in its philosophical ancestry and is, to varying degrees, cognate with poststructuralism, feminism, and other emancipatory ideologies (Wilmot, 2021). Critical theory is a social and political school of thought that analyzes and challenges systemic power relations, arguing that knowledge, truth, and social structures are shaped by power dynamics between dominant and oppressed groups, aiming for social transformation. Critical theory is thus considered "a comprehensive" academic framework that critiques societal power structures, frequently addressing issues of inequality and oppression (Moisio, 2013). Postcolonialism anchors on the critical theory and represents a branch of critical theory that analyzes colonialism's cultural, political, and economic impacts, particularly on the lives of individuals from formerly colonized nations. It examines how the power dynamics established during colonial rule continue to influence contemporary societies. Essentially, postcolonialism utilizes critical theory to explore the enduring legacy of colonialism. Thus, they have been described as mutually complementing projects (Višić, 2023).

Despite this seemingly comprehensive nature of postcolonial theories, D'Souza (2010) argues that they fail to (1) emphasize the importance of grounding their critique in the material reality of the formerly colonized, (2) acknowledge the significance of class, class struggles, and social divisions, and the specific manifestations of capitalism and imperialism in the formerly colonized, (3) examine how imperialism and colonialism have transformed the relationships between nature, society, and people in the formerly colonized, (4) critique the dismissal of the potential for emancipation, freedom, and liberation, (5) highlight the tendency of postcolonial theory to address inequities and hopelessness in the face of new forms of imperialism enforced by neocolonialism, and (6) expose the elitist nature of the postcolonial project on a national and global scale (D'Souza, 2010). These weaknesses of the postcolonial theory gave me the impetus to consider an alternative meta-theoretical position that will underpin my understanding of global health and research colonization and imagine a possible route to decolonize global health.

Despite the above-mentioned weaknesses of postcolonial theories, they can be credited for shedding light on certain forms of dependencies and exclusions fomented by colonialism (Felsch, 2023). While postcolonial and decolonial traditions have the potential to unsettle and reconstitute standard perspectives and processes of knowledge production on colonialism and decolonization, they have done little to explain or predict the causal role of colonialism (coloniality) and, by extension, decoloniality in contemporary society. As Ochoa puts it:

> If coloniality and its resultant thought promote binary stereotypes and validate the values of the colonizers over those of the subaltern, then one would suppose that postcolonial thinking should offer an alternative way of viewing a world no longer divided into colonizers and colonized.
>
> (Ochoa, 1996, p. 224)

He thus argued that we should be able to envision postcolonial writing as that space where new possibilities are presented for consideration beyond promoting binary stereotypes between the colonizer and the colonized. For instance, Naidu et al. (2024) propose viewing (de)coloniality as a "theory and debate around socio-historical, geopolitical, and economic perspectives on gender, race, and hetero paternalism" (p. 53). Notably, postcolonial theories are limited in their ability to adequately explain the complexities of colonialism at the level of the causal nature of coloniality and the need for decoloniality to achieve decolonization. Consequently, Patomäki (2002) proposed critical realism as an alternative philosophical position to understand social phenomena such as colonialism.

Critical theory, which underpins postcolonial theories, seems to share some congruence with critical realism. The overlapping nature of these two philosophical positions can be identified from their shared common Marxist origin underpinned by the need to unveil the "real state of affairs" in society (Whelan, 2019). Critical theory and critical realism are interested in understanding phenomena in their socio-historic context when examining existing structural relationships. The shared use of "critical" across both metatheoretical traditions is not merely a terminological overlap but signals a careful conceptual consideration. This consideration is fundamentally oriented toward deconstructing hegemonic systems, with the dual objectives of interrogating entrenched power dynamics and advancing transformative agency for subaltern communities. While both traditions focus on the critical component in their analytical value, critical realism further identifies the underlying structures and causal mechanisms responsible for social change. It systematically exposes how entrenched power systems—rooted in these structural foundations—shape social actions, thereby highlighting pathways for necessary systemic transformation.

Owing to the congruence between critical realism and critical theory (the foundation of postcolonial theories), regarding unpacking the social processes, I sought to explore the integration of these two traditions to formulate a cogent philosophical metatheory to engage with colonialism and its cognates. Kwete et al. (2022) observed that the current decolonizing global health movement requires us to take a postcolonial perspective on the research and practice of global health. It is thus fitting to adopt a critical realist philosophical approach to reflect on (de)coloniality as a valuable contribution to fostering the agenda of decolonizing global health while retaining the value of a postcolonial engagement. To this end, I considered building on the work of Tinsley (2021), who proposed "postcolonial critical realism" as a critical realist perspective to engaging with colonialism and its cognates. Based on Bhaskar's conceptualization of critical realism, Tinsley (2021) proposed an ontological framework that explains the structuring relationship between racialized, colonial discourses and the social world.

Bhaskar divided his theoretical development of critical realism into three phases: (i) basic critical realism, (ii) dialectical critical realism, and (iii) the philosophy of meta-reality (Bhaskar, 2020). These three phases contribute to understanding society and guide social actions to redress social ills, obtain freedom, and foster human emancipation. Basic critical realism focuses on understanding society and how social events occur, focusing on the structures and mechanisms and their social effects. By articulating the roles of structures and agency to explicate social reality, basic critical realism effectively addresses several crucial philosophical dualisms such as structure/agency, individualism/collectivism, body/mind, causes/reasons, and facts/values (Hartwig, 2015). However, basic critical realism is inadequate to resolve the most significant dualism that impacts human freedom and well-being: the contradictory existence of (inherent) freedom and (existing) slavery. Bhaskar developed the phase of dialectical critical realism to address the dualism of human freedom and well-being. The third phase, meta-reality, adds a transcendental stratum or spiritual infrastructure to critical realist philosophical ontology (Hartwig, 2015).

Owning to my focus on decolonizing global health, the scope of my engagement and contribution to developing a postcolonial critical realism is adequately covered by the first two phases of Bhaskar's three phases of the critical realist philosophy of science—basic critical realism and dialectical critical realism. I have thus allocated separate chapters to engage with each of the phases of critical realism concerning the decolonization of global health. In this chapter, I focus on the contributions of the first theoretical development of critical realism, basic critical realism, and how these tenets contribute to understanding various aspects of colonialism and how they can inform decolonization. According to Bhaskar (2008), in terms of understanding injustice and oppression in all their forms, basic critical realism helps to understand the social mechanisms and structures that produce these power forms and their social effects. Therefore, this chapter considers applying the basic critical realist philosophical principles to unpack coloniality and decolonization.

A Scientific Ontology of Postcolonial Critical Realism

Postcolonial theories have been successfully used for colonial reflections, documenting anticolonial thoughts and addressing the experiences and perceptions of formally colonized communities (Felsch, 2023). While acknowledging the usefulness of postcolonial theories, it has also been highlighted that these theories have their drawbacks, such as ideological bias, the application of blurred and one-sided concepts, the preference for anecdotal evidence over empirical evidence, and ignorance of the major social and political trends of our time (Felsch, 2023; Ochoa, 1996). Owing to these ontological weaknesses, it is argued that postcolonial theories contribute to a distorted perception of colonial reality and their role in shaping modernity. Contrary to postcolonialism, which offers a distorted perception of reality, critical realism, which emphasizes the existence of underlying causal mechanisms that operate beneath the surface of observable phenomena, offers a robust philosophical grounding to explain social events. In search of a more robust ontological position to guide my reflections on the (de)colonization of global health, I found postcolonial critical realism (a blend of the two) most suitable.

Bhabha (1994) contends that "we must not merely change the narratives of our histories but *transform* our sense of what it means to live" (p. 256). To achieve this goal in global health practice and research, we must understand the different powers, ideologies, and mindsets (bundle of underlying causal mechanisms) operating as coloniality to decolonize global health. Because critical realism focuses on understanding the causal entities involved in orchestrating and maintaining social events, postcolonial critical realism can provide a robust meta-theoretical framework for achieving (de)colonialization. My contribution to developing postcolonial critical realism is informed by my desire to be able to (1) explain the manifestations of capitalism and imperialism in the Global South as the overarching social structures, (2) engage with the colonial ideologies and mindsets such as racism, religious paternalism, hegemony, white supremacy, and white saviorism that underlie and interact with social and material structures (colonial matrix of power) and (3) explore the emancipatory potential of value and the formulation of concrete utopias through decolonial reflexivity.

My contribution to establishing the postcolonial critical realist ontology departs by unpacking relevant basic critical realist tenets of the existence of a mind-independent reality, concept dependence of the social world, (in)transitive entities, generative causation, stratified reality, emergence, open systems, and retroductive theorizing and how they contribute to understanding colonialism. Using the ontological features of basic critical realism, I conceptualize five tenets of postcolonial critical realism:

1) Coloniality continues to shape systems, and old colonial beliefs influence and connect to real-world structures like laws, economies, and practices.
2) Colonialism's global impact: Its effects are worldwide but differ depending on existing structures, cultures, and agencies and how people experience them.
3) Marginalized voices matter: The struggles of oppressed groups reveal deeper truths (generative mechanisms) about how society works.
4) Coloniality is hidden: It is deeply rooted, hard to remove, and often operates invisibly.
5) Decolonize everything: To undo coloniality in global health, we must address its ideas, actions, evidence, and practices—and how they all interact (decoloniality).

I think that information obtained through adopted empirical methods using the postcolonial and decolonial lenses can be used to formulate theories about colonialism's impact on the formerly colonized and the continued influence of colonialism through coloniality on the practice of global health. These postcolonial and decolonial theories are unlikely to have the nature of mechanism-based causal theory as the critical theory informs them. Using the critical realist view of scientific knowledge described by Zhang (2023), I developed a scientific ontology of postcolonial critical realism (Figure 3.1).

Postcolonial critical realism is a cogent theory that integrates postcolonialism and tenets of critical realism. Their integration was anchored at three main points:

1) While the tenets of critical realism offer the ingredients of understanding colonialism as a social event, the perspectives of postcolonial discourse maintained the spotlight on the marginalized groups, highlighting their experiences and perspectives while challenging the historically dominant narratives.
2) Critical realism also focuses on the relationship between social structures (capitalism and imperialism) and agency and how their interactions and actions produce, maintain, or change events and structures. Postcolonial discourses contribute in this way by providing a critical lens to examine and challenge the legacies of colonialism, allowing for a deeper understanding of power imbalances, racialized identities, and the experiences of marginalized communities. It examines how colonialism shaped identities and cultural representations, leading to a deeper understanding of hybridity and cultural intersections.
3) Through its dialectical approach, (postcolonial) critical realism advocates addressing social ills and empowering the subjugated to seek emancipation. To this end, postcolonial discourses also contribute to achieving social justice for the colonized by advocating for inclusivity and amplifying "subaltern" voices and perspectives from the colonized world.

Postcolonial theories also help to deconstruct the dominant narrative and create space for diverse voices to be heard. By exposing the historical injustices of colonialism, postcolonial theory informs contemporary social movements advocating for equity and equality. These complementary components provide postcolonial critical realism, a synergistic ontology for tackling colonial-based inequities and injustices.

Principles of Basic Critical Realism

Transcendental realism is a philosophy of science that argues that reality is layered and that scientific knowledge can only be possible if it includes hidden parts of reality. Transcendental realism emerged during the paradigm wars of the 1970s to 1990s, when contestations began surfacing between proponents of

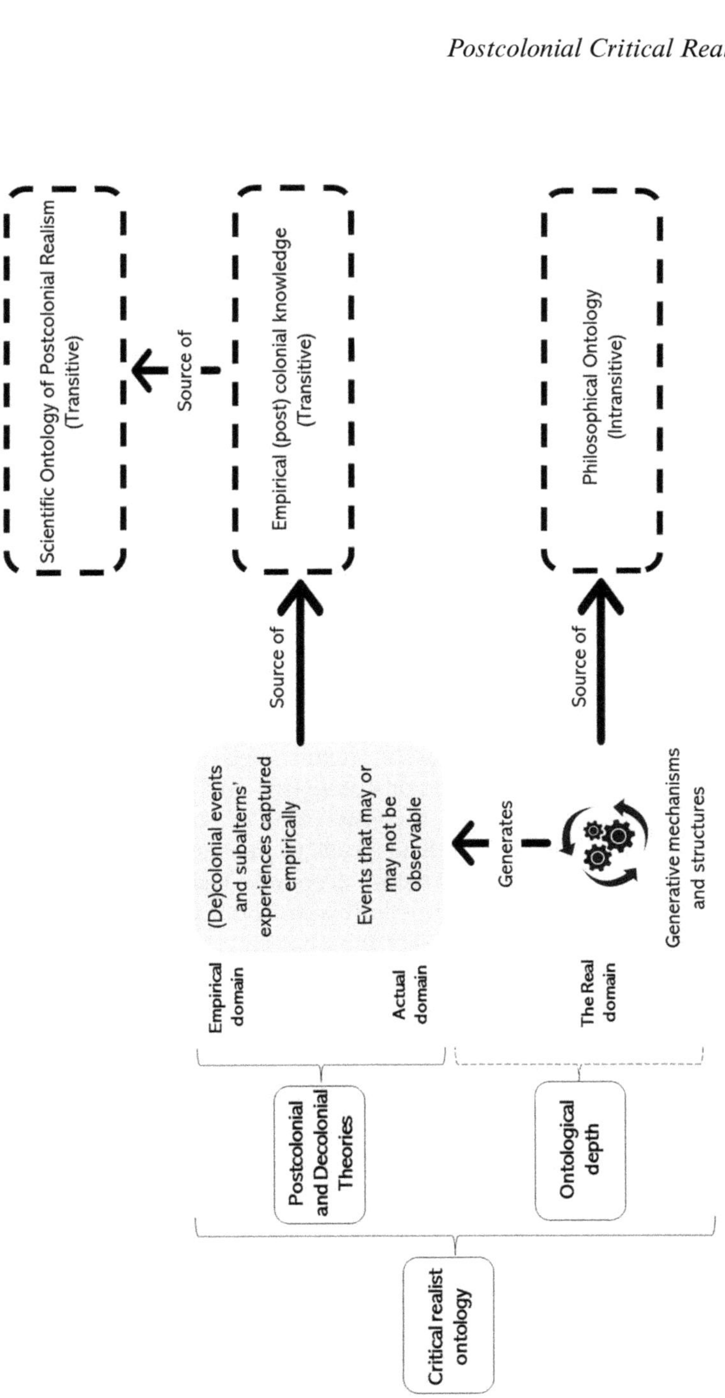

Figure 3.1 A scientific ontology of postcolonial critical realism.

the different schools of philosophical thought on which would be more practical to inform research practice (Gage, 1989; Oakley, 2010). Roy Bhaskar (1975a, 1975b, 1998, 2008, 2016) is credited with establishing transcendental realism, which he later developed as critical realism along with other social scientists like Archer (1995), Sayer (2000), Lawson (2001), Danermark et al. (2019), Dean et al. (2006), Elder-Vass (2008), and more who made telling contributions.

Realism is a philosophical position which claims that reality exists and is knowable. Ontologically, it shares similarities with positivism in that an objective reality exists independent of our perception, meaning there is a "real world" out there to be studied, and both approaches aim to generate knowledge based on this reality. This shared ontological position is described as "ontological realism." However, critical realism diverges from positivism by asserting that causal explanations should not solely rely on empirical regularities but also consider unobservable structures and mechanisms (Cruickshank, 2012). On the other hand, critical realism and constructivism share some common epistemological principles, with both recognizing the significance of ideas, experiences, narratives, and discourses in understanding social phenomena.

Nevertheless, to align with its ontological grounding, critical realism utilizes these forms of expression to explore causal explanations (McEvoy & Richards, 2006). This common epistemological grounding shared between critical realism and constructivism is known as "epistemic relativism." What sets critical realism apart from positivism and constructivism is its acknowledgment that the world is an open system with a constellation of structures, mechanisms, and contexts (Kazi, 2003), which lends itself to open systems theorizing and the possibility of competing explanatory accounts. Therefore, critical realists accept multiple perspectives or competing claims about the nature of the social world (epistemic relativism) but reject the possibility that there are multiple realities (ontological realism).

Bhaskar developed his notion of critical realism in the book *A Realist Theory of Science* (Bhaskar, 1975a) for the sciences and his book *The Possibility of Naturalism* (Bhaskar, 2014) for the social sciences. His goal of developing critical realism was to provide an understanding that a "real social world" can be observed objectively (using our senses) while the observation is simultaneously shaped by personal, social, historical, and cultural frames (Mukumbang, 2023). Critical realism was thus proposed as a philosophical foundation to understand the social world as a function of the interactions between social structure—an organized set of social institutions and patterns of institutionalized relationships—and agency—thoughts and actions taken by people (Archer, 1995; Bhaskar, 1975b). Nevertheless, society is not reducible to the people that comprise society, and these individuals are not passive recipients of the social and cultural forces imposed by society. According to Bhaskar (2008), other social structures like imperialism and capitalism must exist for any intentional act, such as practices enabling global health inequities and injustices. Agency speaks to the ability of individuals to reproduce or transform the structure of society, intentionally or unintentionally (Archer, 1995, p. 255). Social agents are those individuals or organizations acting within a society who can change or transform social structures through their actions at any time. In global health, these social agents will be the interest holders[2] involved in agenda setting, research, policy making, strategy development, interventions, and program designing and implementation, as well as those using or taking up these programs or interventions. These stakeholders can change or transform various aspects of global health practice in their different capacities.

Critical realism is an ontology position (philosophy of science) within the philosophy of social sciences and a research paradigm. Its ontological aspect offers a theory regarding the nature of reality, which can be used to understand social reality. In its epistemological function, critical realism makes it possible to generate knowledge in context and build robust theories and models about the social world (Bhaskar, 2016). While my focus in this book is on the ontological aspect of critical realism, it is worth noting that the ontological and epistemological principles guiding the realist philosophy of science share the same tenets: the existence of a mind-independent reality, concept-dependence of the social world, (in)transitive entities, generative causation, stratified reality, emergence, open systems, and retroductive theorizing (Mukumbang et al., 2023). In the following section, I will dwell in as much detail as possible on the relevant tenets of basic critical realism to facilitate the reader's understanding of (de)colonization through a critical realist perspective.

Mind Independence of Global Health Decolonization

Mind independence is a fundamental critical realist principle stipulating that reality exists whether we experience it or not. There are two ways of thinking about mind independence, which can appear contradictory but are not. The first perspective considers realism as something like a river or a factory. In this case, the interpretation of mind-independence is quite straightforward: the river or the factory exists independently of whether we think it does. Relating this to colonialism means that the existence of colonialism does not depend on whether it was perceived or not. The mind-independent nature of reality applies not only to the physical dimensions but also to the social and cultural aspects (Sturgiss & Clark, 2020). It is, therefore, difficult to talk about colonialism without referring to the way people experienced it because this experience has given the word several connotations. Nevertheless, when triggered under certain conditions, everyone can only partially explain colonialism, which is informed by their encounters and experiences. Reality also does not depend on the different languages and conceptualizations we use to understand a phenomenon; they do not determine what is real.

The second perspective is that the world, including the social world, is intransitive—they exist even when humans cannot interpret them. Social structures like (de)colonialism are concept-dependent, relating to how we define, describe, or understand something and how a group agrees to conceptualize it.

As Sayer (2000) puts it, "a socially constructed world means that social phenomena are concept-dependent" (p. 18). Let us use the concept of money to illustrate this aspect of mind-independence. A banknote is only money if a group agrees to treat it as such. Its very existence as money, as opposed to its existence as a piece of paper, depends on the concepts people ascribed to it. If people stopped believing it was money, it would not be money anymore. So, its existence does depend on what we think about it.

Concept dependence has real consequences for social practices and is accurate and relevant for the decolonization literature. For instance, colonialism has been conceptualized as "a dirty business engaged in by evil people, or a praiseworthy endeavor undertaken by fine gentlemen for the noble purpose of saving the wretched, the savage, the unfortunate" (Horvath, 1972, p. 45). Similarly, decolonization means different things to different people, and the meaning of decolonization also changes based on the context within which it is applied. Decolonization has been used to refer to a country achieving political or legal independence—like how many African countries gained their political independence from their European colonial masters for self-governance (Decolonization$_1$). Decolonization has also been applied to undoing colonization's structural, cultural, and social impacts within different spaces and institutions. Indigenous activists often use the term to mean the restitution of an indigenous community's language, land, culture, and way of life (Decolonization$_2$). Therefore, an essential part of critical realist social science is exploring these different social constructions of a social phenomenon.

The way to reconcile the two perspectives of mind-independence discussed above is to recognize that they apply to different relationships with the phenomenon being considered (money or factory). The first claim concerns the epistemic relationship between an observer and a phenomenon. For the observer, the status (or not) of a piece of paper as money in a certain community is independent of what the observer believes about it. If Americans treat dollar notes as money, an African sociologist may think its status has no impact on whether that is true. For me, the moneyness of dollar notes is just as (my-) mind-independent as the existence of a river or a factor. Using the colonialism thoughts, for countries that were not colonized, their perception of what colonialism is does not matter much if those who were colonized conceptualize it as unfair, discriminatory, and brutal. The second claim concerns the constitutive relationship between a community of participants and a social phenomenon. For the participants, collectively, if they believe the dollar note is money, that makes it money; if they do not, it is not. Hence, its money-ness is not mind-independent for these people in this context. This can be similarly applied to colonialism. If those who were colonized collectively agree that what happened was colonialism, then they were colonized.

Because reality is mind-independent, it can only be captured partially or imperfectly using theories and models. This partial and imperfect understanding of reality can be attributed to four conditions:

1) Our understanding of reality is based on observations and experiences, which are inherently abstracted from our complex perceptions and then interpreted through language, constructs, and existing conceptual frameworks (Danermark et al., 2019). The effects of colonialism reported in Chapters 1 and 2 are the observations and experiences of political colonialism and neocolonialism by different (groups of) individuals.
2) Our knowledge is derived from observing, experiencing, and interacting with an infinitely intricate and constantly evolving universe from a specific contextual standpoint at a given time frame (Brunson et al., 2025). Consequently, after applying our best research and analytic methods, the theories we obtain are only estimates of reality. As applied to global health decolonization, I aim to develop theories or explanations explaining coloniality's role in perpetuating inequities and injustices in global health practice. For instance, using a proposed postcolonial critical realist ontological lens, Tinsley (2021) theorized that colonial discourses underlie and interact with material structures to perpetuate neocolonialism and that coloniality is visible through differential events and experiences. Based on her proposed postcolonial critical realist perspective, her theory represents how neocolonialism is sustained in climate change.
3) Our ability to represent and communicate knowledge depends on symbols, language, and technology, implying that our representation of reality is concept-dependent—using a set of rules that connect the elements of the model to explain observations (Sayer, 2000). Being concept-dependent in the decolonization discourse relates to how we define, describe, or understand coloniality and decoloniality, and such conceptualization has real consequences for decolonizing global health. Using a postcolonial critical realist causal lens allows us to appreciate the ontological reality of coloniality and decoloniality and propose practical processes through which equity and justice can be achieved in global health.
4) Finally, our knowledge sharing occurs through imperfect social processes, whereby any body of knowledge emerges through a social process of evaluating and adopting specific knowledge claims and dismissing others. For example, postcolonial and decolonial dialogues have been used to understand colonization, but they use different lenses, with postcolonialism inclined towards the cultural aspects of decolonization and decolonial dialogues focusing on world systems theory and scholarly research. Adopting different approaches to unpacking decolonization makes its knowledge imperfect, partial, and fallible.

Although reality is independent of human thought, language, conceptual activity, and perceptual experience, critical realists believe it can be captured using theories and models. Critical realism, as a philosophical position, focuses on a transcendental approach to scientific discovery —X is a necessary condition for the possibility of Y. This framework is crucial for scientific discovery, as it seeks to understand the underlying structures and mechanisms that give rise to observable phenomena. It also provides a fresh perspective for understanding society and international relations, offering the potential for a new approach to social investigations to understand the nature and relationships between structure, agency, and culture. Tinsley (2021) proposed postcolonial critical realism as an ontological framework to unpack the notions of racism, colonialism, and the social world and suggested that the framework can be used to understand decolonization. For instance, theories can be used to explain why and how decoloniality can lead to the decolonization of global health and, by extension, how and why the decolonization of global health can lead to equity in the practice of global health. Still, our best and most credible scientific theories represent only an estimation of reality. After applying our best research methods and using the appropriate research tools, whatever theories we obtain are considered only an approximation of the reality of colonization and decolonization of global health. Our elicited theories only approximate how and why decoloniality would lead to decolonization and how decolonization will lead to equity in healthcare globally.

If we accept that reality is mind-independent and that our knowledge of that reality is always partial, then what? How do we know if what we are describing is reality? To answer this question, critical realists advocate for "judgmental rationality," meaning that we need to judge—among the current accounts of reality—which is the best, or at least serves as a better description of reality. According to Bhaskar (2009), Tc is preferable to Td if Tc can explain a wider range of phenomena, including some significant ones that Td cannot explain, even if the theories are incommensurable. Additionally, the selected theory should be capable of explaining a deeper level of reality or achieving a higher order of epistemic integration (Bhaskar, 2009). Our judgment of what theory could best describe realists can be achieved by conceptualizing social reality as having a stratified ontology.

Global Health Reality Is Stratified

Why is reality stratified? Cruickshank (2010) explains that reality, of which global health is a part, is stratified because causal mechanisms, considered inherently unobservable, exist "beneath" the realm of constantly changing empirical events. One of the reasons our theories can only estimate reality is that not everything that exists manifests itself as events, and not all the events that occur are experienced by human agents. Consequently, three levels of reality are identified in critical realism, indicating a stratified reality—empirical, actual, and real (the boundaries are not distinct). The "empirical" is represented as a subset of the "actual," which is also a subset of the "real." The empirical represents events that are experienced and measured empirically. Empirical activities warranted by facts, measurable data, and observable phenomena are predominantly used to capture those events that were experienced.

For events to be empirically captured, they must have been experienced. According to Elder-Vass (2006, p. 6), experiences are social products, and they "are not simply a set of sense-data, but rather the result of our application of a socially influenced conceptual framework to the interpretation of that sense-data." Experiences are the outcomes of events they might appear to reflect and the product of combining them with our prior knowledge or conceptual frameworks (Elder-Vass, 2006). At the level of the empirical, our experiences, despite being interpreted, are constructed based on our sense of perceptions and augmented by any artificial research tools that are available. For instance, the socioeconomic deprivation index has been used to evaluate equity changes over time in low- and middle-income countries. Ferreira et al. (2024) used index-based routine household survey data to analyze the coverage of maternal and child interventions by socioeconomic deprivation status. They found that the coverage of skilled attendants at delivery showed large inequalities, where coverage among the socioeconomically deprived was substantially lower in almost all countries. The data for this study were obtained from national household surveys, which were the reported experiences of participating families. While extensive approaches using quantitative methods, such as the one adopted by Ferreira et al. (2024), can indicate the breadth of the problem, intensive approaches, such as qualitative methods, are used in global health to understand the root causes of health inequities and the experience of various populations of health inequities (Salisu et al., 2023).

Events are situated at the next level, the "actual," as they represent things that "actually" happened, even though not all are experienced. Entities found in the "real" cause events to occur. These entities possess structures and causal powers that can generate an outcome (event) when activated under various conditions. Causal powers exist as emergent properties of the entities that possess them (Elder-Vass, 2006). For instance, we have argued in Chapter 2 that the coloniality in global health perpetuates health inequality with higher burdens of disease experienced by countries in the global south. These inequalities in health outcomes can be empirically measured using research methods at the level of the "empirical" occurring as events and "absences"—such as the non-presence of Global South actors in governance structures at the "actual." One such event can be the limited participation of Global South experts and community representatives in the governance structures and advisory bodies of organizations focusing on improving health in the Global South. However, these events arise because of the interaction between structures and mechanisms with causal powers such as hegemonic power hierarchy in global health, white supremacy, racism, and religious paternalism operating in the "real."

The "real" is everything existing in the universe, tangible or intangible, both at the natural and social level, including entities (structures created in the past that are setting conditions for how present-day events occur) that possess generative powers and wait for the right conditions to manifest in the actual and the empirical. The reality of colonialism in global health, especially in the Global South, is inequity in health outcomes (higher disease burdens) and inequitable distribution of healthcare resources (human and material) compared to the Global North. These components can be measured at the "empirical" level. These global health outcomes are an expression of colonialism in global health, manifested as a limited representation of the local authority in health priority settings and limited considerations of the cultures of the local indigenes ("actual"). This plateau is underpinned by coloniality characterized by white supremacy, hegemony, patriarchy, saviorism, and racism ("real"). Elder-Vass (2006) insisted that structures and mechanisms existing in the real are distinct from the patterns of events that they generate. Similarly, events are real and distinct from the experiences in which they are apprehended. The iceberg metaphor (Figure 3.2) is often used to illustrate the three domains of reality identified by Bhaskar as it provides visual clarity to the conceptualization (Fletcher, 2017).

In the same way that not all events are experienced at the "actual" and thus not captured at the "empirical," causal entities located at the "real" do not always produce the events (outcomes) they tend to produce—demi-regularities (when they are not triggered). Because strict regularities (expected outcomes) are less likely to occur all the time, especially in open and complex systems characterized by various prevailing and countervailing conditions, other unintended or alternative behaviors could be observed—contrastives (Lawson, 2001). Also, because every event is co-determined by multiple interacting causal powers, they will sometimes be inhibited by other conflicting powers

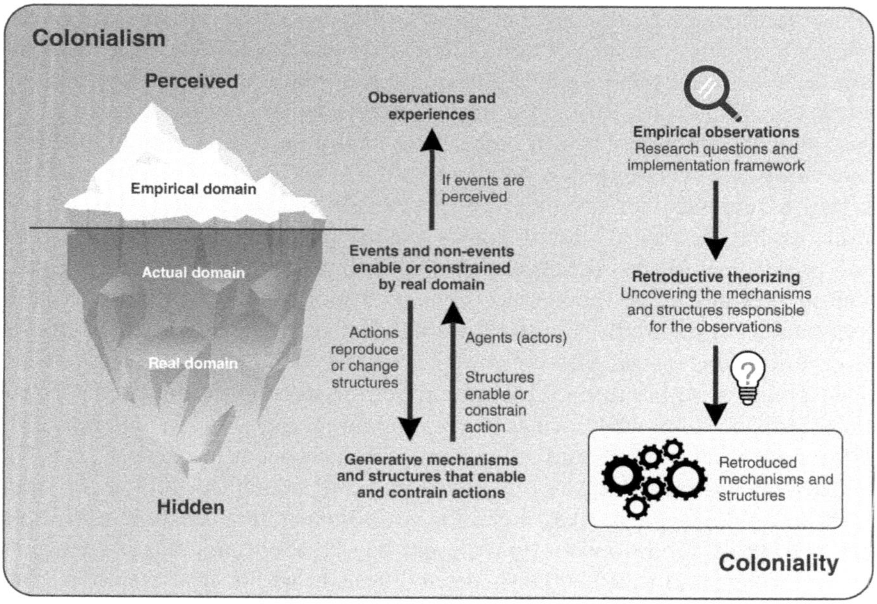

Figure 3.2 A layered ontological representation of reality.

(Elder-Vass, 2008). Causal entities combining in different ways, depending on other conditions and interactions, to form new outcomes is known as emergence. The emerging outcomes are not the sum of the parts of the interacting entities from a lower stratum. Consequently, the emerging outcomes cannot be reduced to the entities that combined to form them. This irreducibility is because the properties inherited from the entities of the lower strata reorganize themselves to obtain a stable set of relations between the parts that constitute them into a new kind of whole (Elder-Vass, 2006). Emergence is a property of open systems, such as the social world within which global health is practiced, with a constellation of structures, mechanisms, and other entities such as obscured relationships, hegemony, religious paternalism, and white saviorism, among others, constantly interacting with each other to form outcomes that favor and sustain the inequities and injustices in the practice of global health. It is not just the complexity of the interactions between various mechanisms that concerns us but the intrinsic contingency of the mechanistic structures themselves (Glynos & Howarth, 2007).

Global Health Is an Open and Complex System

Ontologically, critical realism conceptualizes the social world as an open and complex system characterized by interdependencies running through the same and different layers, with the absence of clear boundaries between causal entities (mechanisms and structures) and the constant emergence of new causal entities and observations (Haigh et al., 2019). Open systems describe a constellation of structures, mechanisms, relationships, and other entities responsible for the observable patterns of events (Fleetwood, 2017). In addition to the constellation perspective, the notion of complexity also emphasizes instability, sudden change, non-equilibrating systems, temporal irreversibility, and sensitivity to initial conditions (Mingers, 2011). The open nature of the social world does not suggest that human capacity and agency are omnipresent and unlimited in their ability to alter their environment; they are restricted by how each role is defined within the structure. The notion of complexity is closely associated with the open nature of the social world (Roux, 2011), engendered through emergence. According to Hill (2011), global health is complex because it has multiple and diverse players with polyvalent and constantly evolving relationships with rich and dynamic interactions. It also deals with a myriad of initiatives requiring multiple networks through which interest holders (re)configure their influence within different contexts in which development for health occurs (Hill, 2011).

As system thinkers, critical realists conceptualize complexity by foregrounding relationships in wholes rather than isolating parts (De Souza, 2022). Complex systems, as open systems, exhibit three critical notions. First, macro-level patterns emerge from the interplay of causal entities at different systems and levels through emergence. For instance, decolonization in global health can be achieved through the interaction and actions of different actors in different contexts tackling different components of coloniality. In his book *The Possibility of Naturalism*, Bhaskar (2014) described emergence as the complex, interactive, and changing domain of society and its agents. Sayer (2000) illustrates this idea by highlighting that "social phenomena are emergent from biological phenomena, which are emergent from chemical and physical strata." Elder-Vass (2006) explained further that higher-level entities emerge from a collection of lower-level entities that are their components or parts. He further explained that "it is the fact that a higher-level entity is composed of a particular stable organization of lower-level entities that gives it the possibility of exerting causal influence in its own right" (Elder-Vass, 2006, p. 4). The exertion of causal influences is also contingent on conditions at the higher "level," a notion that Navarrete and Fryer (2024) describe as "contextual emergence." While mechanisms may emerge from lower strata, they are not reducible to those strata and, therefore, still usually need to be researched in the strata in which they operate to explain their operation. Recognizing that the health of individuals and populations is the manifestation of a system in which biology interacts with environments and individuals interact with each other and with environments over time typifies the operation of complex causal relationships in global health. For instance, the health impact of the COVID-19 pandemic disproportionately affected the Global North. These health concerns prompted these nations to prioritize the development of COVID-19 vaccines and treatment protocols to prevent and manage the COVID-19 pandemic among this population (macro-level causality). Through active vaccination campaigns in high-income countries, a stark disparity in vaccination rates between high- and low-income economies was established, which led the UN to call for vaccine equity on a global scale. With new, more infectious variants complicating responses to outbreaks (contextual emergence), the Global North faced the dilemma of hoarding the vaccines for their population or making them available for other nations, especially in the Global South. This dilemma resulted in high-income countries hoarding many vaccines, while low-income countries could not access enough vaccines, causing vaccine inequity.

Second, individuals or groups of individuals (agents) have the potential to contribute to changing social structures. Social structures depend on human activities, so in some sense, the activities they engage in can influence the direction in which social structures are elaborated. The notion of agent-agent interaction leading to emergence is relevant to global health as a complex system laden with dependencies between individuals (i.e., situations in which the outcome for one individual is affected by the outcomes in other individuals) can lead to new outcomes. For instance, using a systematic methodology and related search functions, Hoffman and Cole (2018) identified 203 global health actor groups and the structure of their social network operating in the global health space with different relationship patterns. Returning to our COVID-19 vaccine illustration, key groups of individuals involved in the COVID-19 vaccine nationalism or hoarding were the policymakers of these nations. The decision of these policymakers to hoard the COVID-19 vaccines in case their population needed it led to the unjust and inequitable distribution of COVID-19 vaccines. Also, considering the vaccine nationalism or hoarding from high-income countries, several African actors, both at the national and regional level, exercised agency by using a range of specific actions to address vaccine shortages (Soulé, 2022). Notably, many African leaders partnered with China and Russia for Sinovac and the Sputnik V COVID-19 vaccines, respectively, for their country's vaccine supply. Other countries like Egypt had the vaccine manufacturing industry constructed in their country (Soulé, 2022).

Third, negating or balancing feedback can regulate a system's behavior to maintain stability or equilibrium over time through the structure-agent and agent-agent interactions. This notion is especially useful for decolonizing global health. Structure and agency are different kinds of emergent entities, possessing different properties and powers. Even though they are crucial for each other's operations, formation, continuation, and development (Archer & Morgan, 2020), their diverse views and expertise are essential in unpacking reality. This last characteristic portrays global health as a complex adaptive system. As applies to global health, the idea of complexity is that changes will continue, whereby "structures will emerge to meet new challenges, and, over time, be shaped by their interface within the system" (Hill, 2011, p 601). Global health predominantly has centers of activity in the Global South and dominant nodes of interaction mainly in the Global North, a dynamic manifesting as a complex system open to influence through the web of communication or reflexivity with the global stakeholders (Hill, 2011). In our COVID-19 vaccine example, the consequence of vaccine hoarding by high-income countries, which is based on the fear of the impact of COVID-19 on their population, is that it leads to inequitable distribution of vaccines, thus reducing vaccine access to low-income countries. To counteract the inequity introduced through vaccine hoarding, the World Health Organization formed programs for the global distribution of COVID-19 vaccines to achieve equitable access to the vaccine. A joint initiative between the World Health Organization, Gavi (formerly the Global Alliance for Vaccines and Immunization), the Coalition for Epidemic Preparedness Innovations, and other non-profits largely funded by the European Union came together to provide two billion vaccines to low-income countries to address poor vaccine access and vaccine distribution inequity.

According to Archer (2024), complexity theories and approaches have often undermined the notion of history and of time. She went on to ask how it is possible to explain how matters came to be the way they are rather than "otherwise" without referencing the preceding social situation. Then, she stated that most social states or occurrences cannot be fully explained or understood without considering their preceding states of affairs. Considering antecedents is particularly relevant to unpacking the agenda and calls for decolonizing global health. How can we discuss decolonizing global health without understanding how global health came to be colonized? What are the historical antecedents and conditions that caused it to be colonized? Archer (2024) argues that our theories of social states or occurrences should accentuate the influence of antecedent structures. These theories should illustrate how, for example, the vested interests of the participants seeking change versus those defending the status quo played a role in the current social states or occurrences. It has been argued that the colonization of global health is due to coloniality—the remnants of the structures and relations of the colonial past—therefore, we cannot fully understand how to decolonize global health if we do not fully understand those antecedents (structures and relationships) that fomented colonialism. Therefore, realist complexity "adopts a relational conception of society, where societal processes occurring in historical time are said to impact our present-day interactions and contribute to emergence and adaptations over time" (De Souza, 2022, p. 79). Archer (2024) says that while considering the history of social events, attention should also be given to agency. While social structures are material rather than agentic, they are still dependent on the activities of people (agents) who decide on carrying out a certain action or not and choose the way by which to carry these actions out, and so on (De Souza, 2022). Therefore, these agents' preceding ideas, decisions, and actions contribute to the current social states or occurrences. With this in mind, Archer (2024) concluded that "history is indispensable precisely because neither structure, culture nor agency can be conceptualized in terms of 'presentism'" (p. 3). As such, outcomes can never be predetermined but are always emergent as they also depend on past interactions between entities of the structures, culture, and agents.

Another important tenet of complexity science relevant to global health and understanding how it can be decolonized is recognizing that social systems are interlinked with other systems at all levels (Knio, 2024). In addition to the understanding that social systems interact with processes that are complex in form, the social systems within which these processes take place interact with other systems at all levels. This level of conceptualization is characteristic of global health operations, which is why some authors have described the global health system as complex and adaptive. Borghi et al. (2022, p. 3) explained that the global health system can be described as a "nested health system comprising all national health systems together with the global health architecture, in which cross-scale interactions influence behaviors." Therefore, other political, economic, and social systems influence the global health systems, which means that what affects one of these interconnected systems can shift the operations of the other systems. For instance, there is now a recognition of the need for prevention and intervention across multiple sectors of the economy to achieve health and planetary goals, which indicates the intersections and links between the economic and global health systems (Petrou & Jakovljevic, 2024). This interlinked and collaborative nature of global health as a complex system means the different structures and mechanisms operating in one system might have effects or produce outcomes that affect other systems. For example, existing inequities in one system can engender inequities in other linked and corresponding systems. The literature, for instance, has consistently linked people in low socioeconomic circumstances with poor access to healthcare services and health outcomes (Fiscella & Williams, 2004; McMaughan et al., 2020). That is to say, the socioeconomic inequities these people experience translate into health inequities. At the biological level, low socioeconomic conditions relate to poor living conditions and food insecurity. Poor eating leads to vulnerability to diseases through poor immune system buildup. Consequently, the same powers and forces perpetuating inequities in one system may be responsible for or introduce inequities in other systems by association. In other words, causal powers stemming from structures or actors from one system can flow into other linked systems and levels. In this paragraph, I have shown how health and illness, while being biological, matter for individuals, and the whole global health system operates on these matters from the structural and agential levels.

Transitive and Intransitive Nature of Entities

Causal entities are characteristically unseen and intransitive—they exist even when humans cannot interpret them. They represent laws and properties of the world independent of our knowledge of (and efforts to understand) them. Nevertheless, through empirical activities, we can formulate theories and develop models to estimate their existence and describe their effects. These models and theories are considered transitive entities because they concern humans and meaning-making (hermeneutics). The theories and knowledge generated through human research activities are considered to be fallible and thus subject to revision and replacement.

The ontological assumptions within the transitive domain may be responsible for making the scientific apparatus functional, but this does not mean that they are infallible (Cruickshank, 2010). This thought suggests that the ontological assumption of critical realism makes it possible to develop explanations about how coloniality engendered the inequities and inequalities observed in global health. Because the theories were obtained through some guiding principles, there is a chance that the theories obtained may be fallible. For this reason, Bhaskar (2014) argues that critical realism considers metaphysics as a "conceptual science" (p. 36). Consequently, realist-informed theories are always provisional and partial, although the entities that cause the observations explained remain unchanged. The task of developing an ontology is to transform the previously implicit assumptions about reality into an explicit set of philosophical definitions that can guide the sciences (Cruickshank, 2010).

Generative Causality in Critical Realism

In the positivist paradigm, causality is understood primarily through Hume's "secessionist" theory (Hausman, 1967). This theory is based on consistently observing events' "constant conjunction" rather than directly perceiving causal relationships. Stroud (1978) further explains that when two events consistently appear one after the other, they are considered causally connected; the former is considered the "cause" and the latter the "effect." While constructivists do not ascribe to causality, they consider uncovering common themes across episodes and contexts. It is important to note that process data can reveal causal relationships that quantitative data alone cannot uncover (Jensen, 2022). Critical realism challenges the Humean account of causality, proposing a more sophisticated account to explain social phenomena. The centrality of causality in critical realism is the consideration of causality through the idea of causal powers (Pratten, 2009). Critical realism considers causality through the lens of open systems with consternation of structures, mechanisms, and other causal entities to provide causal explanations that account for various social phenomena. In the critical realist's conceptualization, structures, mechanisms, and other causal entities can combine in different ways, depending on other conditions and interactions, to form new outcomes, such as emergence.

The concept of mechanisms is central to critical realist ontology and explication of causality. All causal powers are produced by mechanisms, which are processes of interaction between the parts of the entity and the power concerned. Archer (2013) proposed that social structures (indeed culture) possess causal powers to generate events under specific conditions. Following this understanding of structures, I will consider capitalism and imperialism as important structures in the grand scheme of colonialism (as an outcome). While they continue to drive the agenda and offer the reason for interaction with formal colonies, other ideologies such as racism, religious paternalism, hegemony, white supremacy, and white saviorism exert more direct influence over the way the formal colonizers continue to operate in these former colonies. I considered these ideologies and mindsets mechanisms because they instill the notion of power imbalance (colonial matrix of power), which triggers decision-making and behaviors based on the side of the power pendulum the actor is standing on.

Capitalism and imperialism are those conditions that underpin the operations of the ideologies mentioned above and thus constitute antecedent social structures with causal influences in their right. According to Danermark et al. (2019), a mechanism is "that which can cause something in the world to happen, and in this respect, mechanisms can be of many different kinds" (p. 55). Mechanisms are generally not directly observable. When examining a phenomenon, the objective is often to uncover the "underlying mechanisms" that give rise to it and comprehend the interplay between them and how they shape the outcome. Critical realist research and evaluation strive to elucidate the mechanisms orchestrating the observed phenomenon and understand their interplay within a specified organizational, institutional, or social structure. It is important to note that some mechanisms may not yield the expected outcomes empirically because they have not been activated or other mechanisms or context conditions have counteracted their effects. Nevertheless, due to their enduring properties and powers, these mechanisms are continuously active in their outcomes, displaying variability in open systems (Archer et al., 2013).

Natural reality comprises distinct strata of emergent properties, manifested in the biological and chemical domains, which cannot be reduced to the physical domain (Cruickshank, 2010). The stratification includes physical, chemical, biological, psychological, psychosocial, behavioral, social, cultural, and economic layers (Danermark et al., 2019; Sayer, 1992). Mechanisms at a lower level can create conditions for unfolding mechanisms at a higher level. Sayer (2000) illustrates this idea by stating that "social phenomena are emergent from biological phenomena, which are emergent from chemical and physical strata." While mechanisms may emerge from lower strata, they are not reducible to those strata. Therefore, they usually need to be researched in the strata they operate to explain their operation. To achieve this, Danermark et al. (2019) proposed that any investigation into social phenomena should consider diverse explanations of phenomena at multiple levels. The implication of this layered ontology for global health researchers is that explaining health outcomes and evidence adoption requires understanding various mechanisms at multiple levels: biological, psychological, interpersonal, and cultural.

The identified social mechanisms cannot operate in a vacuum. They occur within social structures—normative institutions and established laws, relationships, and regulations. Merton explained that social mechanisms have designated consequences for designated parts of the social structure (Merton, 1968). His thoughts are supported by Elder-Vass (2010), who argues that social structures are "causally effective in their own right, with generative powers distinct from those of individuals" (p. 6), although their operations are complex. As Bhaskar (2009) stated, the individual's generative powers interact with those of the social structures to determine an individual's action. For example, a pregnant woman's agency (motivation and willingness) to attend all her maternity appointments and deliver at the health center is based on the available resources and maternal and child health policies in the local health systems. In the agential movement, an individual's actions (the individual as actor and agent is a social self that participates in collectives) contribute to reproducing and transforming the structure(s) concerned—again interacting with other generative powers (Elder-Vass, 2008). For instance, pregnant women can continue to use traditional birth attendants as opposed to using health centers for delivery. This practice may cause the local health system to consider integrating traditional birth attendants as part of their health system, and their services become regulated by the health system.

Sayer (2000) provided a very useful conceptualization of causality informed by the critical realist philosophy of science (Figure 3.3). In Sayer's conceptualization of causality based on critical realist principles, structures are integral to the operations of mechanisms as mechanisms are embedded within the social structure. Therefore, realist-informed explanations rely on comprehending the structure of natural and social objects, which involves identifying causal mechanisms, understanding their functionality, and determining if and when they are activated.

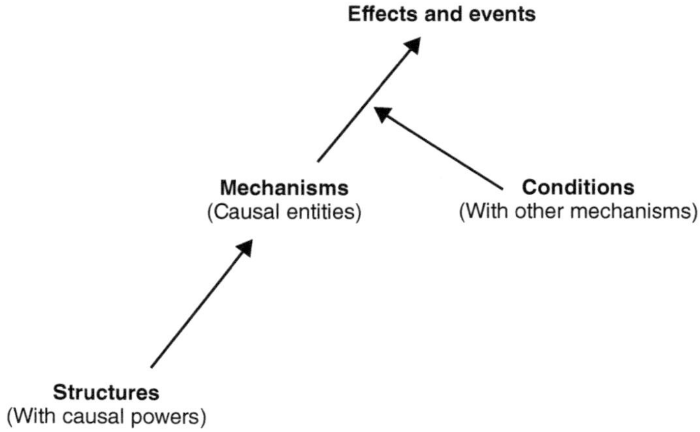

Figure 3.3 A critical realist conceptualization of causality.

This approach is outlined in Figure 3.3, which presents a framework for understanding how causality is conceptualized within the context of critical realism. According to this framework, structures possess causal powers that trigger causal mechanisms under specific conditions, resulting in the occurrence of events.

Critical realists argue that a meta-theory that defines social reality in terms of agents interacting with structural emergent properties is required to underpin social explanations. Therefore, in formulating realist-informed theories, identifying the agent–agent, and agent–structure relations are essential in explaining social behavior (Connelly, 2001). These relationships lead to identifying and conceptualizing structures, generative mechanisms, and demi regularities (anticipated and emergent outcomes). Critical realism's focus on structures, actors, causal mechanisms, and events accommodates a pluralist approach to causation, which acknowledges multiple forms of causality (Cartwright, 2004). These forms of causality include linear causality based on "a straightforward, direct chain of events that characterizes simple phenomena" and also complex causalities, which are used by scholars who "believe that the social world is complex, characterized by path dependence, tipping points, interaction effects, strategic interaction, two-directional causality or feedback loops" (Geels, 2022, p. 6).

Retroductive Theorizing

Formulating theories based on the critical realist philosophy of science is achieved through retroduction or retroductive theorizing. Retroduction is a form of retrospective theorizing (working backward), which entails working from observations to unveil the mechanisms and structures responsible for the observation (Figure 3.2). It entails developing explanations using information obtained from the "Empirical" through interpreting particular actions and events situated in the "Actual" to uncover the structures and mechanisms that will account for the outcome in the "Real" (Jagosh, 2020; Mukumbang, 2023). Retroductive theorizing thus involves a transcendental production of ontological categories to generate concrete explanations of empirical phenomena. Retroductive explanations presuppose the discovery of underlying causal or generative mechanisms from empirical data, and the logic of explanation is based on the contingent interaction of necessary structures, causal mechanisms, and other causal entities (Glynos & Howarth, 2007, 2019). Critical realists thus embrace retroduction as a form of reasoning essential to the activity of hypothesis formation and explanation to capture social reality.

The application of retroduction for goal setting is against its standard application—starting from observation and working backward to identify the causal generative mechanisms. Brown et al. (2002) suggested that rather than retroduce structures and mechanisms responsible for a social phenomenon, researchers should unearth mechanisms by studying similar social events over long periods to see how these mechanisms and structures have actualized. Schoppek (2021) describes the application of retroduction for goal setting, such as decolonizing global health, as "ex-ante" retroduction.

Envisaging a decolonization utopia and setting decolonizing goals require predicting the structures and mechanisms that should exist and how they would interact to produce the desired objective. Ex-ante retroduction is proposed instead of post-ante explanation because ex-ante retroduction theorizing is predictive. Ex-ante retroduction in the context of decolonizing global health asks questions such as, "Under which conditions and through which mechanisms may decolonization initiatives lead to decolonization?" Schoppek (2021) argues that retroduction can be employed in "an ex-ante fashion to investigate what must be the case for a particular result to occur" (p. 6).

Of course, the expected objective has not yet happened or has not been achieved (and perhaps will never be achieved). Therefore, no "direct" empirical data can be used to inform the explanation. Schoppek (2021) suggests using a thought experiment based on theoretical knowledge to identify the mechanisms and structures of transformation. For instance, we know that coloniality sustains hegemony, racism, and white supremacy in global health in modern times, as was in the time of political colonization to perpetuate inequity and injustice in global health. We should be able to hypothesize mechanisms that could be at play to achieve decolonization—decoloniality. Nevertheless, what is key in Schoppek's ex-ante method is drawing parallels from other comparable cases rather than simply speculating about possible mechanisms. Therefore, if we study other projects with similar goals, we can, for instance, examine how decolonization has been achieved in other fields or aspects of life.

Abstraction is a key tool in this process of retroduction, allowing researchers to focus on specific aspects while temporarily setting aside others (Lawson, 1997). Abstraction serves two main purposes. Firstly, it helps identify particular aspects of social reality by identifying partial or demi-regularities[3]—patterns that emerge from contrasting seemingly similar examples. These demi-regularities can range from mundane observations to scientifically puzzling phenomena. They provide a starting point for scientific investigation, directing researchers toward potentially identifiable mechanisms. The second stage of abstraction involves uncovering the "real essence" of the social phenomenon of interest. Guided by the previously identified demi-regularities, researchers formulate hypotheses about underlying social structures and mechanisms. This movement from manifest social phenomena to deeper social structures allows us to focus on aspects of social phenomena beyond their appearances. By abstracting from deeper causal factors, researchers can hypothesize about the powers embedded in specific social structures, which may manifest as demi-regularities at the surface level (Brown et al., 2002).

Brown et al. (2002) contend that, while critical realism may help expose undisclosed aspects of the social sphere, freeing the mind such that an alternative (progressive) image future may be contemplated, retroduction alone is not enough to achieve this feat. They argued that systematic abstraction—the necessary ordering of historical categories from the relatively abstract to the ever more concrete—constitutes a radical addition to retroduction, which mostly focuses on uncovering the mechanisms and structures responsible for a specific phenomenon—movement from the apparent (event) to the real domain.

As Lawson (1997) emphasizes, abstraction's purpose is to understand better one or more aspects, components, or attributes of a social phenomenon and their relationships to reintegrate them into a concrete (concrete utopia). Once this understanding is achieved, it may be possible to combine or synthesize the separate understandings into a comprehensive understanding of the concrete (Lawson, 1997, p. 227). Abstraction's role is to individualize real phenomena, and the integration of revealed "forms" and "essences" comes after in reconstructing the concrete as a whole. In this sense, the synthetic or totalizing moment of critical realism is separate from the actual process of abstraction. The former aims to combine abstractions to reveal potential internal connections in the social world. Lawson (1997) states that features or aspects of an internally related set of structures or dynamic processes cannot be seen as isolated momentary phenomena, like punctiform events. Each feature must be seen as expressing the remaining features or whole to which it is related, as well as its history.

In decolonizing global health, possible demi-regularities would be the outcomes of decolonizing efforts in other areas of life. According to Adhikari et al. (2023) a decolonized global health is:

> a utopian future wherein healthcare providers and researchers, regardless of country of residence or origin, receive equal opportunities in recognition, research, and publishing; training; access to international travel for conferences and work; and salaries and incentives, so that every LMIC expert is considered equivalent to their high-income country (HIC)

> counterparts. We ultimately hope for a future in which people from every country have equal access to quality health care, fulfilling the aspiration of universal health coverage proposed by WHO.

The World Health Organization can help raise awareness among key actors of the interface between global and domestic/local health issues and health and foreign policy. This approach could be done through a regional conference on global health diplomacy. The World Health Organization can draw attention to trends at the regional and global levels. The role of the World Health Organization country offices in health diplomacy needs to be strengthened. A regular meeting of health attachés could be explored.

Conclusion

In this chapter, I focused on establishing postcolonial critical realism as an ontological position that can allow me and other scholars to engage with the literature on (de)colonialism and their variant concepts based on the principles of critical realism. This engagement provides a robust foundation on which I will base my arguments on understanding how global health became colonized and how the colonization of global health was sustained through coloniality. Most importantly, this proposed ontological perspective should guide decolonizing global health providing robust approaches that will successfully dismantle the colonial matrix of power that currently drives global health practice and research. In the next chapter, I will focus on the bundle of generative mechanisms unpacked as colonial matrix of power embedded in coloniality and how these mechanisms perpetuate the outcomes of inequity, knowledge colonialism, and systemic and epistemic injustices in global health.

Notes

1 In this book I will use the term "postcolonial theories" to include the different conceptualization and operationalizations—postcolonial theory, postcolonial studies, postcolonial thought, decolonial thought, and neo-colonial theory.

2 I have adopted the term "interest holders" in this book instead of "stakeholders." The word stakeholders is said to have a colonial foundation. It is explained that it originates from the historical practice of European settlers literally "staking" claims on land they were taking from indigenous peoples, effectively signifying a power dynamic where the colonizers held primary ownership and control, thus making it disrespectful to use the term when referring to indigenous communities or situations where power imbalances exist due to colonization (see further Reed et al., 2024).

3 Real utopias and concrete utopias were used as synonyms. Erik Olin Wright used the term real utopia while Roy Bhaskar used the term concrete utopia. In *Envisioning Real Utopias*, Erik Olin Wright wanted to provide arguments against the notion of radical social transformation, to which end he proposed "real utopias," which might appear oxymoronic. Wright suggested that real utopias are not fantasies, or not only fantasies. Rather, they are "hard-nosed proposals for pragmatically improving our lives" or utopian ideals grounded in reality.

References

Adhikari, S., Torres, I., & Oele, E. (2023). The way forward in decolonising global health. *The Lancet Global Health*, 11(7), e982. https://doi.org/10.1016/S2214-109X(23)00275-9

Archer, M. (1995). *Realist social theory: The morphogenetic approach*. Cambridge University Press.

Archer, M., Bhaskar, R., Collier, A., Lawson, T., & Norrie, A. (2013). Critical realism: Essential readings. In *Critical realism: Essential readings*. Routledge. https://doi.org/10.4324/9781315008592

Archer, M. S. (2013). *Social morphogenesis*. Springer.

Archer, M. S. (2024). Can complexity add anything to critical realism and the morphogenetic approach? *Journal for the Theory of Social Behaviour*. https://doi.org/10.1111/JTSB.12419

Archer, M. S., & Morgan, J. (2020). Contributions to realist social theory: an interview with Margaret S. Archer. *Journal of Critical Realism*, 19(2), 179–200. https://doi.org/10.1080/14767430.2020.1732760

Balandier, G. (2020). The colonial situation: A theoretical approach. In G. Balandier, *The new imperial histories reader*, 23–40. Routledge. https://doi.org/10.4324/9781003060871-3

Bhabha, H. K. (1994). *The location of culture*. Routledge.

Bhambra, G. K. (2014). Postcolonial and decolonial dialogues. *Postcolonial Studies*, 17(2), 115–121. https://doi.org/10.1080/13688790.2014.966414

Bhaskar, R. (1975a). *A realist theory of science*. Leeds Books.

Bhaskar, R. (1975b). Forms of realism. *Philosophica*, 15(1), 99–127.

Bhaskar, R. (1998). *Critical realism and dialectic* (M. Archer, Ed.). Routledge.

Bhaskar, R. (2008). *Dialectic: The pulse of freedom*. Routledge. https://doi.org/10.4324/9780203892633

Bhaskar, R. (2009). *Scientific realism and human emancipation*. Routledge.

Bhaskar, R. (2014). *The possibility of naturalism: A philosophical critique of the contemporary human sciences* (4th ed.). Routledge.

Bhaskar, R. (2016). *Enlightened common sense*. Routledge. https://doi.org/10.4324/9781315542942

Bhaskar, R. (2020). Critical realism and the ontology of persons. *Journal of Critical Realism*, 19(2), 113–120. https://doi.org/10.1080/14767430.2020.1734736

Borghi, J., Ismail, S., Hollway, J., Kim, R. E., Sturmberg, J., Brown, G., Mechler, R., Volmink, H., Spicer, N., Chalabi, Z., Cassidy, R., Johnson, J., Foss, A., Koduah, A., Searle, C., Komendantova, N., Semwanga, A., & Moon, S. (2022). Viewing the global health system as a complex adaptive system: Implications for research and practice. *F1000Research*, 11, 1147. https://doi.org/10.12688/F1000RESEARCH.126201.1

Brown, A., Slater, G., & Spencer, D. A. (2002). Driven to abstraction? Critical realism and the search for the "inner connection" of social phenomena. *Cambridge Journal of Economics*, 26(6). https://about.jstor.org/terms

Brunson, L., Lauzier-Jobin, F., Olson, B., & Côté, L. P. (2025). Seven key insights from critical realism and their implications for ecological thinking and action in community psychology. *Journal of Community Psychology*, 53(1), e23054. https://doi.org/10.1002/jcop.23054

Cartwright, N. (2004). Causation: One word, many things. *Philosophy of Science*, 71. https://doi.org/10.1086/426771

Connelly, J. (2001). Critical realism and health promotion: effective practice needs an effective theory. *Health Education Research*, 16(2), 115–120. https://doi.org/10.1093/her/16.2.115

Cruickshank, J. (2010). Knowing social reality: A critique of Bhaskar and Archer's attempt to derive a social ontology from lay knowledge. *Philosophy of the Social Sciences*, 40(4), 579–602. https://doi.org/10.1177/0048393109340664

Cruickshank, J. (2012). Positioning positivism, critical realism and social constructionism in the health sciences: a philosophical orientation. *Nursing Inquiry*, 19(1), 71–82. https://doi.org/10.1111/j.1440-1800.2011.00558.x

D'Souza, R. (2010). Introduction to the special issue. *Journal of Critical Realism*, 9(3), 263–275. https://doi.org/10.1558/jcr.v9i3.263

Danermark, B., Ekström, M., & Karlsson, J. C. (2019). *Explaining society: Critical realism in the social sciences* (2nd edition). Routledge. https://doi.org/10.4324/9781351017831

De Souza, D. E. (2022). A critical realist approach to systems thinking. *Evaluation*, 28(1), 72– 90. https://doi.org/10.1177/13563890211064639

Dean, K., Joseph, J., Roberts, J. M., & Wight, C. (2006). *Realism, philosophy and social science*. Palgrave Macmillan. https://doi.org/10.1057/9780230502079

Elder-Vass, D. (2006). Re-examining Bhaskar's three ontological domains: The lessons from emergence. In C. Lawson, C. Latsis, & N. Martins (Eds.), *Contributions to social ontology* (pp. 160–176). Routledge.

Elder-Vass, D. (2008). Searching for realism, structure and agency in actor network theory. *The British Journal of Sociology*, 59(3), 455–473. https://doi.org/10.1111/J.1468-4446.2008.00203.X

Elder-Vass, D. (2010). The causal power of social structures: emergence, structures and agency. In D. Elder-Vass, *Structure*. Cambridge University Press. https://doi.org/10.1017/CBO9780511761720

Felsch, M. (2023). The scientific shortcomings of postcolonial theory. *International Studies*, 60(1), 113–130. https://doi.org/10.1177/00208817221142485

Ferreira, L. Z., Wehrmeister, F. C., Dirksen, J., Vidaletti, L. P., Pinilla-Roncancio, M., Kirkby, K., Ricardo, L. I. C., Barros, A. J. D., & Hosseinpoor, A. R. (2024). A composite index; socioeconomic deprivation and coverage of reproductive and maternal health interventions. *Bulletin of the World Health Organization*, 102(2), 105. https://doi.org/10.2471/BLT.23.290866

Fiscella, K., & Williams, D. R. (2004). Health disparities based on socioeconomic inequities: Implications for urban health care. *Academic Medicine*, 79(12), 1139–1147. https://doi.org/10.1097/00001888-200412000-00004

Fleetwood, S. (2017). The critical realist conception of open and closed systems. *Journal of Economic Methodology*, 24(1), 41–68. https://doi.org/10.1080/1350178X.2016.1218532

Fletcher, A. J. (2017). Applying critical realism in qualitative research: methodology meets method. *International Journal of Social Research Methodology*, 20(2), 181–194. https://doi.org/10.1080/13645579.2016.1144401

Gage, N. L. (1989). The paradigm wars and their aftermath a "historical" sketch of research on teaching since 1989. *Educational Researcher*, 18(7), 4–10. https://doi.org/10.3102/0013189X018007004

Geels, F. W. (2022). Causality and explanation in socio-technical transitions research: Mobilising epistemological insights from the wider social sciences. *Research Policy*, 51(6), 104537. https://doi.org/10.1016/J.RESPOL.2022.104537

Glynos, J., & Howarth, D. (2007). *Logics of critical explanation in social and political theory*. Routledge. https://doi.org/10.4324/9780203934753

Glynos, J., & Howarth, D. (2019). The retroductive cycle: The research process in poststructuralist discourse analysis. In T. Marttila (Ed.), *Discourse, culture and organization: Inquiries into relational structures of power* (pp. 105–125). Palgrave Macmillan.

Gordon, L. R. (2019). Decolonizing philosophy. *The Southern Journal of Philosophy*, 57, 16–36. https://doi.org/10.1111/sjp.12343

Haigh, F., Kemp, L., Bazeley, P., & Haigh, N. (2019). Developing a critical realist informed framework to explain how the human rights and social determinants of health relationship works. *BMC Public Health*, 19(1), 1–12. https://doi.org/10.1186/S12889-019-7760-7

Hartwig, M. (2015). MetaRealism. *Journal of Critical Realism*, 14(4), 339–349. https://doi.org/10.1179/1476743015Z.00000000073
Hausman, A. (1967). Hume's theory of relations. *Noûs*, 1(3), 255. https://doi.org/10.2307/2214532
Hill, P. S. (2011). Understanding global health governance as a complex adaptive system. *Global Public Health*, 6(6), 593–605. https://doi.org/10.1080/17441691003762108
Hoffman, S. J., & Cole, C. B. (2018). Defining the global health system and systematically mapping its network of actors. *Globalization and Health*, 14(1), 1–19.
Horvath, R. J. (1972). A definition of colonialism. *Anthropology*, 13(1), 45–57.
Jagosh, J. (2020). Retroductive theorizing in Pawson and Tilley's applied scientific realism. *Journal of Critical Realism*, 19(2), 121–130. https://doi.org/10.1080/14767430.2020.1723301
Jensen, R. (2022). Exploring causal relationships qualitatively: An empirical illustration of how causal relationships become visible across episodes and contexts. *Journal of Educational Change*, 23(2), 179–196. https://doi.org/10.1007/S10833-021-09415-5
Kazi, M. (2003). Realist evaluation for practice. *British Journal of Social Work*, 33(6), 803–818. https://doi.org/10.1093/bjsw/33.6.803
Knio, K. (2024). Special issue on realist complexity: An introduction. *Journal for the Theory of Social Behaviour*. https://doi.org/10.1111/JTSB.12425
Kwete, X., Tang, K., Chen, L., Ren, R., Chen, Q., Wu, Z., Cai, Y., & Li, H. (2022). Decolonizing global health: what should be the target of this movement and where does it lead us? *Global Health Research and Policy*, 7(1), 1–6.
Lacertosa, M. (2025). Philosophical challenges of decolonial options, resistance, and combat. *Metaphilosophy*, 56(1), 52–68. https://doi.org/10.1111/META.12710
Lawson, T. (1997). *Economics and reality*. Routledge.
Lawson, T. (2001). Economics and explanation. *Revue Internationale de Philosophie*, 55(217), 371–393.
Maldonado-Torres, N., Vizcaíno, R., Wallace, J., & We, J. E. A. (2018). Decolonising philosophy. In G. K. Bhambra, D. Gebrial, & K. Nişancıoğlu (Eds.), *Decolonising the university* (pp. 64–90). Pluto Press.
McEvoy, P., & Richards, D. (2006). A critical realist rationale for using a combination of quantitative and qualitative methods. *Journal of Research in Nursing*, 11(1), 66–78. https://doi.org/10.1177/1744987106060192
McMaughan, D. J., Oloruntoba, O., & Smith, M. L. (2020). Socioeconomic status and access to healthcare: Interrelated drivers for healthy aging. *Frontiers in Public Health*, 8. https://doi.org/10.3389/FPUBH.2020.00231
Merton, R. (1968). *Social theory and social structure*. The Free Press.
Mingers, J. (2011). The contribution of systemic thought to critical realism. *Journal of Critical Realism*, 10(3), 303–330. https://doi.org/10.1558/jcr.v10i3.303
Moisio, O.-P. (2013). Critical theory. *Encyclopedia of Sciences and Religions*, 558–560. https://doi.org/10.1007/978-1-4020-8265-8_1642
Mukumbang, F. C. (2023). Retroductive theorizing: A contribution of critical realism to mixed methods research. *Journal of Mixed Methods Research*, 17(1), 93–114. https://doi.org/10.1177/15586898211049847
Mukumbang, F. C., De Souza, D. E., & Eastwood, J. G. (2023). The contributions of scientific realism and critical realism to realist evaluation. *Journal of Critical Realism*, 22(3), 504–524. https://doi.org/10.1080/14767430.2023.2217052
Naidu, T., Gingell, G., & Zaidi, Z. (2024). Decolonial framework for applying reflexivity and positionality in global health research. *Global Health Promotion*, 31(2), 52–58. https://doi.org/10.1177/17579759241238016
Navarrete, C., & Fryer, T. (2024). Redefining emergence: Making the case for contextual emergence in critical realism. *Journal for the Theory of Social Behaviour*, 54(2), 167–184. https://doi.org/10.1111/JTSB.12414

Oakley, A. (2010). Paradigm wars: Some thoughts on a personal and public trajectory. *International Journal of Social Research Methodology*, 2(3), 247–254. https://doi.org/10.1080/136455799295041

Ochoa, P. (1996). The historical moments of postcolonial writing: Beyond colonialism's binary. *Tulsa Studies in Women's Literature*, 15(2), 221–229.

Patomäki, H. (2002). *After international relations: critical realism and the (re)construction of world politics*. Routledge.

Petrou, S., & Jakovljevic, M. (2024). Reimagining the relationship between economics and health– WHO "Health for all" provisions. *Cost Effectiveness and Resource Allocation*, 22(1), 1–4. https://doi.org/10.1186/s12962-024-00512-9

Pratten, S. (2009). Critical realism and causality: Tracing the Aristotelian legacy. *Journal for the Theory of Social Behaviour*, 39(2), 0021–8308.

Reed, M. S., et al. (2024). Reimagining the language of engagement in a post-stakeholder world. *Sustainability Science*, 19, 1481–1490. https://doi.org/10.1007/s11625-024-01496-4

Roux, A. V. D. (2011). Complex systems thinking and current impasses in health disparities research. *American Journal of Public Health*, 101(9), 1627. https://doi.org/10.2105/AJPH.2011.300149

Salisu, M., Blackwell, T., Lewis, G., Hoglund, M. W., DiVittis, A., Chahal, K., Samuels, C., Boutin-Foster, C., Montgomery, D., & Afable, A. (2023). Community perceptions of health equity: A qualitative study. *Journal of Primary Care & Community Health*, 14. https://doi.org/10.1177/21501319231211439

Samuel-Mbaekwe, I. J. (1986). Colonialism and social structure. *Trans-African Journal of History*, 15, 81–95.

Sayer, A. (2000). *Realism and social science*. Sage. https://doi.org/10.4135/9781446218730

Sayer, R. A. (1992). *Method in social science: a realist approach*. Routledge.

Schoppek, D. E. (2021). How do we research possible roads to alternative futures? Theoretical and methodological considerations. *Journal of Critical Realism*, 20(2), 146–158. https://doi.org/10.1080/14767430.2021.1894908

Soulé, F. (2022). Addressing vaccine inequity: African agency and access to COVID-19 vaccines. *China International Strategy Review*, 4(1), 156. https://doi.org/10.1007/S42533-022-00105-2

Stroud, B. (1978). Hume and the idea of causal necessity. *Philosophical Studies*, 33, 39–59.

Sturgiss, E. A., & Clark, A. M. (2020). Using critical realism in primary care research: An overview of methods. *Family Practice*, 37(1), 143–145. https://doi.org/10.1093/fampra/cmz084

Talabi, J. M. (2021). Philosophical discourse on the decolonisation of the African mind. *AIPGG Journal of Humanities and Peace Studies*, 2(2). https://papers.ssrn.com/abstract=3919433

Tinsley, M. (2021). Towards a postcolonial critical realism. *Critical Sociology* https://doi.org/10.1177/08969205211003962

Tobi, A. T. (2020). Towards a plausible account of epistemic decolonisation. *Philosophical Papers*, 49(2), 253–278. https://doi.org/10.1080/05568641.2020.1779602

Višić, M. (2023). Marcuse's brand of critical theory and postcolonialism. *Interdisciplinary Description of Complex Systems*, 21(3), 230–246. https://doi.org/10.7906/indecs.21.3.2

Whelan, J. (2019, February 19). How does critical realism relate to critical theory? *Social Theory Applied*. https://socialtheoryapplied.com/2019/02/26/how-does-critical-realism-relate-to-critical-theory/

Wilmot, S. (2021). Postcolonial theory and Canada's health care professions: bridging the gap. *Medicine, Health Care, and Philosophy*, 24(3), 433. https://doi.org/10.1007/S11019-021-10019-2

Wolfe, P. (2006). Settler colonialism and the elimination of the native. *Journal of Genocide Research*, 8(4), 387–409. https://doi.org/10.1080/14623520601056240
Young, R. J. C. (2021). *Postcolonialism: A very short introduction* (2nd edition). Oxford University Press.
Zhang, T. (2023). Critical realism: A critical evaluation. *Social Epistemology*, 37(1), 15–29. https://doi.org/10.1080/02691728.2022.2080127

4 Colonial Matrix of Power in Global Health

Introduction

Coloniality is considered the hidden darker side of modernity (Quijano, 2007), including the current practice of global health. Global health partnerships and practice are undergirded by the relics of colonialism and historical dynamics that exclude specific populations from power, engineering an inequitable and unjust global health tableau. This assertion suggests that coloniality is at the heart of the injustices and inequities experienced in global health, such as higher disease burden and fewer resources to address the health challenges in the Global South. Epistemologically, we can also infer that coloniality operationalizes through the colonial matrix of power—pervasive ideologies or mentalities. In this chapter, I will explore the nature of the power structures that constitute the colonial matrix of power, their causal nature, and how they underpin the events or effects of coloniality on global health. Furthermore, using Sayer's conceptualization of causality based on the critical realist philosophy of science (introduced in Chapter 3), I will examine how these power structures continue to inform global health practice today. The advantage of this approach is that I will explore the conditions under which these power structures operate and their role in transforming social structures in global health practice. Therefore, in addition to viewing these power structures as the relationship between the dominant and the dominated, I will explore them more structurally.

I found Hedström and Swedberg's (1996) classification of the effects of social mechanisms at three levels to help unpack how the identified causal mechanism of coloniality works (Figure 4.1). Their conceptualizations of the effects of social mechanisms start at the macro level (society or organization), and their effects are felt by the individual at the micro level (psychological and psychosocial engagements). They explain further that based on the effects felt at the individual level, collective individual action mechanisms linked to desires and beliefs with action opportunities at the micro level are formulated (macro-to-micro transition). These collective desires and beliefs constitute the transformational mechanisms linking individual actions into wider intended or unintended effects at the macro level—micro-to-macro transition (Hedström & Swedberg, 1996). This conceptualization aligns with Archer's

DOI: 10.4324/9781032700786-4

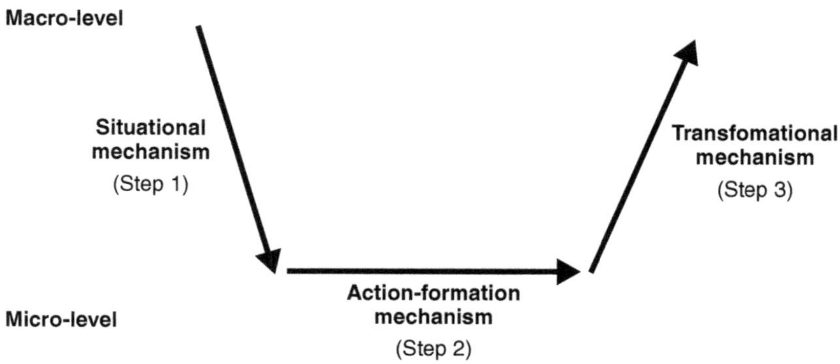

Figure 4.1 Classification of operational levels of social mechanisms.

agency-structure interaction where individual choices and actions (agency) are understood as both influenced by and capable of transforming broader social systems, norms, and constraints (structure).

The proposed conceptualization model of social mechanisms enables social scientists to explain how macro-level events affect the individual, how the individual assimilates the impact of the macro-level events, and how a group of individuals generate macro-level outcomes through their actions and interactions. Therefore, discussing the different mindsets and mentalities that informed and emanated from colonialism, I considered Hedström and Swedberg's (1996) conceptualization of generative causal mechanisms.

Generative Mechanisms of Coloniality (Colonial Matrix of Power)

My identification and discussion of the colonial matrix of power as generative mechanisms of coloniality follow Bhaskar's notion of multiple determinations. By multiple determinations, Bhaskar suggests that some observations have "dual control," "multiple control," or "multiple determination." He argues that different causal mechanisms and their interactions account for different aspects of the events and that no single law or entity "determines" the whole. Patomäki and Morgan (2023) unpacked this as the plurality of causes in any given context, which is a key part of the idea of causal complexity. The ideas of plurality of causes or multiple determination recognize that "the [actual] ordinary phenomena of the world" are inherently multi-layered, that we need to bring to bear different (real) single-layered causal mechanisms to explain different aspects of them (Elder-Vass, 2006).

Colonization and its enduring consequences stem from a mentality (or ideologies) that enabled the colonizers to rationalize their actions (Binagwaho et al., 2022). Mentality and ideologies inform how people think, perceive the world, and act. Owing to their abilities to dictate the way people perceive reality and consequently act as informed by their perception, ideologies constitute the driving force of an event, in this case, colonialism. These mentalities or ideologies constitute the matrix of power that not only perpetuated colonialism but also emerged due to colonialism. Their ability to continue to define the culture, labor, intersubjectivity relations, and knowledge production of formerly colonized countries well beyond the limits of formal colonialism gives them causal tendencies. Because of their causal tendencies, they are considered generative mechanisms, trans-empirical but real existing entities explaining why observable events occur (Blom & Morén, 2011). For example, racism is identified as one of the drivers of colonialism, and although political colonialism has ended, racism continues to influence the distribution of health care services, thus the observed health inequities among different racial groups.

In this chapter, I will focus on five main ideologies (colonialism-led power patterns) commonly cited in the literature as drivers of colonialism, which have maintained the colonized state of global health through coloniality. These ideologies include racism, white supremacy, hegemony, religious paternalism, and white saviorism. For instance, Ndlovu (2017) described coloniality as "a racist global power structure," implying that coloniality adopted the racist traits that were embedded in the practice of colonialism. Taiwo (1993) also argued that with colonization came the exclusion of individuals from the Global South from knowledge-generating bodies and the erasure and abandonment of knowledge and expertise produced in the Global South. The undermining of knowledge from the Global South and erasure gave prominence, credence, and importance to the knowledge generated by the formal colonizers and scholars from the Global North. It has been argued that this epistemic injustice is related to white supremacy and hegemony over knowledge (Binagwaho et al., 2022). Tarusarira (2020) has also demonstrated how various contemporary public/global health-related policy issues, such as gender equality, sexuality, and reproductive rights, are tied to religious influences emanating from the legacies of colonialism. Tarusarira (2020) also reported on the prevailing perception in contemporary global political relations that modern (Euro-American) civilization sees itself as the most advanced and superior civilization. This belief in superiority makes the Global North feel obligated to "develop" (civilize, uplift, educate) the less developed civilizations predominantly in the Global South. The ideology in which a white person, mostly from the Global North, acts from a position of superiority to save or assist a community or individual who is black, indigenous, or a person of color (BIPOC) is also pervasive in contemporary global health practice with colonial roots (Banerjee et al., 2023). I will explain how these ideologies and mentalities (racism, hegemony, religious paternalism, white supremacy, and white saviorism) constituted colonialism-led power patterns and social mechanisms driving the colonized state of global health.

Racism (Racial Ideology)

Racism and white supremacy are two interrelated power-related colonial constructs when it comes to colonization. The ideology of race emanates from

European colonialism (Cox, 1948). Consequently, many people believe that racism was the cause of the conquest of Native Americans and the enslavement of Africans. They think that racial phenomena are regarded as the "normal" outcome of the racial structure of a society (Bonilla-Silva, 1997, p. 475). However, scholars like Cox (1948) and Fredrickson (2002) argue the contrary: that it was conquest and slavery that gave rise to racism. They argue that following the backlash from the colonization of other nations, usually characterized by hostilities and violence, there was a strong need—psychological, sociological, economic, and political—for people with disproportionate power and resources to justify their positions and actions. Consequently, "racism" was used to describe the hostile or negative feelings of one ethnic group or "people" toward another and the actions resulting from such attitudes. Following this line of thinking, it was suggested that "the myth of race is, at its heart, about power relations … a rationale for brutality" (Jones, 2013; p. 309). Since capitalism arose first in Western Europe, black–white racialization became the dominant form of racism (Bagchi, 2021).

Despite the debate on whether racism emanated from colonialism or informed colonialism, what is clear is that there is an established relationship between them. What is also well documented is that there were interconnected social, political, economic, and ideological systems that created, maintained, and exacerbated stratification in access to opportunities and resources based on a group's or individual's location in a socially constructed racial hierarchy (Bonilla-Silva, 1997; Michener & LeBron, 2022). Consequently, Bonilla-Silva (1997, p. 469) proposed that the concept of racism can be best understood as a racialized social system referring "to societies in which economic, political, social, and ideological levels are partially structured by the placement of actors in racial categories or races." I argue that the racialized social system construct describes the nature of global health nowadays.

Racism refers to prejudiced attitudes, biases, and intolerance between racial groups. Racial discrimination involves policies and systems that create unequal opportunities and outcomes based on ethnicity or race. The concept of "race" became a powerful tool to support the social, political, and economic structures of colonialism. The extant literature suggests that two forms of racism were instrumental in perpetuating colonialism: systemic and structural racism. Braveman et al. (2022) explained that "systemic and structural racism are forms of racism that are pervasively and deeply embedded in and throughout systems, laws, written or unwritten policies, entrenched practices, and established beliefs and attitudes that produce, condone, and perpetuate widespread unfair treatment of people of color" (p. 171). Structural racism focuses on the role of the structures (laws, policies, institutional practices, and entrenched norms) in perpetuating the unfair discrimination and unfair treatment of people of color. Systemic racism, which is informed by Bonilla-Silva's (1997) racialized social system, emphasizes the involvement of whole systems, like political, legal, economic, health care, school, and criminal justice systems—including the oppressive structures that uphold the systems. Consequently, they are sometimes described as systemic racism, one of the social determinants of health that Farmer calls "structural violence" (Farmer, 2009).

The health impacts of racism can take many forms and can result from racialized acts of violence between people or institutional and structural racism (Devakumar et al., 2024). This conceptualization of "race" and "racism" speaks to its causal tendency and thus its consideration as a causal mechanism operating at the level of the "real" to orchestrate behaviors such as discrimination. The term "social construct" has been used to describe racism and applied in varying contexts and forms. Other terms, such as "power" and "control," have been used to qualify what racism is all about. These terms have been used to indicate the nature of racism (social construct) and its causal tendency (power and control). Therefore, racism, as applies to colonialism, is an invisible force with causal tendencies and is associated with social structures (laws, policies, institutional practices, and entrenched norms). Social racism, for example, emphasizes the role of the structures in scaffolding racism (Braveman et al., 2022). Using the iceberg analogy, Gee et al. (2009) represented systemic and structural racism as the unseen aspect of the iceberg, which is synonymous with the illustration of structures and mechanisms in Bhaskar's classification of reality (see Figure 3.2). Braveman et al. (2022), reflecting on the iceberg conceptualization, explained that systemic and structural racism represents "societal systems and structures that expose people of color to health-harming conditions and that impose and sustain barriers to opportunities that promote good health and well-being" (p. 172). This analogy certainly aligns with the critical realist understanding of the representation of structures and mechanisms and their role in orchestrating events and observable outcomes. To concretize this conceptualization of racism, Emerson and Smith (2000) referred to the unequal distribution of resources in the US (outcomes) as the "racialization" of the society (mechanism), suggesting that racism plays a role in discrimination.

Not only was colonization driven by racism, but the colonial transfer of wealth and racial oppression created a legacy of social, economic, cultural, and political exclusion, the effects of which are being felt after several generations and on the practice of global health. As with many other social constructs, the notion of racism has also evolved. In contemporary times, racism is operationalized as "a system of structuring opportunity and assigning value based on the social interpretation of how one looks" (Jones, 2018, p. 231). Sabado-Liwag et al. (2022) argued that racism is an ever-evolving system of power and a driving force of health inequities. Indeed, the disproportionate burden of morbidity and mortality among racial minorities has been linked to racism (Gee & Ford, 2011; Williams et al., 2019).

While racism targets a group of people, it affects the personal lives of the individuals towards which it is directed, influencing their racial self-image, self-worth, thoughts, emotions, and behaviors. The process of influencing how individuals think of and perceive themselves based on consistent exposure to racial biases is described as internalized racism. Internalized racism is the acceptance, belief, and conviction that one is inferior based on the racial hierarchy (Adhikari et al., 2025). This self-discrimination arises from the belief that one deserves the prejudice projected by other racial groups. It involves internalizing and underestimating oneself and others who share similar physical characteristics. Individual behavior and actions are influenced by personal choices and preferences and their position within a social structure. The development of internalized racism can be explained by Pierre Bourdieu's concept of habitus (Bourdieu, 1984). Habitus develops during socialization through interactions with social circumstances and relations (Bourdieu, 1984). Consistent exposure to racial treatments and encounters generates choices and practices with subjective meaning within specific contexts.

Self-discrimination may stem from an inferiority complex caused by systemic and structural racism. This long-term impact can result in individuals desiring to imitate the perceived superior race, such as whites or their culture. In doing so, they may unintentionally or intentionally harm their self-esteem and the esteem of others in their community. Akbar's (1996) concept of psychological slavery can be adopted to explain the nature and effects of internalized racism. He argues that internalized or psychological slavery, which captures the mind and restricts motivation, perception, aspiration, and identity with negative self-images, is even more cruel than physical shackles. Akbar contends that psychological slavery invades the soul and destroys loyalty to oneself, establishing allegiance to destructive forces.

Following Akbar's (1996) reasoning, internalized racism can also be considered a consequence of both overt and covert racism that can create feelings of inferiority and self-hatred over time and destroy a person's loyalty to themselves. Similarly, Cort et al. (2009) found that internalizing negative stereotypes like internalized racism constitutes stressors that require strong coping skills. Therefore, victims of racism face stressors that not only shape their way of life but also their perspective on life. Internalized racism can, therefore, harm a person's self-esteem and have a spillover effect (Feagin & Sikes, 1994). While it can lead to a range of perceived inferiority, self-harm, discrimination, and harassment towards individuals of the same race, it can also influence the way one interacts with others. Of relevance to global health practice, perceived inferiority diminished self-esteem and self-efficacy, and perceived incompetence can reduce one's confidence as a knower, thus prioritizing the knowledge of the Global North (epistemic injustice). These psychological processes imply that they interfere with an individual's ability to contribute to goal formulation and agenda-setting, leading to social injustice and health inequities in global health.

Internalized racism also leads to perceived inferiority, self-hate, discrimination, and harassment towards individuals of the same race. A glaring example of how internalized racism leads to negative actions towards individuals of the same race plays out in South Africa in the form of Afrophobia. "Afrophobia" is used to describe the negative attitudes of black South Africans towards

African immigrants (Dube, 2018). Some authors have highlighted how Afrophobia is rooted in the legacy of apartheid and racism (Addae & Quan-Baffour, 2022; Ndlovu, 2017). Ndlovu (2017) argued that Afrophobia instigates black-on-black violence in South Africa, which is a product of colonialism (apartheid). He argued further that coloniality resulting from the experiences of apartheid in South Africa orchestrates incidents of "non-revolutionary violence" among the oppressed black subject.

The practice of racism was institutionalized in May 1948 in South Africa, but its origins date back to the seventeenth century. A deep hatred and violence towards black and colored South Africans characterized apartheid in South Africa. This prolonged practice resulted in internalized racism and self-hate. Many scholars refer to xenophobia in South Africa as a form of black-on-black violence or Afrophobia. Consequently, black African immigrants in contemporary South Africa are often labeled as "illegal," "job stealers," "criminals," and "diseased." In contrast, immigrants of other racial backgrounds are seen as job providers and tourists. This negative labeling has justified violence against black African immigrants in the post-apartheid era, illustrating how the acceptance and internalization of dominant white culture can manifest in harmful actions and beliefs towards black people. These actions have been described as a new form of racism in South Africa. It is important to note that xenophobia, like apartheid, is not always expressed through violence but also discrimination in service delivery. While violence against black African immigrants has been observed, discrimination in access to healthcare services and social services, such as food parcels, has been particularly evident during the COVID-19 pandemic. Mukumbang et al. (2020) have systematically examined the discrimination experienced by black African immigrants during the pandemic, including limited access to healthcare and social services, exacerbating the existing issues of hunger among the general population. These findings highlight the implications of internalized racism on public and global health. The relationship between overt racism, internalized racism, and engagement in global health is captured in Figure 4.2.

My conceptualization of internalized racism in Figure 4.2 leads me to consider internalized (racism) as a generative mechanism of the colonized nature of global health as it is practiced. Of course, my conceptualization does not suggest that there is a direct relationship between overt racism and colonized global health. There are other critical psychological processes through which overt racism operates to exert its effects on global health. I have identified these psychological processes (perceived inferiority and diminished self-esteem and self-efficacy) as micro-mechanisms that have a cumulative effect as a macro-mechanism for colonized global health. Therefore, oppressive structures that continue to sustain structural racism also continue to trigger internalized racism and, consequently, the participation of individuals with perceived racism in global health activities.

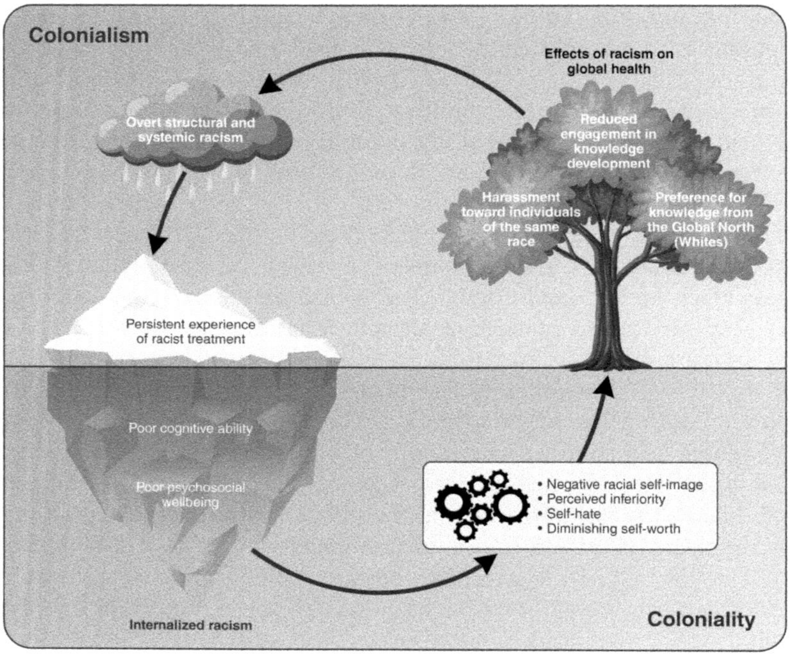

Figure 4.2 An ecosystem representation of (internalized) racism as a generative mechanism.

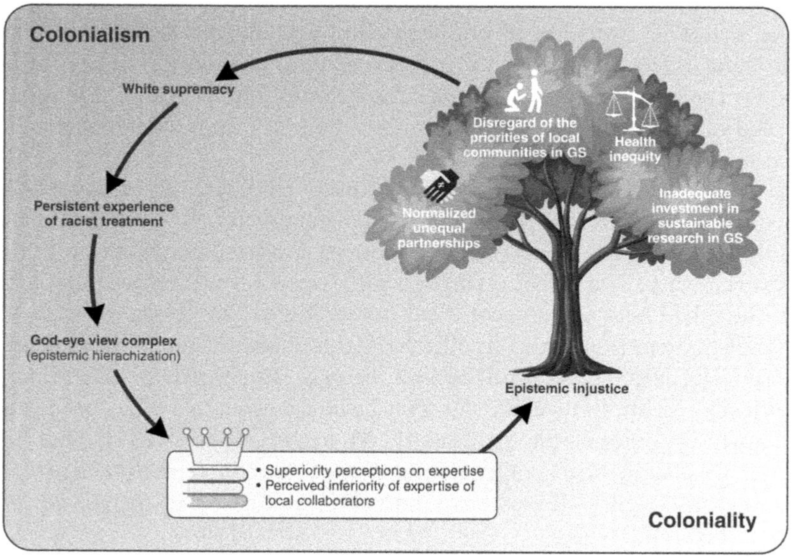

Figure 4.3 The causative potential of white supremacy to inequitable global health.

White Supremacy

Racism is the mindset and practice of downgrading people of color to "inferior" status and opportunities. This mindset and practice are based on unfounded beliefs about innate "inferiority" (Braveman et al., 2022). The use of the word *inferior* in defining the notion of racism is intentional. It emphasizes that the allocation of the inferior status and perpetuation of inferior treatment is along race lines. This argument is suggestive that white people see themselves as superior to people of color. Consequently, white supremacy can be described as a mindset and a way of thinking. Functionally, white supremacy describes a political, economic, and cultural system in which white people overwhelmingly control power and material resources as well as conscious and unconscious ideas of entitlement and development. Following the functional definition, a strong connection is made between white supremacy and systemic racism. They are connected in that they elevate whiteness as dominant and racial "otherness" as submissive and enforce each other. Their "supremacy" is used to justify the subjugation of "inferior beings and territories," and this becomes a driving force of colonialism.

European countries with predominantly white populations used their perceived superiority as a justification for the colonization of the Global South, where most non-white individuals reside (Binagwaho et al., 2022). This assertion suggests that white supremacy was at the heart of colonialism and consequently sustained the agenda of the colonizers in the Global South. For example, framing indigenous and other knowledge systems as uncivilized and illegitimate was and continues to be a part of a racialized agenda to distinguish colonizers and colonial ways as inherently superior (Bwire et al., 2022). Consequently, white people are considered the civilized teacher (the "definer"), and the colonized, mostly from the Global South, as the black/brown primitive student (the "defined") in global health (Daffé et al., 2021, p. 558).

White supremacy endorses the idea that the Global North continues to produce knowledge from the Western man's "point zero" God-eye view (Grosfoguel, 2007, p. 214). With the God-eye complex, Global North researchers consider their knowledge the only one capable of achieving a universal consciousness. Consequently, non-Western knowledge has often been disregarded as particularistic and incapable of attaining universality (Grosfoguel, 2007). This understanding translates to excluding local and marginalized groups in research and other knowledge practices (Koum Besson, 2022; Shiffman, 2014) and claiming the right of unlimited access to data from other countries, especially in the Global South (Galtung, 1967). Such a perspective or ideology lends itself to an epistemic hierarchy that privileges Western knowledge and cosmology over non-Western knowledge and cosmologies and is institutionalized in the global university system (Grosfoguel, 2007). Such epistemic hierarchization, which was born in the colonial era, continues to perpetuate what is known as helicopter, parachute, or parasitic research—researchers from Global North conducting research in the Global South without involving local researchers

(McIntosh et al., 2023). The practice of helicopter research enforces historical power imbalances, disregards the priorities of communities in the Global South in favor of the interests of the Global North researchers or funders, and leads to inadequate investment in sustainable research infrastructure in the Global South (McIntosh et al., 2023; Lancet Global Health, 2018).

Hegemony

White supremacist mindset and racist ideologies engendered power asymmetries between the colonized and the colonizers, which led to an established dominance and subordination relationship—the elementary aspects of master-servant relationships. The power asymmetry that white supremacist and racist mindsets ushered during colonialism required a persuasion and collaboration exchange relationship. Persuasion flows from the master to the servant, and collaboration flows from the servant to the master. While dominance relates to the complex of persuasion and coercion, subordination includes elements of collaboration and resistance (Chaudhury, 1994). Nevertheless, driven by capitalist and imperialist agendas, the colonial rule required the formation of colonial hegemony—a form of control exercised by a dominant class—after the end of political colonialism.

Gramsci's *Prison Notebooks* provides insights into the concepts of hegemony. In his writings, he attempts to map the political strategies employed by elites to influence social groups through their ideological projects (Dahlan, 2014). Gramsci coined the term "apparatus" to analyze the practices of institutions and collective agencies throughout history. Since then, Gramsci's theory of hegemony has been widely used to examine the dynamic interaction between class relations, the state's form and role, changing ideological beliefs and norms, and the hegemonic apparatuses present in civil society. Explanations of hegemonic influence in (mainly North American) literature focus on how a hegemon can garner consent and support from other states—coercion, incentives, and references to shared norms or "soft power" (Kentikelenis et al., 2023, p. 352). In its simplest form, hegemony relates to leadership exercised by a dominant group over subordinate groups. In its more complex form, hegemony deals with issues such as the elaboration of political projects, the articulation of interests, the construction of social alliances, the development of historical blocs, the deployment of state strategies, and the initiation of passive revolutions (Joseph, 2001).

In his book *Hegemony: A Realist Analysis*, Joseph (2002) presented a critical realist account of hegemony and its relation to societal processes. He explained that political forces use hegemony to conserve (ascertain the unity and cohesion of the social system) to promote their interest (Joseph, 2001, 2002). In Gramsci's theory of hegemony, he explored how the apparatus of a political society can strongly lead various strata of society to accept the status quo through legal institutions (Dahlan, 2014). After the end of political colonialism, the colonial hegemonic project was sustained through the signing of treaties and agreements between the colonizers and the formal colonies to ground coloniality. In this sense, Joseph (2002) argues that hegemony is fundamental to establishing human societies, including modern society. Consequently, we see hegemony being used as an apparatus to maintain the status quo of global health practice.

For any form of collaboration to occur, in the need to maintain some level of control after the end of political colonization, there was a need for a forum of engagement. Such engagement was made possible by continuing the hegemonic project, which had been established during colonization. While hegemonic influence was direct during the height of political colonization, the transition to postcolonial relations required that the former colonizers exerted influence over the former colonies using more clandestine approaches. In other words, there needed to be a change in the hegemonic power dynamics that existed during the political colonization era. Therefore, Western nations had to create a cultural space within which the complex of persuasion and collaboration could occur. Chaudhury (1994) termed this new form of control as synthetic hegemony. He described synthetic hegemony as transmitting modified persuasive principles from the master to the servant, who receives these principles in the form of modified collaborative principles (Chaudhury, 1994).

It is argued that hegemony's (post)colonial or neocolonial nature is that the developed capitalistic states persuade, and the underdeveloped countries collaborate. Modern hegemony is the "master persuades; the servant is persuaded and therefore collaborates" (Chaudhury, 1994, p. 47). Hegemony is, therefore, embedded in neo-patrimonial structures of power (Rubongoya, 2019). For instance, the adoption and use of language reinforce the hegemony of the Global North over the Global South by defining nations by economic status set to Euro-American indices of prosperity and development as an expression of the neo-patrimonial structures of power.

Kentikelenis et al. (2023) argue that global health norms are established in the "shadow of hegemony." These global health norms are established through global health expertise, whereby experts and professionals provide the knowledge on which global health initiatives are based. Kentikelenis et al. (2023) contend that global health expertise lies in the shadow of global-level hegemonic dynamics. Global North weaponizes it to replicate its dominance by favoring global governance initiatives compatible with its public and private interests. A conspicuous representation of this idea of global health is the setting of global health agendas and goals. However, the Global South is expected to collaborate with the Global North to achieve these goals. Hegemonies, therefore, diminish consent in favor of effectiveness, opt for consensus at the expense of participation and competition, and subordinate representation to governability (Rubongoya, 2019).

Synthetic hegemony in global health occurs in situations such as having a larger participation of Global North experts but limited participation of Global South experts and community representatives in the governance structures and advisory bodies of organizations focusing on addressing health concerns in the Global South. For instance, the Global Health 50/50 report showed that almost all global organizations (87% of nonprofit and 98% of for-profit) are headquartered in high-income countries, with most of their board seats (65% of nonprofit and 89% of for-profit) held by people from high-income countries (Global Health 50/50, 2024). This report indicates that the "Tyranny of experts" often subjugates local knowledge and leadership (Easterly, 2015). Funding, predominantly obtained from (financial) institutions from the Global North, is a form of power (synthetic hegemony) used to dictate agendas and priorities of global health. A study to explore the dynamics of power and its sources and how it shapes policymaking and implementation within the Nigerian health systems offered clear examples of how global health funding-supported policies sustain or exacerbate existing inequities in local contexts (Lassa et al., 2022). They explained that hegemony is achieved through the monopolization of the processes of knowledge production and practice. Hegemony is, therefore, a reference to the nature and character of specific modes of power (Rubongoya, 2019), an invisible entity with causal tendencies having the potential to affect how global health is practiced. The Global North applies synthetic hegemony to maintain a colonized global health, fomenting colonized global health practice.

I have argued in Chapter 2 that one of the areas impacted by white supremacy in global health relates to what constitutes an "expert in global health," which is informed by the hierarchization of knowledge and, consequently, expertise. Kentikelenis et al. (2023) illustrated strong connections and interactions between epistemic injustice and hegemonic interests. They argued that these interactions produce four types of epistemic consensus between the Global North and the Global South in setting global agendas. They classified this epistemic consensus into supportive (compatible and strategic) and opposed (incoherent and conflictual), with issue areas moving across these types over time. The negative impact of hegemony on global health occurs through the pathway of the opposed (incoherent and conflictual) epistemic consensus (Figure 4.4).

According to Kentikelenis et al. (2023), hegemonic support entails prioritizing an issue and driving its agenda through policies, while opposition involves ignoring or downgrading the issue's importance. The first component of opposed epistemic consensus, incoherence, represents a situation where the hegemon does not provide support, and there is a low level of agreement among experts on an issue; it opens opportunities for other actors to contribute to shaping global norms. For example, a study conducted in South Africa showed that most community members in the Eastern Cape of South Africa consult traditional healers before or simultaneously visiting the hospital. Despite this evidence, traditional healers are still not acknowledged or integrated into the mainstream health system (Mutola et al., 2021). The authors concluded that the lack of integration of traditional healers into the main healthcare system suggests the continued hegemony of biomedicine as institutionalized by the apartheid system of governance in South Africa (Mutola et al., 2021). At the global

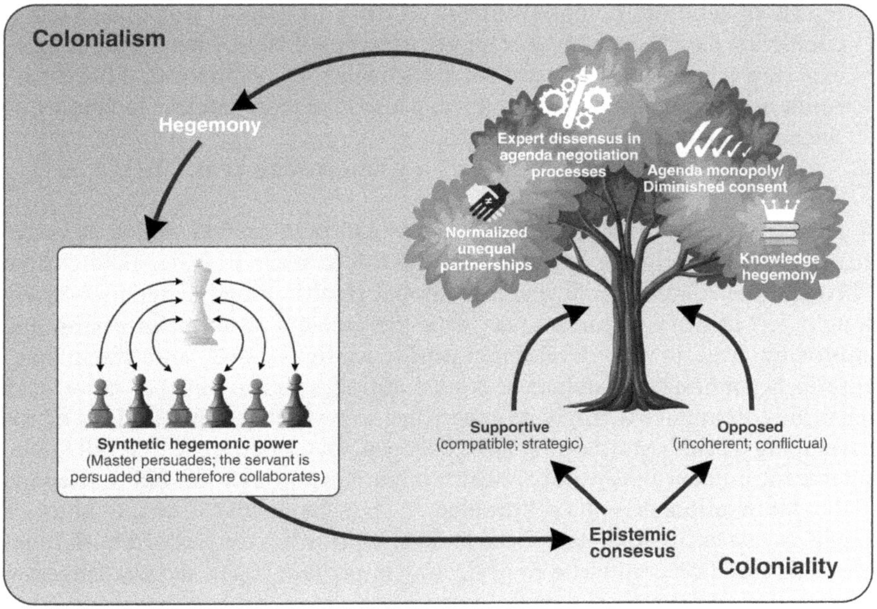

Figure 4.4 Hegemony as a generative causal mechanism for health inequity and injustice.

level, while the World Health Organization has long advocated the use of traditional medicine, particularly in developing countries, that endorsement is limited to scientifically supported traditional remedies (Sifuna & Sifuna, 2022). This position is scaffolded by arguments suggesting that the drugs we take to treat almost all health conditions have been manufactured by pharmaceutical companies, emanating from large-scale, sustained investment in research and development amounting to billions of dollars annually. The institutionalization of traditional medicines then presents a complex dilemma, as the lack of scientific evidence often undermines the credibility of many traditional medicinal practices. At the same time, pharmaceutical companies continue to whirl their power and commitment to scientific methods to develop medicine, which further undermines the consideration of traditional medicines for health care globally. This situation creates the conditions under which expert dissensus in agenda negotiation processes and agenda monopoly/diminished consent occurs.

Conflictual engagement constitutes the second component of opposed epistemic consensus. According to Kentikelenis et al. (2023):

> When manifest hegemonic interests and high epistemic consensus are at odds, we term this relationship conflictual. This means that norm-making is marked by battles between expertise drawing on scientific consensus and attempts by hegemonic powers to institutionalize a different set of

> norms or fend off potential threats to the normative status quo. Such conflicts typically develop over longer stretches of time, where competing expertise is mobilized to advance a particular set of interests. This can result in continued stalemate, but it can also lead to key states—including the hegemon—changing its policy.
>
> (Kentikelenis et al., 2023, p. 355)

A glaring example of hegemonic powers in action in agenda setting in global health can be seen in the operations of the Bill & Melinda Gates Foundation. Through their Grand Challenges for Global Health initiative, the foundation sought to "identify research areas with the greatest promise for saving and improving lives in the developing world; to fund novel, interdisciplinary approaches among researchers seeking solutions; and to get the 'rich-world' scientific community to apply its experience to pivotal health questions of the developing world" (Matthews & Ho, 2008, p. 410). Critics argue that Bill Gates' significant influence over global health initiatives through the Bill & Melinda Gates Foundation presents a "problem." They claim that it largely allows a single private entity to dictate the agenda and priorities for global health funding. This situation could lead to neglecting important issues and challenges, as the foundation prioritizes specific interventions based on its metrics and interests, often with limited accountability and transparency (Stirling, 2024). As a result, there are concerns about excessive influence on government policies and research agendas, which may overlook the needs of local communities and the complex social determinants of health. Conflictual relationships in the agenda-setting process for the benefit of global health thus constitute a generative mechanism for expert dissensus in agenda negotiation processes. The lack of consensus generated by hegemonic interests and epistemic consensus leads to disagreements on which direction to take for the greater good of the world's populations.

White Saviorism

To a greater extent, global health practice takes the form of (white) saviorism, an idea in which a (white) person, or (white) culture, "rescues" people of color from their situation. The term "white savior" can refer to any person or group, regardless of race, possessing an imbalance of power or privilege (Agarwal et al., 2020). In global health, these tropes include attitudes that researchers and health practitioners from the Global South have the right to do whatever they want because their intentions are good. Therefore, white saviorism is "not about justice." Rather, "it is about a big emotional experience that validates privilege" (Agarwal et al., 2020, p. e342).

In 2020, an estimated 85% of global health organizations had headquarters in Europe and North America (Global Health 50/50, 2024). The predominant existence of global health organizations in the Global North feeds the imbalance of power that maintains the colonial status quo. Consequently, working and training younger generations on global health occurs predominantly based on visions, agendas, and a culture of saviorism in institutions in the North. According to Banerjee et al. (2023), irrespective of where the individual is originally from, those who work in global health and are based in the Global North (me included) benefit from an imbalance of power perpetuated by this culture of saviorism that maintains inequity and consequently an entrenched divide in global health. Therefore, non-whites can also perpetuate white saviorism by their proximity to whiteness, power, or privilege because they rely on these structures to maintain inequality (Mirpuri, 2022). Similarly, not only do countries found in the Global North have colonial mindsets and systems that perpetuate power imbalances, but there are organizations in the Global South that also perpetuate power imbalances through these systems (Khan et al., 2021).

The practice of saviorism in global health exhibits (neo)colonial-(neo)colonized processes, enhancing the complexity of the power dynamics and the medical and cultural contexts that providers and researchers experience when entering these roles. The complex nature of these interactions makes saviorism very pervasive but also complicated and challenging to recognize, especially from the perspective of the global health practitioner. Indeed, the nature of the relationships between institutes of the Global North and those of the Global South in tackling global health issues also has a white saviorism undertone. The culture of white saviorism is so pervasive that after efforts to generate images that show black doctors providing health care services to poor white children in global health, instead, unwittingly created hundreds of visuals representing white saviorism and black suffering tropes (Alenichev et al., 2023). In essence, generative artificial intelligence proved incapable of avoiding the perpetuation of inequality and prejudice in global health.

The operations of these mechanisms and structures manifested at the level of the "actual" and captured empirically at the level of the empirical. The "actual" level captures activities and events such as agreements and cooperations being formed to allow the colonizers to continue exploiting their colonized nations' natural resources. For example, through the France-backed CFA franc created in December 1945, the French Treasury guaranteed the currency under a fixed currency rate dependent on the deposit of 50% of CFA franc into the French central bank. This arrangement allowed France to print money and control the economies of these nations, which prevented their economic development. What was observed at the level of "empirical" is that domestic production lapsed in these Francophone countries, and these countries increasingly relied on imported goods and services. CFA countries' public debt increased, and central banks exceeded statutory ceilings, leading to significant fiscal imbalances.

Moreover, participants from the Global South who travel to the Global North often become more deeply entrenched in a colonial mindset, as they are not encouraged to question the root causes of the inequalities they witness in the Global South. The white saviorism mindset, therefore, constitutes an important mechanism for the perpetuation of colonialism in global health.

Religious Paternalism

Apart from the use of race and the inferiority of people of color (white supremacy), it is widely acknowledged that religion (specifically Christianity) was used to justify the exploitation and conquest of many nations in the Global South. The spread of the Christian religion has been put forth as a justification for the colonization and exploitation of other parts of the world. For instance, it is said that European nations such as Great Britain, France, and the Netherlands sought to educate and reform African culture by disseminating Christian doctrine. Christianity represented Western civilization in the early eighteenth century and was the basis for Anglo-Saxon morality. During the late nineteenth century, Christianity was a major force in Africa's partition and eventual colonization (Boahen, 1990). Because Europeans were unfamiliar with Africa's diverse cultures and practices, and because of racism, their explorers considered these cultures and practices less than theirs and savage. Therefore, "Mid- and late-nineteenth-century Europeans were generally convinced that their Christian, scientific, and industrial society was intrinsically far superior to anything that Africa had produced" (Fage, 1995, p. 322).

Paternalism, in general, is the assertion of epistemic and moral authority over another, likened to a father's authority over their children. Ruth Slade (1960), author of *The Belgian Congo*, explained that the Congolese often used the phrase "You are my father and my mother" when addressing a European administrator when they were colonized. This phase captures their sense of dependence upon the colonizers who were changing the old patterns of tribal society. The Belgian government at that time "found it necessary to concentrate thousands of men around the mines, tearing them away from their traditional tribal backgrounds. It was good business to provide accommodation for their families, to give them food, clothing, medical care, and social amenities, the pastoral solicitude of a Catholic mission, and an educational system for their children" (Slade, 1960, p. 4). The actions of the Belgian government during the colonial times were described by Slade (1960) as paternalist. According to Hershey (1985), an action is paternalistic if "(1) the paternalistic action is primarily intended to benefit the recipient, and (2) the recipient's consent or dissent is not a relevant consideration for the initiator" (p. 171). Archard (1990) further refined Hershey's definition, suggesting that an action must fulfill three conditions to be paternalistic. Archard (1990) thus proposes that P behaves paternalistically towards Q if:

1. P aims to bring it about that concerning some state(s) of affairs which concern Q's good, Q's choice or opportunity to choose is denied or diminished.
2. P's belief that this behavior promotes Q's good is the main reason for P's behavior.
3. P discounts Q's belief that P's behavior does not promote something.

I applied the notion of paternalism to describe the religious contribution to colonialization and identified religious paternalism as a generative mechanism of colonialism. Following the conditions offered by Hershey (1985) and Archard (1990), I describe religious paternalism as interfering with the liberty of the colonized states, based on religious beliefs, for the good of the colonized, often to protect and promote their social and moral welfare. When European missionaries started their missions, especially the Christian missionaries, their mission was to spread Christianity, and the Church leaders believed colonization was necessary to save souls. To achieve these goals, they used "charity" or "philanthropy" to address some of the social needs of the local community. The political and capitalistically driven colonizers harnessed the knowledge of their "good works" or strategies to achieve their political and economic agendas. Consequently, reshaping the indigenous religious beliefs of the nations they colonized, originally the religious missionaries' goal, became a part of the Western imperialist agenda in the late nineteenth century. Therefore, European nations like Great Britain, France, and the Netherlands sought to educate and reform African culture by spreading Christian doctrine to promote morality among the indigenes, as their own cultures and traditions were considered salvage and uncouth; however, as Césaire (2000) explained:

> [T]he motives of the colonizers were neither evangelization, nor a philanthropic enterprise, nor a desire to push back the frontiers of ignorance and tyranny, nor a project undertaken for the greater glory of God, nor an attempt to extend the rule of law.
>
> (Césaire, 2000, p. 32)

According to Saunders (1920), the Bible was used to enforce the agendas of the West and a force of pacification that helped to enable colonization and the cultural assimilation of Africans. Religion was, therefore, sometimes used as a front to achieve the hidden agendas of the colonizers. For example, King Leopold II of Belgium wrote a letter to the missionaries in the now Democratic Republic of Congo in 1883 to ensure that the natives of Congo and their knowledge remained undermined and for the Indigenes to become less willing to empower themselves towards financial independence. The excerpt below indicates how King Leopold II weaponized religion to enforce paternalism among the Congolese people so they would not focus on their territory's riches:

> Your knowledge of the gospel will allow you to find texts ordering and encouraging your followers to love poverty, like "Happier are the poor because they will inherit the heaven" and "It is very difficult for the rich to enter the kingdom of God." You have to detach from them and make them disrespect everything, which gives courage to affront us. I reference their Mystic System and their war fetish—warfare protection—which they pretend not to want to abandon, and you must do everything in your power to make it disappear.
>
> (Leopold, 1883)

This excerpt from King Leopold II's letter to the missionaries to the Congo in 1883 illustrates religion's paternalist and imperial power and how the colonizers used it to dominate the local populations. Culled Biblical verses were advertently used to manipulate the locals into believing that it was the will of God that they remained poor and led modest lives. At the same time, the colonizers told the colonized that the secret of their success and development lies in the Bible (Saunders, 1920) while exploiting their raw materials to enrich the West. Religion was thus used to brainwash the natives of Congo into believing that what is most beneficial to them as Christians is to remain impoverished financially but made sure that they also encouraged them to be morally upright. The impoverished mindset constitutes a generative mechanism that enhanced the colonization of the Democratic Republic of Congo. This gospel of salvation, or focusing on salvation over the riches that the world had to offer, diminished the sense of prosperity of the Congolese people, thus reducing their ability to examine and consider their own beliefs and experiences.

Religious missionary work was strongly paternalistic, which continues to prevail today (Saunders, 1920; Williams, 2021). To achieve its imperialist agenda, religion in the Global South took on many faces, from the overflowing seminaries and Marian shrines of the Catholic church to Pentecostalist movements. The proliferation of different religious movements and denominations in the Global South subsequently made religion a central part of the lives of the people in the region during colonialism and in contemporary times. For example, in 1900, only 18% of Christians lived in the Global South, but by 2020, that number had increased to two-thirds (Zurlo et al., 2020). Religion has been aggressively instilled in the Global South, acculturating the indigenous traditions that had existed for centuries. With acculturation taking a foothold in the Global South scaffolded by other political and economic structures, religious establishments took on a paternalist approach to assert their imperialist agenda. Indoctrination in a religious tradition reduces the examination of a significant part of belief and experience, decreasing one's agency to seek solutions to their problems.

In addition to the agenda of using Western religion to change the world views of the colonized nations, some colonizers, such as Britain and France, relied on different sets of actors to organize their colonial empires after World War II, owing to the war's devastation on human resources. They relied on pre-existing local arrangements, such as religious missions, to establish schools and hospitals and to address various social concerns. For instance, England gave colonial administrations greater leeway and collaborated more intensely with other actors, especially religious organizations, described as colonial administrators (Becker, 2020). This approach gave the religious organizations the authority to insert their agendas into the local populations, thus giving them paternalistic control over the local population while serving to achieve the colonial agendas of control.

Regarding the coloniality of religion in contemporary global health practice, Walker (2022) showed that the religious features of colonial state architecture are still in operation in the Global South. He argued that many states in the Global South, particularly in Africa, have created their health services through the amalgamation of international humanitarian interventions provided by religious organizations (paternalism), government services, local communities, and the involvement of numerous other foreign powers. Beyond their creating and participating in service-providing structures, religious organizations are also involved in working on public/global health policy matters like gender equality, sexuality, and reproductive rights, which are connected to religious influences rooted in colonial legacies. Sometimes, religious beliefs conflict with public health initiatives, especially in areas such as reproductive health and gender equality, such as opposition to contraception, emanating from doctrinal stances on sexual morality (Ala et al., 2025). In this way, religion legitimizes some forms of thought, morality, and behavior while marginalizing others (de Vries & Sullivan, 2006) as a father would when raising their children. As a result, public and global health policies sometimes respond to perceptions and prescriptions of religion and not necessarily to reality as experienced by communities in these regions—religious paternalism (Tarusarira, 2020). For example, Lucero (2024) explained that in Mexico, discourses of salvation foreground some of today's most urgent reproductive injustices, including the spiritual, legal, and medical prioritization of the unborn over women. Sometimes, the poor and racially marginalized women preferred for their children to be born healthy than for them to survive the birth process. Consequently, religion influences individuals' perspectives on whether or how they access healthcare services. These motivations also include how physical health and self-discipline are viewed using the religious lens in the context of colonialism. Therefore, religious indoctrination potentially reduces scrutiny of a significant portion of belief and experience, decreases the likelihood of self-initiated remedies, and violates individuality requirements.

Religious paternalism, therefore, through its religious beliefs and dogmas, limits the autonomy or freedom of choice of those practicing the religion, often by making decisions for them under the justification that it is in their best interest. What makes paternalism wrong is that the paternalist disregards or fails to respect the rational will of the paternalized, which is done by substituting their own "superior" judgments about what ends should the paternalized pursue, or how should they pursue them (Cholbi, 2017). This means that religious paternalism undermines the agency—the capacity to make their own choices and exercise control over their actions—of the paternalized. Agency directly contradicts paternalism's idea by prioritizing personal agency; paternalism undermines agency by taking decision-making power away from paternalized. When paternalistic actions consistently override someone's choice, it can diminish their sense of self-efficacy and ability to make independent decisions (Cholbi, 2017). The diminished agency of the Global South through religious paternalism can lead to health inequities, epistemic injustice, and agenda monopoly through diminished agency (Figure 4.5).

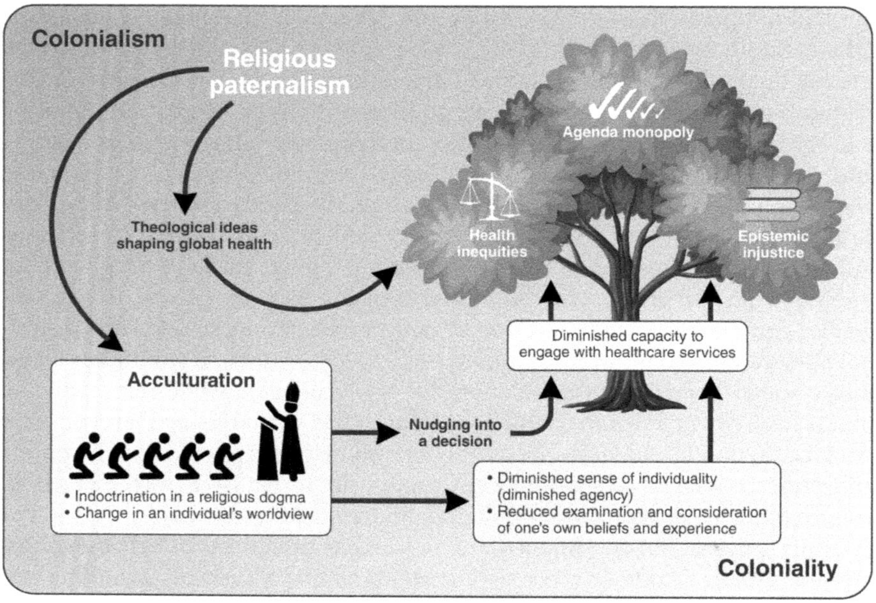

Figure 4.5 Religious paternalism.

An example of how religion has impacted individuals' agency to seek healthcare can be seen in its role in seeking treatment and care for HIV. A recent study showed that some Pentecostal pastors tend to persuade and nudge their Christians to rely more on faith and spiritual healing at the expense of adherence to antiretroviral treatment (Azia et al., 2025). They use religious arguments such as taking medication as a sign of unbelief in God or faithlessness. Owing to these religious persuasions, studies have reported that some people living with HIV preferred to rely on religious rituals (laying on of hands, prayers, and using anointing water from bottles) and prayers as well to be healed from HIV (Azia et al., 2023). The consequence of this is an increased risk of HIV transmission to others, accelerated disease progression, higher mortality rates, development of drug-resistant strains, and potential damage to the immune system, ultimately impacting the overall health and life expectancy of the individual living with HIV (Desta et al., 2020). Religious indoctrination and beliefs thus restrict the individuals' beliefs and limit their exposure to other potential remedies (reduced agency).

A Causal Understanding of Coloniality

We are following the explication of the causal tendencies of the mindsets, ideologies, and logic that form the basis of coloniality and orchestrate the colonial practice of global health. Colonialism is an economic, social, and political system that relies on the principles of cultural hierarchy and supremacy as justification for the multifaceted domination of a group of people. Mindsets and logics of racism, white supremacy, hegemony, (systemic) racism, and culture of saviorism, constituting the colonial matrix of power, were used as social mechanisms of control to sustain material structures for capitalism and imperialism—coloniality. Coloniality is, therefore, the application of mindsets and logic as tools for sustaining (advertently or inadvertently) colonialism in global health (Marsh et al., 2022). These mechanisms and structures of control establish asymmetric power dynamics related to the history and conception of global health and observed inequities that place institutions and practitioners in the Global North above those in the Global South (Daffé et al., 2021). This colonial matrix of power constitutes the oppressive structures and mechanisms scaffolding coloniality and operate at the level of "Real," which have produced the blend of modernism and traditional values in most nations in the Global South.

Thus far, I have focused on identifying and conceptualizing the generative social mechanisms in propagating global health inequities and injustices. To a lesser extent, I have engaged with a causal explanation of how these inequities and injustices are causally possible. To this end, I found Sayer's representation of causality (see Figure 3.2 in Chapter 3) based on critical realist principles to conceptualize the causal tendencies of racism, hegemony, white supremacy, white saviorism, and religious propaganda (Sayer, 2000).

This bundle of mechanisms operates within structures such as the political, economic, and sociocultural systems and the associated policies governing their operations. The interactions of these structures and mechanisms with causal tendencies and conditions such as capitalism and imperialism orchestrate a global health practice characterized by unequal Global North to Global South partnerships, Global North knowledge hegemony, agenda monopoly, Global South dependency syndrome, epistemic injustice, and health inequity (Figure 4.6).

A common trait between the five identified mindsets, ideologies, and logics (mechanisms) is that they each seek to create a power differential—situations in which one person is perceived or has more authority, agency, or knowledge than the other/s—between the former colonizers and the colonized. These five ideologies, hence described as social power, cause social groups to act differently based on one person or group who has more power exercising that power over another individual or group. Owing to the potential of these social powers to instigate a pattern of behavior, they are identified as mechanisms of colonialism, which form the basis of coloniality. Ndlovu-Gatsheni (2013) calls them "matrices of power." Ndlovu-Gatsheni (2013) explained that colonialism and, indeed, the current practice of global health "is a world that is overseen and controlled remotely by global coloniality through invisible colonial matrices of power" (p. 12). I operationalized the different forms of power that make up the colonial matrix of power as mechanisms operating in a complex and open system to remain faithful to the critical realist philosophy (Chapter 3).

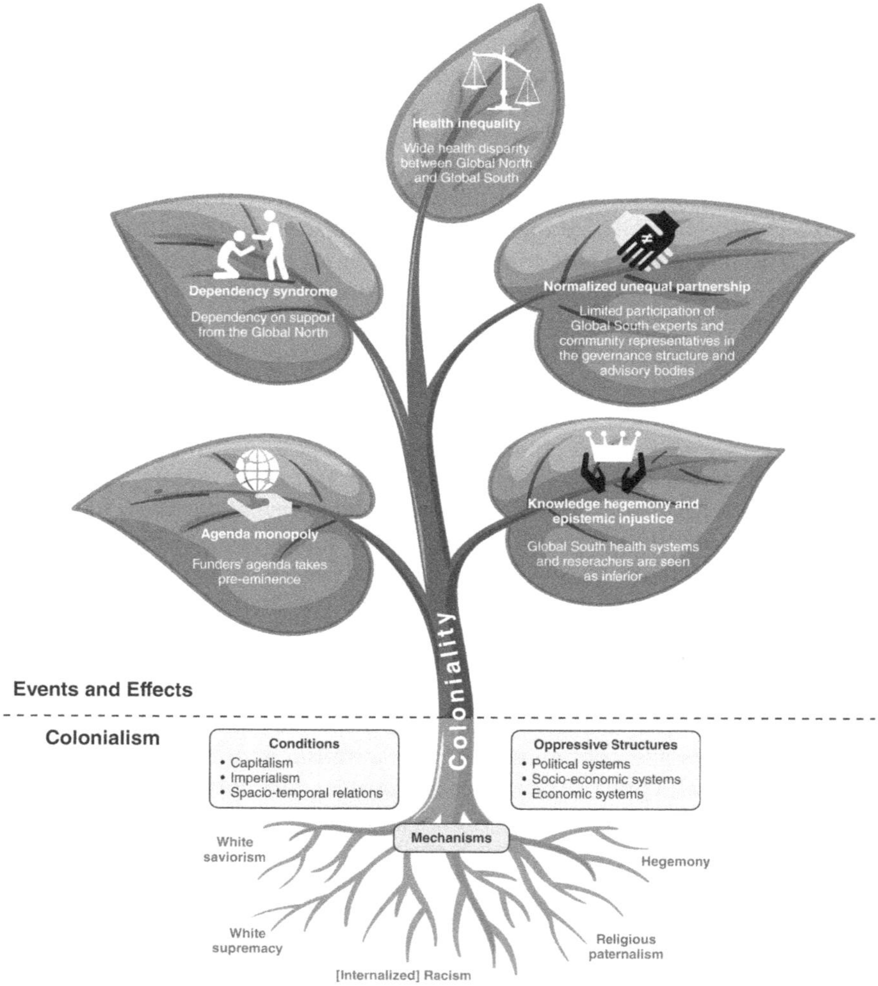

Figure 4.6 Critical realist-informed causality of colonial practice of global health.

I build the concept of the causal complex in global colonization based on John Mackie's idea of how causes can be investigated. Mackie (1965) coined the term INUS to express the idea of "insufficient but non-redundant part of an unnecessary but sufficient condition" (p. 245). For example, a short circuit is not a sufficient part of the condition "short circuit and flammable material" to cause a fire, but it is a necessary part. Fires can also be started by arson or lightning. Tracing the actions and effects of each generative mechanism can show how each of the identified generative mechanisms was necessary for colonizing global health. However, colonization does not depend solely on that mechanism to have happened but rather occurs as interdependent causal agents.

While each of these generative mechanisms might be necessary but not sufficient to orchestrate the colonization of global health, I am arguing that an amalgam or interdependence of these causal mechanisms was sufficient and necessary for the colonization of global health.

The amalgam and the causal interactions of different ideologies and mindsets were necessary and sufficient to perpetuate colonialization through coloniality and thus conceptualized as the colonial matrix of power. For instance, the ideology of being superior because of one's race, such as white supremacy, which could be expressed through hegemony, engenders the notion of white saviorism while at the same time enforcing racialization. Opara (2021) argues that coloniality operationalizes through narratives of "interdependent causative relationship" that drives the inequitable distribution of global wealth—wealth of Europe and North America and the under-development and poverty of their past and present colonies. Streamlining each generative mechanism of global health colonization also shows how their contribution was sufficient to contribute to colonization. To this end, my goal in this chapter is to unravel the nature of each of the generative causal mechanisms embedded in the notion of coloniality [involved in] orchestrating the unjust and inequitable nature of global health as seen today. My second goal is to show that these generative causal mechanisms, which underpin the construct of coloniality, form the colonial matrix of power driving the colonized nature of global health.

Using Sayer's conceptualization of causality, I argue that the colonial matrix of power is responsible for the coloniality processes leading to the observed colonial practices in global health. Sayer (2012) identified some instances in which power differential is causally linked to unfair treatment of other groups considered to be inferior. For example, he contends that we should not hesitate to argue that the methods used to handle asylum seekers, for example, can lead to humiliation. We should also acknowledge that systemic domination is likely to result in feelings of inferiority and shame among those who are dominated. He added that it is important to recognize that racism hinders minority ethnic groups from reaching their full potential.

My conceptualization of colonial practices in global health, informed by Sayer's causality framework, proposes a multidirectional, causal relationship between political, sociocultural, and economic structures and tangible global health events and experiences through the colonial matrix of power embedded in coloniality. Other important causal conditions relevant to perpetuating colonial practices in global health include capitalist and imperialistic ideologies and spatial-temporary relations such as colonizer and colonized relationships between the nations involved in the engagement. "[I]mperialism and colonialism brought complete disorder to colonized peoples, disconnecting them from their histories, their landscapes, their languages, their social relations and their ways of thinking, feeling and interacting with the world" (Smith, 2012, p. 782). The interactions between social structures with causal tendencies and social mechanisms enable us to recognize and reconcile their causal contributions and the emergentist nature of (neo)colonialism.

References

Addae, D., & Quan-Baffour, K. P. (2022). Afrophobia, "black on black" violence and the new racism in South Africa: the nexus between adult education and mutual co-existence. *Cogent Social Sciences*, 8(1). https://doi.org/10.1080/23311886.2022.2130458

Adhikari, B., Amaratunga, C., Mukumbang, F. C., & Mishra, S. R. (2025). Why should we be concerned by internalised racism in global health?. *BMJ Global Health*, 10(6), e016740. https://doi.org/10.1136/bmjgh-2024-016740

Agarwal, A., Crawford, N., Nguyen, V., & Walker, A. (2020). The white savior industrial complex in global health. BMJ Global Health: Blog. https://blogs.bmj.com/bmjgh/2020/03/11/the-white-savior-industrial-complex-in-global-health/

Akbar, N. (1996). *Breaking the chains of psychological slavery*. Mind Productions & Associates.

Ala, A., Touray, M. M. L., Shafi, S., Egan, B., Dar, O., Essa, F., Flores, N. L. C., Ocama, P., Parker, S., Maeurer, M., & Zumla, A. (2025). Harnessing faith-based organisations for global health equity. *The Lancet*, 405(10472), 10–13. https://doi.org/10.1016/S0140-6736(24)02614-X

Alenichev, A., Kingori, P., & Grietens, K. P. (2023). Reflections before the storm: the AI reproduction of biased imagery in global health visuals. *The Lancet Global Health*, 11(10), E1496–E1498. https://doi.org/10.1016/S2214-109X(23)00329-7

Archard, D. (1990). Paternalism defined. *Analysis*, 50(1), 36–42. www.jstor.org/stable/3328207

Azia, I. N., Nyembezi, A., Carelse, S., & Mukumbang, F. C. (2023). Understanding the role of religious beliefs in adherence to antiretroviral therapy among Pentecostal Christians living with HIV in sub-Saharan Africa: a scoping review. *BMC Public Health*, 23(1), 1–12. https://doi.org/10.1186/S12889-023-16616-5

Azia, I. N., Nyembezi, A., Carelse, S., & Mukumbang, F. C. (2025). Beliefs of Pentecostal pastors on the use of antiretroviral treatment among Pentecostal Christians living with HIV in a suburb of Cape Town-South Africa: a community health systems lens. *Health Policy and Planning*, 40(1), 13–22. https://doi.org/10.1093/HEAPOL/CZAE089

Bagchi, A. (2021). On capitalist colonialism and imperialism. *Social Scientist*, 49(9), 19–28.

Banerjee, A. T., Bandara, S., Senga, J., González-Domínguez, N., & Pai, M. (2023). Are we training our students to be white saviours in global health? *The Lancet*, 402(10401), 520–521. https://doi.org/10.1016/S0140-6736(23)01629-X

Becker, B. (2020). Colonial legacies in international aid: Policy priorities and actor constellations. In C. Schmitt (Ed.), *From colonialism to international aid: External actors and social protection in the Global South* (pp. 161–185). https://doi.org/10.1007/978-3-030-38200-1_7

Binagwaho, A., Ngarambe, B., & Mathewos, K. (2022). Eliminating the white supremacy mindset from global health education. *Annals of Global Health*, 88(1). https://doi.org/10.5334/AOGH.3578

Blom, B., & Morén, S. (2011). Analysis of generative mechanisms. *Journal of Critical Realism*, 10(1), 60–79. https://doi.org/10.1558/JCR.V10I1.60

Boahen, A. A. (1990). *Africa under colonial domination 1880–1935*. University of California Press.

Bonilla-Silva, E. (1997). Rethinking racism: Toward a structural interpretation. *American Sociological Review*, 62(3), 465–480.

Bourdieu, P. (1984). *Distinction: A social critique of the judgement of taste*. Routledge & Kegan Paul.

Braveman, P. A., Arkin, E., Proctor, D., Kauh, T., & Holm, N. (2022). Systemic and structural racism: Definitions, examples, health damages, and approaches to dismantling. *Health Affairs*, 41(2), 171–178. https://doi.org/10.1377/HLTHAFF.2021.01394

Bwire, G., Ario, A. R., Eyu, P., Ocom, F., Wamala, J. F., Kusi, K. A., Ndeketa, L., Jambo, K. C., Wanyenze, R. K., & Talisuna, A. O. (2022). The COVID-19 pandemic in the African continent. *BMC Medicine*, 20(1). https://doi.org/10.1186/S12916-022-02367-4
Césaire, A. (2000). *Discourse on colonialism* (J. Pinkham, Trans.). Monthly Review Press.
Chaudhury, A. (1994). On colonial hegemony: Toward a critique of brown orientalism. *Rethinking Marxism*, 7(4), 44–58. https://doi.org/10.1080/08935699408658122
Cholbi, M. (2017). Paternalism and our rational powers. *Mind*, 126(501). https://doi.org/10.1093/mind/fzv205
Cort, M. A., Tull, E. S., Gwebu, K., Dlamini, P., Pinkney, E., Gramby, E., Cuthbertson, S., Daniels, A., Luu, S., & Gwebu, E. T. (2009). Education and internalized racism in socio-political context: Zimbabwe and Swaziland. *The Social Science Journal*, 46(4), 644. https://doi.org/10.1016/J.SOSCIJ.2009.08.001
Cox, O. C. (1948). *Caste, class, and race: A study in social dynamics* (1st ed.). Monthly Review Press
Daffé, Z. N., Guillaume, Y., & Ivers, L. C. (2021). Anti-racism and anti-colonialism praxis in global health—reflection and action for practitioners in US academic medical centers. *American Journal of Tropical Medicine and Hygiene*, 105(3), 557–560. https://doi.org/10.4269/ajtmh.21-0187
Dahlan, A. (2014). The "American" hegemonic culture: Its roots, features and implications to world culture. *Rubikon*, 1(1), 19–30.
de Vries, H., & Sullivan, L. E. (2006). Political theologies: Public religions in a post-secular world. *Political Theologies*. https://doi.org/10.5422/FSO/9780823226443.001.0001
Desta, A. A., Woldearegay, T. W., Futwi, N., Gebrehiwot, G. T., Gebru, G. G., Berhe, A. A., & Godefay, H. (2020). HIV virological non-suppression and factors associated with non-suppression among adolescents and adults on antiretroviral therapy in northern Ethiopia: a retrospective study. *BMC Infectious Diseases*, 20(1), 4. https://doi.org/10.1186/S12879-019-4732-6
Devakumar, D., Gram, L., English, S., Deivanayagam, T. A., Huq, M., & Das, P. (2024). Racism and health inequity: a global syndemic for children. *The Lancet*, 0(0). https://doi.org/10.1016/S0140-6736(24)02358-4
Dube, G. (2018). Afrophobia in Mzansi? Evidence from the 2013 South African Social Attitudes Survey. *Journal of Southern African Studies*, 44(6), 1005–1021. https://doi.org/10.1080/03057070.2018.1533300
Easterly, W. (2015). *The tyranny of experts: Economists, dictators, and the forgotten rights of the poor*. Basic Books.
Elder-Vass, D. (2006). Re-examining Bhaskar's three ontological domains: The lessons from emergence. In C. Lawson, C. Latsis, & N. Martins (Eds.), *Contributions to Social Ontology* (pp. 160–176). Routledge.
Emerson, M. O., & Smith, C. (2000). *Divided by faith: Evangelical religion and the problem of race in America*. Oxford University Press.
Fage, J. D. (1995). *A history of Africa* (3rd edition). Routledge.
Farmer, P. (2009). On suffering and structural violence: A view from below. *Race/Ethnicity: Multidisciplinary Global Contexts*, 3(1), 11–28.
Feagin, J. R., & Sikes, M. P. (1994). *Living with racism: The black middle-class experience* (1st ed.). Beacon Press. https://psycnet.apa.org/record/1994-97653-000
Fredrickson, G. M. (2002). *Racism: A short history* (1st ed.). Princeton University Press.
Galtung, J. (1967). Scientific colonialism. *Transition*, 30, 10–15.
Gee, G. C., & Ford, C. L. (2011). Structural racism and health inequity: Old issues, new directions. Du Bois Review: *Social Science Research on Race*, 8(1), 115–132. https://doi.org/10.1017/S1742058X11000130
Gee, G. C., Ro, A., Shariff-Marco, S., & Chae, D. (2009). Racial discrimination and health among Asian Americans: evidence, assessment, and directions for future research. *Epidemiologic Reviews*, 31(1), 130–151. https://doi.org/10.1093/EPIREV/MXP009

Global Health 50/50. (2024). Gaining ground? Analysis of the gender-related policies and practices of 201 global organisations active in health. https://doi.org/10.56649/OVWL4422
Grosfoguel, R. (2007). The epistemic decolonial turn: Beyond political-economy paradigms. *Cultural Studies*, 21(2–3), 211–223. https://doi.org/10.1080/09502380601162514
Hedström, P., & Swedberg, R. (1996). Social mechanisms. *Acta Sociologica*, 39(3), 281–308. https://doi.org/10.1177/000169939603900302
Hershey, P. T. (1985). A definition for paternalism. *The Journal of Medicine and Philosophy: A Forum for Bioethics and Philosophy of Medicine*, 10(2), 171–182. https://doi.org/10.1093/jmp/10.2.171
Jones, C. P. (2018). Toward the science and practice of anti-racism: Launching a national campaign against racism. *Ethnicity & Disease*, 28(Suppl 1), 231.
Jones, J. (2013). *A dreadful deceit: the myth of race from the colonial era to Obama's America*. Basic Books.
Joseph, J. (2001). A realist theory of hegemony. *Journal for the Theory of Social Behaviour*, 30(2), 179–202.
Joseph, J. (2002). *Hegemony: A realist analysis*. Routledge.
Kentikelenis, A., Seabrooke, L., & Sending, O. J. (2023). Global health expertise in the shadow of hegemony. *Studies in Comparative International Development*, 58(3), 347–368. https://doi.org/10.1007/S12116-023-09405-z
Khan, M., Abimbola, S., Aloudat, T., Capobianco, E., Hawkes, S., & Rahman-Shepherd, A. (2021). Decolonising global health in 2021: a roadmap to move from rhetoric to reform. *BMJ Global Health*, 6(3), e005604. https://doi.org/10.1136/BMJGH-2021-005604
Koum Besson, E. S. (2022). How to identify epistemic injustice in global health research funding practices: a decolonial guide. *BMJ Global Health*, 7(4), 8950. https://doi.org/10.1136/BMJGH-2022-008950
Lancet Global Health. (2018). Closing the door on parachutes and parasites. *The Lancet Global Health*, 6(6), e593. https://doi.org/10.1016/S2214-109X(18)30239-0
Lassa, S., Saddiq, M., Owen, J., Burton, C., & Balen, J. (2022). Power dynamics among health professionals in Nigeria: A case study of the global fund policy process. *International Journal of Health Policy and Management*, 11(12), 2876. https://doi.org/10.34172/IJHPM.2022.6097
Leopold. (1883). Letter From King Leopold II to colonial missionaries heading to Africa, 1883. www.africanglobe.net/africa/letter-king-leopold-ii-colonial-missionaries-heading-africa-1883.
Lucero, B. A. (2024). Religious paternalism and racial prejudice in obstetric surgery in Mexico. *História, Ciências, Saúde-Manguinhos*, 31, e2024069. https://doi.org/10.1590/S0104-59702024000100069
Mackie, J. L. (1965). Causes and condition. *American Philosophical Quarterly*, 2(4), 245–264.
Marsh, T. E. J., Wright, J., Khalifa, M., & López, G. R. (2022). Coloniality, educational leadership, and white supremacy: The other global pandemic. *Educational Administration Quarterly*, 58(5), 679. https://doi.org/10.1177/0013161X221136728
Matthews, K. R. W., & Ho, V. (2008). The grand impact of the Gates Foundation. Sixty billion dollars and one famous person can affect the spending and research focus of public agencies. *EMBO Reports*, 9(5), 409. https://doi.org/10.1038/EMBOR.2008.52
McIntosh, K., Messin, L., Jin, P., & Mullan, Z. (2023). Countering helicopter research with equitable partnerships. *The Lancet Global Health*, 11(7), e1007–e1008. https://doi.org/10.1016/S2214-109X(23)00278-4
Michener, J., & LeBron, A. M. W. (2022). Racism, health, and politics: Advancing interdisciplinary knowledge. *Journal of Health Politics, Policy and Law*, 47(2), 111–130. https://doi.org/10.1215/03616878-9517149

Mirpuri, S. (2022). Racism, systemic racism, & white supremacy: What's the difference? https://www.nrpa.org/contentassets/f6a2fb863afc41e584e6b1f52cba3ba8/220602.racism_systemic_racism_and_white-supremacy.pdf

Mukumbang, F. C., Ambe, A. N., & Adebiyi, B. O. (2020). Unspoken inequality: how COVID-19 has exacerbated existing vulnerabilities of asylum-seekers, refugees, and undocumented migrants in South Africa. *International Journal for Equity in Health*, 19(1), 1–7. https://doi.org/10.1186/s12939-020-01259-4

Mutola, S., Pemunta, N. V., & Ngo, N. V. (2021). Utilization of traditional medicine and its integration into the healthcare system in Qokolweni, South Africa: Prospects for enhanced universal health coverage. *Complementary Therapies in Clinical Practice*, 43, 101386. https://doi.org/10.1016/J.CTCP.2021.101386

Ndlovu, M. (2017). Manufacturing black-on-black violence in Africa: A decolonial perspective on Mfecane and Afrophobia/xenophobia in South Africa. *International Journal of African Renaissance Studies*, 12(2), 97–109. https://doi.org/10.1080/18186874.2017.1401768

Ndlovu-Gatsheni, S. J. (2013). The entrapment of Africa within the global colonial matrices of power. *Journal of Developing Societies*, 29(4), 331–353. https://doi.org/10.1177/0169796X13503195

Opara, I. N. (2021). It's time to decolonize the decolonization movement—Speaking of medicine and Health. https://speakingofmedicine.plos.org/2021/07/29/its-time-to-decolonize-the-decolonization-movement/

Patomäki, H., & Morgan, J. (2023). World politics, critical realism and the future of humanity: An interview with Heikki Patomäki, part 1. *Journal of Critical Realism*, 22(3), 562–603. https://doi.org/10.1080/14767430.2023.2188527

Quijano, A. (2007). Coloniality and modernity/rationality. *Cultural Studies*, 21(2–3), 168–178. https://doi.org/10.1080/09502380601164353

Rubongoya, J. B. (2019). Hegemonic political regimes in Africa. *Oxford research encyclopedia of politics*. https://doi.org/10.1093/ACREFORE/9780190228637.013.1325

Sabado-Liwag, M. D., Manalo-Pedro, E., Taggueg, R., Bacong, A. M., Adia, A., Demanarig, D., Sumibcay, J. R., Valderama-Wallace, C., Oronce, C. I. A., Bonus, R., & Ponce, N. A. (2022). Addressing the interlocking impact of colonialism and racism on Filipinx/a/o American health inequities. *Health Affairs*, 41(2), 289–295. https://doi.org/10.1377/HLTHAFF.2021.01418

Saunders, K. (1920). The passing or paternalism in missions. *The Journal of Religion*, 2(5), 466–475.

Sayer, A. (2000). *Realism and social science*. Sage Publications. https://doi.org/10.4135/9781446218730

Sayer, A. (2012). Power, causality and normativity: a critical realist critique of Foucault. *Journal of Political Power*, 5(2), 179–194. https://doi.org/10.1080/2158379X.2012.698898

Shiffman, J. (2014). Knowledge, moral claims and the exercise of power in global health. *International Journal of Health Policy and Management*, 3(6), 297–299. https://doi.org/10.15171/IJHPM.2014.120

Sifuna, N., & Sifuna, N. (2022). African traditional medicine: Its potential, limitations and challenges. *Jouornal of Healthcare*, 5(1), 141. https://doi.org/10.36959/569/475

Slade, R. (1960). *The Belgian Congo: Some recent changes*. Oxford University Press. https://doi.org/10.2307/2610116

Smith, L. T. (2012). *Decolonizing methodologies: research and indigenous peoples* (2nd ed.). Palgrave Macmillan.

Stirling, A. (2024). The "Bill Gates problem": do billionaire philanthropists skew global health research? *Nature*, 626(7999), 477–479. https://doi.org/10.1038/D41586-024-00394-0

Taiwo, O. (1993). Colonialism and its aftermath: The crisis of knowledge production. *Callaloo*, 16(4), 891–908.
Tarusarira, J. (2020). Religion and coloniality in diplomacy. *The Review of Faith & International Affairs*, 18(3), 87–96. https://doi.org/10.1080/15570274.2020.1795442
Walker, B. B. (2022). *Religion in global health and development: The case of twentieth-century Ghana*. McGill-Queen's University Press.
Williams, A. L. (2021). Religion and paternalism: International relief and development organization mission statements. https://cdn.ymaws.com/www.istr.org/resource/resmgr/working_papers_virtual_2021/andrew_williams_-_religion_a.pdf.
Williams, D. R., Lawrence, J. A., & Davis, B. A. (2019). Racism and health: Evidence and needed research. *Annual Review of Public Health*, 40, 105–125. https://doi.org/10.1146/annurev-publhealth-040218-043750
Zurlo, G. A., Johnson, T. M., & Crossing, P. F. (2020). World Christianity and mission 2020: Ongoing shift to the Global South. *International Bulletin of Mission Research*, 44(1), 8–19. https://doi.org/10.1177/2396939319880074

5 Decoloniality

Countering Coloniality in Global Health

Introduction

I will start this chapter by recounting a story by Galtung (1967) in his paper "Scientific Colonialism," about a painting that used to hang in the ante-room of former President Kwame Nkrumah of Ghana. This is what he said about the painting:

> The painting was enormous, and the main figure was Nkrumah, fighting and wrestling with the last chains of colonialism. The chains are yielding, thunder and lightning are in the air, and the earth is shaking. Out of all this, three small figures are fleeing: white men and pallid. One of them is the capitalist. He carries a briefcase. Another is the priest or missionary, who carries the Bible. The third, a lesser figure, carries a book entitled *African Political Systems*: he is the anthropologist or social scientist in general.
>
> (Galtung, 1967, p. 13)

My interpretation of this painting, as Galtung (1967) describes it, is that this was the ultimate dream or vision of President Kwame Nkrumah. This should remain the vision of today in the Global South if we strive to achieve equity and justice, not only in global health but in every aspect of life in the Global South. This painting represents a reversal of the colonization process illustrated in Figure 1.1 (see p. 5), which had key actors of imperialism and capitalism (politicians, economists, and religious figures). In addition, the anthropologist represents epistemic injustice or knowledge colonialism, as Galtung (1967) prefers to describe it. The painting in President Kwame Nkrumah's office would be a better representation of the decolonization process, especially as it pertains to global health as it accounts for addressing epistemic injustice, at least, as it considers ousting the foreign researcher who conceptualizes the Global South based on western epistemic foundations. Figure 5.1 seeks to illustrate the dream or the idea of decolonization—the antonym of colonization.

DOI: 10.4324/9781032700786-5

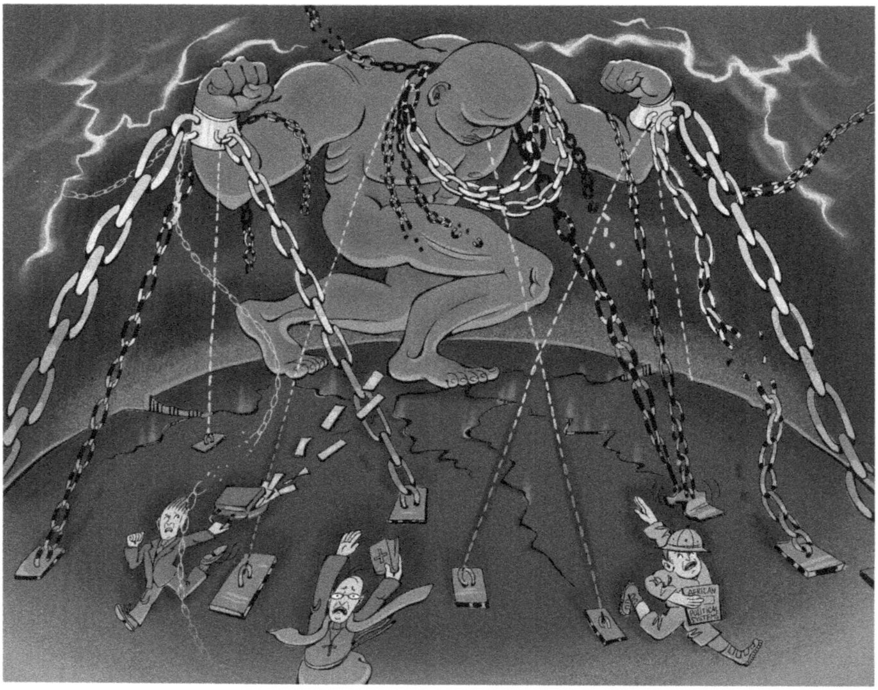

Figure 5.1 My pictorial representation of the image that was in President Kwame Nkrumah's office. After an elaborate search of the extant literature, I could not find the original picture that Galtung (1967, p. 13) described. Nevertheless, based on his description, I worked with an artist to come up with this visual representation. Of course, we do not think it is like the original painting in presentation, but we hope that it captured the same message the original painting wanted to portray.

The straightforward and obvious definition of decolonization is the process by which colonies become independent of their colonizers. In the context of political colonization, decolonization entailed a calculated military disengagement and diplomatic negotiation between the colonized and colonial countries (Betts, 2012). Nevertheless, the consideration that decolonization was a straightforward affair has been challenged by other authors suggesting decolonization was a process that began before the colonizers officially "left." Although it was described as a process, the understanding was that decolonization occurred with a "force of inevitability" (Betts, 2012). After World War II, some colonized nations started resisting the control that the colonizers had over them following the weakened state of the colonizers through their participation in World War II. The first record of colonizers leaving was the United States leaving the Philippines in 1944. Resistance to colonial rule grew successfully worldwide, including among the colonizers' populations. Despite the momentum to decolonize the colonized nations gaining traction over the years, sufficient vestiges of colonial domination remained until the General Assembly declared "the international decade for eradicating colonialism" in the 1990s.

Decolonization is predominantly driven by nationalist consciousness or anti-colonial sentiments and self-determination. Political decolonization is predominantly considered a national liberation project and is organized along with nationalism to challenge the colonial powers and dismantle their empires. For many new nation-states, political decolonization (independence) was achieved through nationalism. However, no such coordination occurred in the African Francophonie zone until recently when Sahel countries (Mali, Burkina Faso, and Niger) displayed a historic regional trend in 2022, requesting the French army to withdraw. The demands to withdraw are expected to trickle to other former French colonies as in recent weeks (at time of writing in March 2025), Senegal and Côte d'Ivoire have announced they want French forces to leave their countries too. This liberation plan seeks "to respect and grant autonomy not only to individuals, but also to, among others, indigenous, black, peasant, women's groups, and social movements" (Beghin, 2022, p. 179). Although the political decolonization process is linked to the current practice of global health today, there remain some fundamental differences between the historical contexts of political decolonization (Decolonization$_1$) in the 1950s and 1960s, and institutional processes in high-income countries to decolonize global health (Decolonization$_2$).

Global health research and practice in the Global South is underscored by morality rather than obligation. Reacting to the United States of America for stopping the United States President's Emergency Plan for AIDS Relief and the United States Agency for International Development grants, Katumba (2025) argued that the Global North has no obligation to support the Global South unless it profits them. This argument aligns with the modus operandi of the colonization agenda of Africa in the early twentieth century. What is distinguishable in Decolonization$_1$ and Decolonization$_2$ is that there are no legally enforceable mandates for the Global North to support Decolonization$_2$. This argument is supported by the fact that apart from various governments and global health actors condemning the actions of the United States, there have been no legal repercussions to their actions. Consequently, there is limited global effort and coordination to decolonize global health, as was the case with political decolonization. Therefore, the Decolonization$_2$ project is an ethical-moral responsibility rather than a mandate from the Global North's perspective. For example, colonial-era psychiatry in Africa pathologized local cultures and institutionalized racial hierarchies, perpetuating stigma and epistemic violence. Ethically, these demands acknowledge historical harm and rectify its modern manifestations. Also, global health remains dominated by institutions and funders from the Global North, reinforcing a "white gaze" in research agendas and resource allocation. The vaccine inequity during COVID-19 exemplified how colonial dynamics prioritize Global North's interests. Morally, this inequity necessitates redistributing decision-making power to marginalized communities and dismantling extractive partnerships.

Many global health authors have argued that decolonizing global health is difficult as it involves undoing colonial systems established over centuries to perpetuate and maintain the unfair practices observed today—coloniality. Because colonization was achieved predominantly through violence, violent insurgencies were also required to force the hands of Western powers to give up their control over their colonies—political pressure and forced hand (Hirsch, 2021). Coloniality, although it is the remnants of colonization, is not achieved through violence but through ideological domination (racism, hegemony, paternalism, superiority, and saviorism). Therefore, decoloniality and $Decolonization_2$ cannot be achieved through violence. It requires a change of mindset or ideological engagements. While $Decolonization_1$ required a complete removal of Western dominance in politics, the economy, and governance in the colonized nations, the calls for $Decolonization_2$ are geared toward achieving equity and justice in international interactions, including global health. Unfortunately, the calls for $Decolonization_2$ do not have the global advocacy and support that $Decolonization_1$ had. $Decolonization_2$ is sometimes relegated to the desires of a few international organizations and institutions as part of their social responsibility. Within some of these organizations, advocacy for $Decolonization_2$ is also entrusted to a handful of people on a fraction of their time. The question is if it is realistic for these global health organizations and institutes to accomplish what began through insurgent action during $Decolonization_1$ (Hirsch, 2021).

It is now no secret that modern global health institutions predominantly based in the Global North continue to operate with colonial vestiges. To overlook their colonial roots, these global health institutions focus on explaining global health inequalities largely through biomedicine and cultural frameworks rather than associating them with colonialism (Hirsch, 2021). Consequently, communities such as decolonization working groups and diversity, equity, and inclusion (DEI) committees working to achieve decolonization within these (global health) institutions in the Global North will always be perfunctory and performative. A keen assessment of the roles of Diversity, Equity, and Inclusion and decolonization committees indicates that they will likely continue to be ineffective in achieving meaningful $Decolonization_2$. Meaningful $Decolonization_2$ cannot be achieved because it is oxymoronic for global health institutions to "decolonize" while retaining their epistemic, political, and financial power. For these global health institutions to achieve meaningful $Decolonization_2$, their commitment to working against the colonial vestiges—ideologies and practices—must focus on fighting the colonial matrix of power, which entails giving up some or all their powers (Hirsch, 2021). In other words, decolonizing global health entails working at a deeper level to undo these forces (ideologies) and systems that continue to drive unfair practices in global health. Kwete et al. (2022) suggest that meaningful $Decolonization_2$ entails adopting systemic reforms that challenge the fundamental assumptions of global health—decoloniality.

Decoloniality

In his book *Against Decolonisation: Taking African Agency Seriously*, Olúfẹ́mi Táíwò differentiates between two forms of decolonization: Decolonization$_1$, which refers to the attainment of political independence and sovereignty, and Decolonization$_2$, a post-independence ideological initiative aimed at eliminating all colonial influences. Eliminating colonial administrations during Decolonization$_1$ did not lead to the "complete" decolonization of the former colonies (Grosfoguel, 2007). While Decolonization$_1$ across various regions was achieved through a mix of conflict, negotiations, and political changes, the calls for Decolonization$_2$ focuses mainly on decoloniality—reflexivity and pleas to change mindsets, ideas, narratives, and practices (McCoy, 2024). For instance, global health researchers are being called upon to reflect on their practices and applied methodologies when conducting indigenous research in formerly colonized nations (Pant et al., 2022). Nevertheless, a core aspiration of Decolonization$_2$ or the "postcolonial project" is recognizing that "change of economic and political structures of domination and inequality requires a parallel and profound change of their epistemological and psychological underpinnings and effects" (Parashar & Schulz, 2021, p. 869). To this end, Erondu et al. (2025) propose decoloniality as a transformative lens for global health reform, emphasizing the need to dismantle colonial hierarchies in knowledge production, funding, and governance. Therefore, the goal of decolonizing global health must address the colonial matrix of power, the legacy of colonization in the field, unethical profiteering within the healthcare industry, and epistemic injustice and create a clear agenda for transformation (McCoy, 2024).

We have seen in the previous chapters that contemporary global health practice is scaffolded by coloniality. Therefore, the foundations of coloniality must be undone to have a decolonized global health practice. Of course, the logical way to undo coloniality is decoloniality. According to Beghin (2022), decoloniality offers those oppressed through coloniality a way to restore their culture, principles, voice, and visibility. The goal of decoloniality is to undo coloniality and its effects. Decoloniality and decolonization are driven by nationalist consciousness or anti-colonial sentiments and self-determination. Anti-colonial nationalists' idea of decoloniality involved filtering colonial ideas to "fashion a 'modern' national culture that is nevertheless not Western." In other words, the goal should be to create its domain of sovereignty. For example, in India, the local intellectual class insisted on using mother tongues over English as the language of school instruction. Anti-colonial nationalist movements are best understood in terms of hybridity: nationalism draws upon Western ideas and vocabularies to challenge the colonial rule and integrated with "indigenous ideas, reading it through their interpretive lens, and even using it to assert cultural alterity or insist on an unbridgeable difference between colonizer and colonized" (Loomba, 2015). Such hybridity guides decoloniality towards self-determination.

While there is a conflation between decoloniality and decolonization, I contend that decolonization can only be possible when decoloniality occurs. The move from the colonial era through the current reality of neo-colonialism sustained by coloniality to achieve the goal of decolonization can only be achieved through decoloniality. Decoloniality, therefore, involves rethinking and deconstructing Eurocentric/Western ideologies and practices that uphold coloniality as the power over people, lands, and knowledge. Decolonial perspectives see the long-lasting effects of colonial power as intersectional, multidimensional, multisystemic, institutional, historical, and self-perpetuating (Naidu et al., 2024). Therefore, unpacking the central mechanisms and structures embedded within the notion of coloniality is critical to unpacking how decolonization can be achieved.

In Chapters 1 and 2, I established the difference between colonization and coloniality. Similarly, decoloniality and decolonization are different. Decolonization refers to the independence process of former colonies, while decoloniality concerns challenging and dismantling the ideological frameworks that justify and maintain colonial power relations. In its simplest definition, decoloniality is about prohibiting or undoing colonialism's domineering effects (Maldonado-Torres et al., 2018). While colonialism was characterized by a paternalistic approach to engaging with the rest of the world, decoloniality proposes a respectful approach. Figure 5.2 illustrates the distinctions between colonialism, coloniality, decoloniality, and decolonization.

A Postcolonial Critical Realist Perspective on Decoloniality

To fully understand decoloniality, it may be best to explore what it is not. Decoloniality is not decolonization. Decolonization refers to the physical and political power shift between colonizing powers and their soon-to-be-former subjects. Decolonization$_1$ occurs when colonized people militarily overthrow an occupying power or, more rarely, negotiate their freedom in some other way and reclaim their country as independent with their sovereignty. Decolonization$_1$ is the legal-political withdrawal of former colonizers from their once-colonized state(s), which was predominantly driven by nationalist consciousness or anti-colonial sentiments and self-determination. The historical event of legal-political withdrawal has been described in Chapter 1.

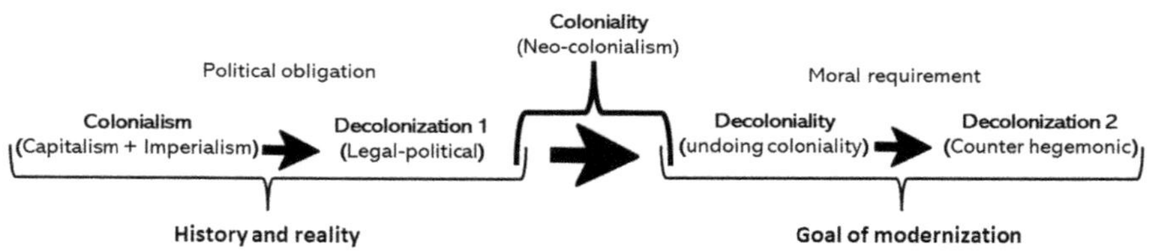

Figure 5.2 A logic model conceptualizing decolonization through decoloniality.

Decoloniality, on the other hand, is a mindset or praxis; it is an orientation toward a culture marked by a commitment to rooting out what remains in culture, education, society, and so on from the colonial era. Decoloniality "disobeys and delinks from [the colonial matrix of power], constructing paths and praxis toward an otherwise of thinking, sensing, believing, doing, and living" (Mignolo & Walsh, 2018, p. 194). Focusing on the generation and use of knowledge in the Global North and South, Galtung (1967) proposed that undoing the colonial mindset on how knowledge is generated and used would contribute to more equality globally by institutionalizing equality in nations' access to knowledge about each other, and, consequently, to a "balance of knowledge" as opposed to a "knowledge hegemony." Ontologically, therefore, decoloniality entails focusing on value and taking the stance of morality and justice. Practically, it entails undoing the mindsets of racism, religious paternalism, knowledge hegemony, white supremacy, and white saviorism.

Values are what we think things should be, for instance, equitable distribution of power and resources to achieve population health, not necessarily how they are—inequitable distribution of resources and power leading to differential health outcomes, which is what decoloniality is meant to change. The fact–value distinction is tantamount to the is–ought distinction—the difference between "what is" and "what ought to be." The fact-value distinction distinguishes between "what is" the case (facts—colonization of global health as argued in Chapter 1) and "what ought to be"—(values—decolonized global health) based on human rights principles, morality, and justice. Facts are mostly presented using descriptive claims (statements about matters of fact), while values are expressed using evaluative claims (judgment about something's value). Descriptive claims make statements about how the world is. They describe the facts of something, what one observes as the case, without any evaluation or judgment. For instance, there is an inequitable distribution of resources, and countries with fewer resources (predominantly in the Global South) have a higher disease burden than those with higher incomes (predominantly in the Global North). Evaluative claims suggest how the world ought to be. They express value judgments: what is good, just, fair, morally right, important, etc. Decoloniality is an evaluative or assessment exercise in global health practice to achieve justice, equity, global solidarity, and collective liberation.

Ontologically, positivism promotes the idea that science is exclusively concerned with "facts" and that it is a fallacy to assume that "ought" can be derived from "is." This assumption poses the challenge of moving from statements of fact (something is) to statements of value (something ought to be). While the positivist tradition suggests that moral judgments (value) are logically independent from empirical beliefs (facts), critical realists do not distinguish between facts and value. Hume argued that "ought" could not be derived from "is" because morality concerns sentiments, not facts. Morality, however, involves expressing sentiments about a factual matter, which is achieved through decoloniality (reflecting on what needs to be done). For example, the agenda to decolonize global health would be considered more of a moral agenda and colonization factual. Elder-Vass (2019) argues that critical social science needs an ontology of values, which recognizes that values are created by human beings in social settings rather than objectively true. Social morphogenesis thus offers a framework through which one can understand how we move from facts to value, in which case, through reflexivity, facts are converted into value. For example, Individuals advocating for decolonization seek to draw attention to the relationship between colonialism and the nature of the practice of contemporary global health. Therefore, contemporary global health practice is viewed as intricately connected to colonial practices and, thus, the calls to decolonize global health. Moral realists deny the fact-value distinction and argue for a more objective concept of morality. Critical realism, as we have seen, assumes that the ground for knowledge is real and has a value base such as "colonization is immoral" (Wong, 2019), from which we can construct more complex critiques through reflexives to establish that decolonization is a legal and moral obligation. The mindset and thought processes guiding these reflexives constitute decoloniality.

Houston and Montgomery (2018) contend that there is a presumption in favor of finding the truth (value) about a phenomenon through what empirical research endeavors indicate. They argue that certain descriptive claims imply an evaluative claim (valuation), especially if the concept of purpose or function links them. In this case, values and valuation are obtained from reflexivity. Consequently, some philosophers, especially critical realists like Connelly (2001), argue that there is no distinction between fact and value. While facts may inform value and valuation, according to Elder-Vass (2019, 2022), value and valuation depend more on social construction as a process in which discursive forces shape the principles or conventions of valuation acceptable to the community of actors and the balance of social power influences those discursive forces themselves. For instance, if colonization is considered to have enhanced inequities between nations through coloniality and consequently the health outcomes of the colonized, then discursive forces like advocacy groups and decolonization movements based on the inequity fact form valuations for decolonization to address coloniality. Decoloniality is thus the process of formulating valuations to address or undo coloniality. These are engagements on "what should be," which are the product of reflexives. Of course, developing values to address the harms found during the fact-finding entails providing alternatives to the harmful situation and asking, "What moral principles should a given alternative share?" (Wright, 2010).

Contrary to moral realists such as Bhaskar, who believe morality is objective (it exists irrespective of our knowledge), Elder-Vass (2019) argues that they are not objective but rather emergent mental properties of human beings developed through social interactions, and those beliefs emerge as values. Applying Elder-Vass's (2019) argument means that we could apply no moral or ethical positions to address decolonization but that through discursive engagements with relevant interest holders, relevant moral and ethical values about (de)colonization could be established. Nevertheless, it is worth noting that existing ethical and moral principles have been established through historical engagement that could be applied to the issue of (de)colonization. For example, the United Nations Declaration of Human Rights is one area where we might argue that this value has been arrived at through a process that conforms with longstanding engagement with different interested parties at the global scale, which can be applied when having a responsible critique on (de)colonization.

Colonialism was portrayed as a moral and civilizing act towards "inferior" cultures and races (McCoy, 2024). On the contrary, the specific moral wrong of colonialism, apart from treating other races as inferior, was undermining and/or removing the agency of communities and people from serving their communities and putting this agency in the service of the interests of colonizers (de Campos-Rudinsky et al., 2024). Decoloniality, from a realist perspective, is, therefore, a process of developing new ideologies and mindsets from the moral standpoint of colonialism being immoral. Having the understanding that colonial practices in global health are sustained by the colonial matrix of power, decoloniality should focus on dismantling the power matrix to promote equitable practice of global health.

Decoloniality and the Practice of Contemporary Global Health

Decolonizing global health means "removing all forms of supremacy within all spaces of global health practice, within countries, between countries, and at the global level" (Abimbola & Pai, 2021, p. 1628). Decoloniality entails collapsing hegemonic influences, which requires fostering dialogue among various stakeholders including funding bodies, policymakers, researchers, implementers, and the public. This dialogue should focus on the contextual injustice that globally funded programs may cause and ways to address this issue. By presenting evidence, such as the study conducted by Lassa et al. (2022), we can advocate effectively for including neglected actors, like frontline workers and community voices, in policy discussions. This inclusive approach can lead to interdisciplinary and equitable engagement with policymaking.

Global health practice entails challenging the mentalities of white supremacy, religious paternalization, racism, hegemony, and white saviorism that underpin global health practice—research and curricula, partnerships, and the attitude that ignores the capacity, knowledge, and contributions of the Global South. Citing Africa as an example of a continent that requires a decolonial mindset, Ndlovu-Gatsheni (2013) suggested that for decoloniality to take place, "What African intellectuals and academics must do is to strive to shift the location from which the hegemonic paradigms are enunciated and, in the process, read and interpret African history from a critical African and Global South perspective" (p. 5).

According to Beghin (2022), "[t]he culture of coloniality is capitalist, racist, patriarchal, and anti-democratic." These ideologies are pervasive in global health, intending to maintain a "power hierarchy that is still predominantly white, cis-gendered, heterosexual, male, and European/American" (Opara, 2021). Coloniality in global health therefore reinforces a superiority complex from the Global North over the societies in the Global South and a hegemonic pattern of knowledge, thus denying or undermining the knowledge of people with low incomes and of blacks, indigenous people, and women (Beghin, 2022).

Counter-Hegemonic and Equity-Based Praxis in Global Health

Having immersed myself in decolonizing global health literature and advocacy through co-authoring various pieces with other colleagues and reading extensively the work of other respectable authors advocating and championing the calls to action to decolonize global health, I have identified five mindsets or processes that must form a part of a counter-hegemonic discourse in global health. Several authors have noted that decoloniality as a radical rethink or reimagination of global health's political and economic structures is impossible. Counter-hegemony discourse refers to the efforts that challenge hegemony's cultural and institutional foundations (Adkin, 2022). Therefore, my argument is that counter-hegemony discourse must form the basis of any decolonial agenda. To this end, I will present a counter-hegemonic praxis for countering the colonial matrix of power towards decoloniality. I conceptualized this counter-hegemonic and equity-based praxis in a triad of (1) epistemic reorientation (decolonizing the mind and centering indigenous knowledge systems), (2) institutional critique (confronting historical erasure and redefining global health expertise), and (3) relational ethics (fostering equitable collaboration while cultivating epistemic self-determination). The counter-hegemonic and equity-based praxis is thus built from six inter-related decolonial reflexivity components: decolonizing the mind, combating colonial amnesia, going beyond traditional mastery (global health expertise), establishing meaningful global health collaborations, valorizing local knowledge, and having a self-reliant mindset (Figure 5.3).

Decolonizing the Mind (Knowing Our History and Valuing Ourselves)

Coloniality has also been conceptualized at the individual level. Decolonizing the mind should occur from two perspectives. The perspectives of individuals from previously colonized states in the Global South, especially those educated in institutions in the Global North and planning to practice in the Global South. For individuals from the Global South, individual-level coloniality appears to be an individual bias and tendencies emanating from a historical and ongoing colonial impact on health equity (Bua & Sahi, 2022).

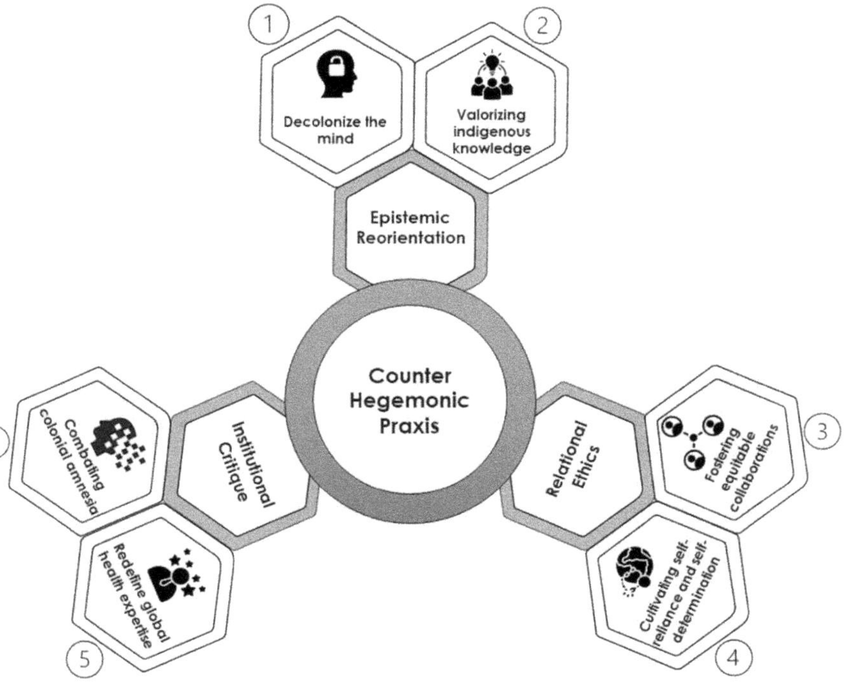

Figure 5.3 Counter-hegemonic and equity-based praxis to decolonize global health.

Steve Biko states, "The most potent weapon in the hands of the oppressor is the mind of the oppressed." The revolutionary idea of starting to undo the effects of colonializing through our reflections and actions was first introduced by Ngũgĩ wa Thiong'o (1986) in his book "Decolonizing the Mind." Decolonization of the mind is a cultural movement that aims to challenge and dismantle the effects of colonialism. Decolonizing the mind means liberating one's consciousness from the limitations of dominant powers while revitalizing indigenous knowledge, language, and culture (Achieng et al., 2024). This transformative process requires a careful and critical re-evaluation of historical events and prevailing narratives. It also serves as a call to action for advancing social justice, equity, and individual agency. Decolonization of the mind is an expedition of self-discovery, empowerment, and reclamation of our identities. By recognizing the narratives imposed upon us, we can actively work to change them. Therefore, it focuses on transforming our minds and reshaping global health practice (Achieng et al., 2024).

Opara (2021) proposes that individuals from the Global South, including global health practitioners from the region, need to thoroughly purge themselves from centuries of psychosocial conditioning and internalized colonization grounded in Western myths, perspectives, and narratives of who we are, our abilities, value, contributions to the world, and how we found ourselves in this current situation. These narratives were designed for us to internalize the delusion of superiority, even while they depended, and continue to depend, on our wealth, resources, intellect, skills, and labor to survive. We need to engage in individual and collective healing practices to address the cumulative trauma of coloniality, racism, patriarchy, ableism, capitalism, homo-transphobia, and all intersecting systems of oppression that have been transmitted intergenerationally and experienced on the levels of the intrapersonal, interpersonal, institutional, systemic, and structural. Without healing from our trauma, we are doomed to reproduce it among ourselves and reinforce the same systems of dominance in our problem-solving processes, which are then rendered impotent.

Coloniality at the individual level is mainly achieved through the curriculums delivered in global health training centers in the Global North. These curriculums offer a hypnotizing colonial gaze to the students—seeing things from the perspectives of the colonizer- and form the foundation of the knowledge base and bias of global health practice in the Global South. These curricula are developed based on colonial ideologies and perspectives and thus foster colonialist power structures, which influence current global health practices, including donor-directed priority setting and the creation of partnerships. According to Scheiner et al. (2020), while global and international health practice may appear to be a win–win situation for the volunteers from the Global North and the hosts (Global South), that is, a pathway to bilateral academic success, it also offers a new platform of colonialism of a Global South country by a country in the Global North. This situation can only be changed through reflexivity and education through curricula designed to decolonize global health (Kalbarczyk et al., 2023).

There is a growing awareness that knowledge generated in the Global North defines practices and informs the thinking of those trained through those curricula, which is usually to the detriment of knowledge systems in the Global South (Bua & Sahi, 2022). Through their curricula, global health training centers in the Global North perpetuate coloniality (Eichbaum et al., 2021). In the same way that global health education can perpetuate coloniality, it also presents an opportunity to redress and redesign these systems by helping the students unlearn the colonial mindsets and receive decolonial mindsets for the equitable benefit of the various partners (Rabin et al., 2021). Education, therefore, offers a great opportunity to decolonize the minds of formally colonized individuals as they can learn more about their history. Education can offer the opportunity for Global North students to reflect on their positionality and its effects on indigenous populations during global health practice and research. Such education should focus on constantly training the imagination—pushing the imagination to learn from historical events. Only in this way do the individuals challenge hegemonic structures and allow themselves to imagine a decolonized global health.

Valorizing Local Knowledge—Local Knowledge Usage Preference

Epistemic injustice or unfair knowledge practice is a flagship characteristic of global health (Abimbola et al., 2024; Koum Besson, 2022). It has also been described as knowledge colonialism (Galtung, 1967), which entails using colonial communicative structures and institutions to produce, distribute and use knowledge. Epistemic injustice in global health assumes power disparities between the global health institutions or actors, for instance, because they rely heavily on certain forms of knowledge and information when designing global health interventions. For example, during the colonial days, many medical departments, such as the Indian Medical Service, relegated indigenous practitioners to a subordinate service (Johnson, 2010). Epistemic injustice in global health is a symptom of coloniality perpetuated by white supremacy and knowledge hegemony. White supremacy and knowledge hegemony foment epistemic injustice by undermining local or indigenous knowledge and its associated structures largely built on oral traditions, which have long been perceived as an aberration (Kolawole, 2022). Epistemic injustice leads to inappropriate or ineffective intervention development, lack of community engagement, and poor intervention uptake or adoption by the local communities. As distal consequences, unfair and unjust communicative structures, institutions, and practices grounded in coloniality can reproduce and exacerbate existing socioeconomic inequalities and injustices (Byskov, 2021) and, indeed, health inequities (Bhakuni & Abimbola, 2021; Koum Besson, 2022).

The concept of core-periphery, developed by the United Nations Economic Commission for Latin America, is often used in the literature on epistemic (in) justice (Kolawole, 2022). The core-periphery model describes a spatial and economic division where "core" regions are dominant, developed, and wealthy (Global North), while "periphery" regions are less developed, dependent, and often exploited for resources and labor (Global South). The central argument of modernists is that the periphery will only experience socioeconomic progress and better health outcomes if they religiously adopt technological "innovations" introduced to them by the core. This implies that knowledge emanating from the periphery is perceived as suboptimal in achieving better health outcomes (Kolawole, 2022; Tobi, 2020). The argument is that knowledge from the core is superior and can transform the periphery and thus must be privileged over local or indigenous knowledge, which constitutes epistemic injustice or unfair knowledge practices.

It is widely understood that local knowledge should be used to identify and understand local challenges and develop local solutions. Nevertheless, there is a history of the reluctance of the core or the Global North to consider knowledge from indigenous or the local community in the Global South. For example, Brazilian, Peruvian, and Colombian indigenous peoples have been using ayahuasca therapeutically for a very long time for the management of depression. Ayahuasca is a tea made from two Amazonian plants: *Banisteriopsis caapi* and

Psychotria viridis. The former contains harmala alkaloids, while the latter is rich in dimethyltryptamine. Indigenous peoples in Brazil, Ecuador, and Peru have utilized this tea for medicinal, spiritual, and cultural purposes since pre-Columbian times (Tupper, 2008). After decades of biomedical research on ayahuasca's molecular compounds and their physiological effects, it is only recently that clinical trials have shown evidence of its therapeutic potential for depression (Schenberg & Gerber, 2022b). This scenario questions why it was only after the confirmation through the trials that the West considered it useful, highlighting the epistemic authority attributed to scientific studies. This situation highlights the possibility that epistemic injustices were committed with practical, cultural, social, and legal consequences. This reluctance has been attributed to implicit or explicit prejudices (McKinnon, 2016), which suggests that they do not know better or understand their situation, and those from the Global North can provide that understanding. Epistemic injustice is, therefore, "a wrong done to someone specifically in their capacity as a knower" (Fricker, 2007) and speaks to the moral wrongs related to the way knowledge is produced, used, or shared (Fricker, 2007; Tobi, 2020).

An individual or a group is considered to suffer from epistemic injustice because they fulfill the following five conditions proposed by Fricker (2007). The periphery experiences epistemic injustice because of their socioeconomic disadvantage compared to the core (the *disadvantage* condition), which leads to discrimination stemming from prejudice (i.e., unfair) sentiments directed at them (the *prejudice* condition). Byskov (2021) argued that there are facets of epistemic injustice that the disadvantage and prejudice conditions do not encompass, leading to the identification of three additional conditions: stakeholder, epistemic, and social justice conditions. The *stakeholder condition* asserts that for someone to be unjustly discriminated against as a knower, they must be affected by decisions from which they are excluded from influencing. The *epistemic condition* states that the discriminated individual or group must possess relevant knowledge about the decisions in which they are excluded. Lastly, the *social justice condition* posits that for epistemic discrimination or inequality to qualify as epistemic injustice, the affected individual or group must simultaneously endure other forms of social injustice. I argue that the Global South or the periphery meets all these conditions, especially regarding global health practices and research.

Abimbola et al. (2024) recently described four categories of unfair knowledge practices pervasive in global health, which align with the conditions for epistemic injustice identified by Byskov (2021) and Fricker (2007). The unique contribution of Abimbola et al. (2024) in this regard is that with each category of unfair knowledge practice, following the realist philosophy of science, they identified the causal mechanisms that trigger each unfair knowledge practice:

1. Credibility deficit related to gaze is identified as one of the unfair knowledge practices in global health and is linked to the epistemic condition. The mechanisms perpetuating the credibility deficit are the periphery's cultural

knowledge, technical knowledge, and "articulation" of knowledge, which do not matter, indicating that the core undermines these forms of knowledge.
2. Credibility deficit related to gaze (mechanisms: "the center's learning needs, knowledge platforms, and scholarly standards must drive collective knowledge-making").
3. Interpretive marginalization related to pose (mechanisms: "the periphery's sensemaking of partnerships, problems and social reality do not matter").
4. Interpretive marginalization related to gaze (mechanisms: "the center's learning needs, social sensitivities and status preservation must drive collective sensemaking").

The mechanisms perpetuating epistemic injustice in global health speak to the perceptions of the Global North and are related to the influence of pose and gaze to highlight the presence of epistemology. To find one's voice within this space, most global health practitioners and researchers from the Global South tend to operate within the epistemic positions of their Global North counterparts, which means that they "are pre-emptively silenced" as they "smother their testimony" and "lactify their scholarly offerings" (Abimbola et al., 2024). Overcoming this situation entails valorizing local and indigenous knowledge and resisting the temptation of aligning with Western epistemic systems especially when they do not fit the narratives.

Decolonizing global health regarding epistemic injustice thus entails valorization or entrenchment of local knowledge in developing theory and practice (Kolawole, 2022). In our example on the globalization of ayahuasca, Schenberg and Gerber (2022a) explained that indigenous people do not lose knowledge when ignored or undermined by biomedical science and that they do not need biomedical sciences to validate their practice. This shows how much they valorize and are confident in their knowledge and practice of ayahuasca. According to Tobi (2020), epistemic decolonization must consider two key principles: relevance and diversity. Relevance involves establishing pathways that allow different social groups to explore knowledge that resonates with them, while diversity refers to creating multiple epistemic centers that aim to achieve epistemic richness through engaging in discourse (Tobi, 2020). These two principles can be ensured by adopting a multi-faceted and multidisciplinary approach to improve the knowledge base and practice to address global health concerns.

Community epistemic systems can be strengthened and blended with evidence-based medicine to harmonize the evidence, secure and expand community buy-in, and ultimately improve its implementation (Chaturvedi et al., 2023). Kolawole (2019) argues that hybridizing knowledge development and adoption processes can be more useful to peripheral societies. This approach means that global health scientists should consciously engage in a broad-spectrum science that simultaneously embraces or focuses its lens on the local realities. Sarmiento et al. (2020) argue that intercultural dialogue can improve the functioning of Western health services for indigenous communities, as they can instill principles of respecting cultural differences and leveraging local resources. This approach will likely engender knowledge decolonization—to even out credibility deficits and reverse interpretive marginalization in global health practice and research (Tobi, 2020).

Fostering Equitable Global Health Collaborations

In Chapter 2, we established that although partnerships are fundamental to the success of global health, the nature of these partnerships is inequitable. According to McCoy (2024), decolonizing global health would require challenging unequal, unfair, or exploitative relationships between actors working within global health. Current reflections in this regard focus on the relationships between the Global North with power and resources and those who are vulnerable to being subjugated and exploited in the Global South. As such, some funders advocate for equitable resource distribution among partner organizations by prioritizing spending in the Global South and appointing principal investigators from that region (Charani et al., 2022; Zaman et al., 2020). However, these efforts are insufficient, as academics from the Global South remain underrepresented in global health literature (Abimbola, 2019; Kaufman et al., 2023).

Equity in global health partnerships entails more than merely creating a level playing field for partners; it also involves recognizing and addressing inherent inequalities to ensure that all participants can fully engage in and benefit from collaborative efforts. McIntosh et al. (2023) propose that Global South researchers should be included in recruiting study participants and present their insights and leadership from study inception to manuscript write-up. The equity principle is especially important when co-creating research questions to address local challenges effectively. For instance, Global South researchers who are based in or familiar with the community where the study is conducted are best placed to formulate research questions with local relevance—being mindful of cultural sensitivities during study design; and to interpret findings within the cultural and research context, such that decision makers receive valid information. Global health researchers can also promote equitable engagement by involving research beneficiaries as both participants and partners. Bharadwaj (2014) proposed a framework (Figure 5.4) and guidance to Global North researchers on establishing respectful and productive partnerships with Global South researchers and communities. Therefore, adopting a Global South-centered research framework for equitable partnership and collaboration is useful for decolonizing global health research.

Fairness is crucial in distributing financial resources and attributing contributions and credit for research outputs. Many funding organizations seek evidence of collaborative development of research questions among all partners. Therefore, funders should prioritize this co-creation process and, whenever possible, facilitate opportunities for potential partners to refine research questions as part of the funding process collectively. Global health researchers who

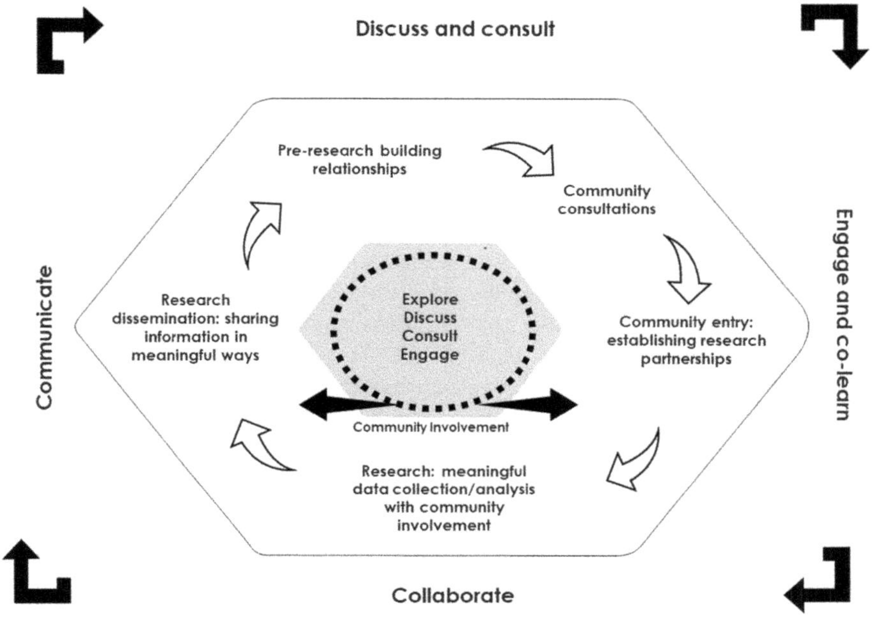

Figure 5.4 Global South-centered research framework for equitable partnership and collaboration.

are involved in this partnership must take the initiative to foster equitable and mutually supportive partnerships. Kaufman et al. (2023) suggest this could be achieved by ensuring that when collaborating on research efforts, they should start their engagements from the initial research concept and continue through project delivery and the dissemination of research outcomes.

Cultivating a Self-Reliant Mindset

Self-reliance encompasses the ability of individuals and communities to meet their needs and improve their well-being using local resources and capabilities, emphasizing autonomy and independence. Hope (1983) defines self-reliance as "autonomy of decision-making and full mobilization of a society's resources under its initiative and direction. It also means rejecting the principle of exploitative appropriation of others' resources" (p. 455). The central emphasis of self-reliance in decolonizing global health is meeting the previously colonized's basic needs and encouraging them to participate in their development process (Hope, 1983). The framework of self-reliance, thus, has two main components: (1) maximization of the use of local resources and values and (2) participation of the locals or indigenes in the development process. For example, members of the 1987 South Commission, led by President

Julius Nyerere and with membership from 27 nations, called for "self-reliant and people-centered development" through both the mobilization of people of "the South" and a transformation of relationships with "the North" (South Commission, 1990).

Self-reliance in the Global South was a predominant mindset between the 1920s and 1980s as a rallying cry for decolonization—the emancipatory frame. Historically, Global South actors adopted a transformational self-reliance perspective, representing a fundamental shift in power distribution concerning priority setting, financial flows, and trade terms within the international system (Neill et al., 2023). Nevertheless, after political decolonization, there was a proliferation of donors in the region, thus establishing the mindset of aid dependency (Muyebe, 2025). Part of the dependency also meant that the notion of self-reliance of the Global South countries depended on the funding bodies. This phase of self-reliance is described as the reformist frame, led by donor agencies. There is a divergence in opinions regarding the extent to which Global North agencies share responsibility for promoting self-reliance (Shawar et al., 2023).

The reformist view of self-reliance differs from the original emancipatory frame of self-reliance in that the latter required enhanced domestic resource mobilization and distribution and prioritized the Global South's agency. Nevertheless, the US Agency for International Development (USAID) most recently advanced its organizational strategy for self-reliance entitled the Journey to Self-Reliance (J2SR), which is conceptualized as a country's capacity to plan, finance, and implement solutions to local development challenges, as well as the commitment to see these through effectively, inclusively, and with accountability (Neill et al., 2023). The J2SR approach was based on the original emancipation framework. Nevertheless, in the advent of President Donald Trump's second term, the US Agency for International Development halted and canceled its support to the Global South under the banner of "America First." These cancellations were made without consulting the implementers—international non-governmental organizations in the United States and the Global South, health ministries, and the millions of people in the Global South who depended on the US Agency for International Development-funded programs for healthcare (Kyobutungi et al., 2025) revealed the flaws in reformist self-reliance approach (Lancet, 2025).

Indeed, Nonvignon et al. (2024), a year earlier, identified that a major flaw in global health grant-financing institutions and initiatives is that they have no end date. The implication of the no-end-date approach of these global health initiatives is that an expectation of indefinite financing for potentially limitless demand is created. Adeyi and Nonvignon (2024) argued that most global health initiatives are based on a flawed design—the externally modeled burden of disease estimate combined with cost-effectiveness estimates often lacking contextual relevance. This design informs externally inspired packages of essential health services marketed as "best buys" and the global health foundation focuses on financing various components of these best buys

(Adeyi & Nonvignon, 2024). Owing to this flawed design, they inherently lack sustained impact and do not strengthen their health systems or improve population health; rather, they create dependency (Kyobutungi et al., 2025).

In global health, self-reliance was most clearly expressed in the 1978 Alma Ata declaration, which identified self-reliance as a key element of comprehensive primary health care (Banerji, 2004). Self-reliance and other associated ideologies, such as resilience and "increasing country voice," gained traction as approaches to improve the participation of the Global South (Shawar et al., 2023). These ideologies are viewed in global health as sustainable development, localization, indigenous participation, and primary health care (Fonchingong & Fonjong, 2002). Consequently, there was advocacy for more community development programs and global health initiatives to enhance self-reliance (Nayar et al., 2004). Over time, over-reliance on aid or health-related support from the Global North, such as the President's Emergency Plan for AIDS Relief, US Agency for International Development, and Gates and Melinda Foundations, metamorphosed through expectations into a mindset. Aid dependency, or more generally, dependency syndrome, as discussed in Chapter 2, evolved from structural dependency. Through the recent halts and cuts of the PEPPFA and USAID funding by President Donald Trump, several countries in the Global South started appreciating or becoming aware of the aid dependency mindset. The early (Lankiewicz et al., 2025) and projected impact of this halt and cuts (Hoan Tram et al., 2025) indicate the level of aid dependence in these parts of the world. Aid dependency will persist if the Global South does not seek to develop the capacity to support itself and meet its economic and health needs. To do this, the Global South must re-emancipate from the dependency syndrome to a self-reliant mindset.

In the wake of the withdrawal and halting of aid funds, the Global South has intensified its examination of current aid models. To this end, the Global South should go beyond the reformist view of self-reliance and strive for genuine sovereignty or self-sufficiency. This new self-reliant mindset should not only offer scope for national development and bargaining power vis-à-vis the Global North but should entail tapping from opportunities for innovation in health systems development and strengthening, training of health care providers, disease surveillance, vaccines, and drug development, which have not been charted before.

Beyond Traditional Mastery (Redefining Global Health Expertise)

Redefining what constitutes "expertise" or who an expert is in Global is an important component of counter-hegemony in global health. This assertion is grounded in the "politics of expertise" coined by Turner (2015), which refers to the power dynamics and influence wielded by individuals with specialized knowledge in decision-making processes. The politics of expertise examines how expert knowledge is legitimized, aggregated, and distributed and how these processes influence the distribution of power (Turner, 2015). Essentially, it explores the interplay between scientific or technical expertise and political agendas, suggesting that the distribution of knowledge and power are connected. According to this understanding, therefore, being grounded in evidence, facts, and science on how diseases are transmitted and affect different population groups should make one an expert in global health. Knowing the culture, human behavior, governance, law, politics, regulations, and community frameworks are equally key aspects of global health (Ojiako et al., 2023). Based on the required wide knowledge base and interdisciplinary nature of global health, there is no consensus on who is an expert in global health. According to Ojiako (2022), this lack of consensus creates a double-edged sword situation. The lack of consensus on what constitutes expertise in global health has created global health experts by default.

Global health experts are created based on the health professionals' nationality or country of residence—predominantly from the Global North (Ojiako, 2022). Most global health multisite trials are often conceived and designed by international research networks based in the Global North, and they subsequently identify country leads at each site whom they will work with to recruit and train researchers for that specific site (Lawrence & Hirsch, 2020). This modus operandi lends itself to view those from the Global North as the experts. Ojiako (2022) quoted a global health practitioner who explained the established consensus of a global health expert: "a white Westerner who studied global health at a prestigious university in the West and is working on large-scale public health projects to improve the health of people in LMICs ..." Owing to these entrenched viewpoints, expertise, therefore, almost exclusively means relying on Global North researchers who have superior understanding about how best to identify, prioritize and solve pressing health problems somewhere else (King & Koski, 2020). These authors explained further that an assumed expertise gradient is created when the superior understanding of disease manifestation and the social, political, and economic complexities around the health problems are given to Global North researchers (King & Koski, 2020), which is informed by the colonial ideologies of white supremacy, knowledge hegemony and saviorism.

Of course, the contemporary nature of a global health expert is informed by colonial epistemologies of expertise developed during colonial times. When Joseph Chamberlain (1836–1914), the Secretary of State for the Colonial Office in the UK, called for the establishment of the London School of Hygiene and Tropical Medicine in 1899, the goal was to train physicians in the field of tropical medicine who were to be deployed to British colonies to support their imperialist agenda (Greenwood, 2022). The tropical medical career was reserved for physicians of the middle class, who were white, masculine, and sporty but not of the top class (Greenwood, 2022). Trained in this then-unique field to provide prevention and disease eradication services, these mediocre physicians were now seen as "experts" in tropical medicine and hygiene. Johnson (2010) provides evidence of how the colonial perspective of a global health expert came to be through his narrative of how England formed the West African

Medical Staff institution at the turn of the twentieth century but insisted that it should be an all-white institution. The goal was to have physicians work under the principles of "modern tropical medicine and hygiene," which we have seen was the nature of global health at the time. Nevertheless, according to Johnson (2010), the West African Medical Staff institution was the only department in the empire that was explicitly racist when it was publicized. It explicitly excluded West Africans—or any physician not being of "European parentage." While West Africans were allowed to work as attorneys, accountants, clerks, and in other professional medical capacities for the colonial state, they were not allowed to join the West African Medical Staff, which provided "global health" expertise to the colonizers working in the colonized states. Predominantly, those trained in the Institutes of Tropical Medicine across Europe were allowed to be part of the West African Medical Staff.

One of the drivers of coloniality that was discussed in Chapter 2 was the establishment of feudal structures. According to Keshri and Bhaumik (2022), feudal structures in global health take the form of "a small group of multilateral entities and [Global North] universities evolved into what we see as the 'Crown' which controls the global health (knowledge and practice) ecosystem" (p. 1). These global health practitioners are usually based in the Global North, but their realm of action is predominantly the Global South, and they are the "experts." These experts primarily enhance their portfolio of work in the Global South but are answerable to their institutions in the Global North "Crown." Decolonizing this type of expertise in global health entails breaking the feudal structure supporting its operation, requiring many global health actors to take cognizance of their positionality within the ecosystem (Keshri & Bhaumik, 2022).

Dismantling colonial epistemologies of expertise can lead to more effective and culturally appropriate solutions for addressing health inequity than relying on "expertise" from individuals in the Global North. A global health practitioner explained further:

> They [global health experts] are the unpaid community health workers who go from house to house to check up on their patients; the midwives at the rural health post who work round the clock to give care to laboring women; and the district health officer who drives hours on their motorbike to provide bedside care. These heroes may not have the academic degrees behind their names, but they are passionate and continue to serve their communities long after the donor project funding dries up and the "Western global health experts" move on to another flashy donor project.
>
> (Ojiako, 2022)

Ojiako (2022) argues that expertise in global health should be based on experience and competence in global health practices and research. What is observed, rather, is that people from the Global North are often appointed as the global health experts to occupy senior positions while those affected by and more proximal to the health issues (the real experts) are side-lined (Weekes-Richemond, 2022). This is because our current perspective of a global health expert excludes the diverse and lived experiences of health professionals working on the front lines and at the community level in the Global South (Ojiako et al., 2023). Weekes-Richemond (2022) explained that "There need to be more Global South-based experts steering the ship as opposed to all-white headquarters senior leadership teams. If this means organizational restructuring to redistribute power to country and regional offices, then so be it." The Global South can reduce reliance on Global North expertise by leveraging experts from the Global South in program management and otherwise to strengthen local ownership and sustainability. I argue, therefore, that our way of viewing who an expert is in global health must change for there to be a true decoloniality of expertise. Decoloniality of expertise will mean the dismantling of the mindsets of knowledge hegemony, white supremacy, and white saviorism, which means addressing white saviorism.

Combating Colonial Amnesia (Confronting Historical Erasure)

The passage of time is a significant obstacle to redressing colonial injustice (Stahn, 2020) and could lead to colonial amnesia. Colonial amnesia (also known as postcolonial amnesia or imperialist amnesia) is a concept in postcolonial studies that describes the phenomenon of forgetting colonial history or selectively remembering it in ways that obscure the experiences of the colonized. It has also been used to describe the romanticization of the colonial past or a sense of nostalgia for it (Stahn, 2020). Fletcher (2012) eloquently describes it as "the fetishistic disavowal of the legacy of European colonization within the contemporary post" (p. 423). He went further to explain that imperialist amnesia is "a tendency on the part of 'agents of colonialism' to either ignore the history of colonial domination in their accounts or to present a sanitized version of colonialism from which evidence of exploitation, persecution, subjugation, and genocide has been effectively effaced" (p. 423). For example, Ejdus (2022) illustrated that colonialism is being erased from official memory at the permanent exhibition House of European History in Brussels. Such is the nature of most (global health) institutions operative from the Global North. Hence, colonial amnesia is always from the colonizer's gaze.

According to Fletcher (2012), international development planners have long been criticized for ignoring colonization's impact on the structure of the "less-developed" societies they aim to modernize. Failure to acknowledge or downplay the influence of colonialism in an organization's operations, which historically has benefited from the colonial operations, constitutes colonial amnesia. Puri (2020) points out that the European Union has its form of amnesia, which entails fixating on its immediate twentieth-century history and largely ignoring the broader patterns of imperial history that have shaped the continent. Consequently, it has failed to grapple adequately with Europe's colonial past and its influence on the European Union's external relations

(Pace & Roccu, 2020). Fletcher (2012) argues that the disavowal of colonialism functions as what Michael Taussig calls a "public secret"—something commonly known but not generally acknowledged to efface the grim realities—helping to efface the grim reality of the colonial enterprise. The "loss" of knowledge and experience related to colonialism can negatively impact an institution's global health practice and research activities, as practice depends heavily on what people recall and what is embedded in facts (Stark, 2019). Ejdus (2022) argues that collective amnesia is a distinct form of anxiety-driven avoidance mechanism in world politics. In global health, institutional amnesia relates to not recognizing or acknowledging the historical foundations and circumstances that led to establishing a global health institution and some medical discoveries and advancements made through unethical research conducted on indigenous populations in colonies.

Several recent studies have established that colonial institutions influence current Global North institutions and their contemporary operations (Jones, 2013). This connection does not only apply to extractive institutions—institutions that allowed them to extract vast amounts of wealth and knowledge "at the expense" of their colonies—but also other institutions that then benefited from the activities of the extractive institutions (Goldstone, 2024). For instance, a doctor trained at a School of Tropical Medicine and Hygiene conducted research in their colonies, but the findings were used to develop medication used by their countries of origin. A good case is that of Dr. Georges Lacapère, a French venereologist, who coined the term "Arab syphilis" in 1923 after publishing research based on his work at a clinic in Fez, Morocco, which he used to describe a form of syphilis found in Morocco, Algeria, and Tunisia (Amster, 2022). Colonial amnesia is quite common in global health institutions, and collective colonial amnesia and disavowal produce unsympathetic (and unemphatic) responses to health problems in the Global South (Affun-Adegbulu et al., 2023). Colonial amnesia in global health institutions matters because these institutions define the "rules of the game" in global health research and practice, thus determining the payoffs associated with global health knowledge production, transmission, and application.

Global North institutions, including governments, banks, and international organizations, significantly benefited from colonialism through resource extraction, the establishment of exploitative trade patterns, and the perpetuation of unequal power dynamics that continue to shape the global economy. Institutional amnesia, in this regard, can hinder decolonization efforts by preventing a comprehensive understanding of colonial legacies and the necessary steps for redress and not acknowledging how colonialism contributed to the prestigious positions that inform their current global (health) operations. It includes failing to recognize or downplaying how coloniality continues to underpin their collaborations with less privileged organizations in the Global South and how they carry out global health initiatives and research activities. Thus, institutional amnesia undermines history's importance and critical role despite its centrality in shaping social structures.

Colonial amnesia often prevails in certain enlightened circles because most of those running in these circles have decided "enough is enough." This phrase relates to the fact that there is enough talk about colonialism and everything that has to do with the Global South being often linked to colonialism. Others suggest that they have done more than enough as reparations—measures that wrongdoers offer to their victims to help repair the harm they inflicted upon them or the colonial damage—so we must move along (Goldstone, 2024). To this end, some former colonial powers question the legality and practicality of reparations, arguing that they cannot be held accountable for actions taken by previous governments (Dunham & Shinard, 2022). Using the European Union and the permanent exhibition in the House of European History in Brussels as a case study, Ejdus (2022) explained that "imperial amnesia" is meant to address the dissonance between the self-proclaimed image of a normative and civilian power on the one hand and imperial-like tendencies in its behavior on the other. I argue that many global health institutions, such as the Schools of Tropical Medicines and Hygiene across Europe, find themselves in a similar situation given their embeddedness in current global (power) structures of coloniality. They are faced with the complex and complicated task of delinking themselves— (re)negotiating, (re)defining, and (re)envisioning their role as agents of the colonial project in the global health space (Affun-Adegbulu et al., 2023).

It is believed that coming to terms with the colonial past and acknowledging one's guilt are vital foundations for decoloniality. Institutional memory (or corporate memory), the opposite of institutional amnesia, is the continued consideration of the ethos and practices that have guided an organization's operations. It points out the positives and negatives of past thought processes and guidelines so that it is helpful to continue with what has worked in delivering the aims in the past and what has not, thereby ensuring that lessons learned are remembered and passed on to the next generation. Institutional amnesia may occur when the training of the next generation of global health practitioners is void of the colonial foundation of global health and lacks meaningful institutional reflexivity of the role of coloniality in global health practices and research. Retaining institutional knowledge should allow an institution to highlight and acknowledge how these institutions and their favorable funding ecosystems exert substantial control over health initiatives and research in the rest of the world.

Gopal (2016) argues that to address colonial amnesia, there is the need to go beyond the reflexivity of the impact of colonialism or a simplistic "inclusion" of the indigenes of the formerly colonized countries. Instead, Gopal (2016) advocates for examining the agency and influence of the struggles of the formal colonies. Therefore, addressing colonial amnesia should inform the goal of decoloniality, focusing on reflexivity to change mindsets, ideas, narratives, and practices constructed to enable and legitimize systemic exploitation. For global health institutions, the components of memories, concepts, experiences, and know-how held within an organization should be a part of the infrastructure of the institutions, and these tools should be used to inform practices that achieve equity in (social and epistemic) justice.

One fundamental premise of global health is that many developing countries do not have a solution to their health problems, which deals with the issue of epistemic injustice. Nevertheless, global health cannot be decolonized using the same logic, dynamics, and paradigms responsible for its origin (Opara, 2021). While there are suggestions that decolonization can be achieved with countries in the Global South engaging with other health organizations based in the Global North with medical technologies in a non-exploitable but symbiotic relationship, others have proposed that the focus should instead be on the South by the South itself—self-reliance or self-sufficiency. The latter scholars argue that events like the United States cuts and European receding funding opportunities on funding to the Global South should prompt a renewed focus on self-reliance, independence, and strategic unity (Katumba, 2025; Kyobutungi et al., 2025; Parashar & Schulz, 2021). They argue that there should not be any reason why the Global South should be looking up to the Global North for salvation (Rahman et al., 2025). In this way, decolonizing allows countries of the Global South to exploit their resources to address the health challenges plaguing their populations. Others contend that Global South countries already have the resources to solve their health issues. It has also been argued that decolonization does not have to adopt only a single approach and that the fluidity of decoloniality allows for a multi-faceted approach to decolonization.

A new relational approach necessitates a broader range of measures to address colonial amnesia, which includes historical inquiry, archival research, public investigation, individual or collective reparations, acknowledgment of wrongdoing, and critical remembrance (Stahn, 2020). Global health research and practice should go beyond compensation or redress; they also consider (postcolonial) identity and the need to reinvent relationships in Global North-South collaborations in global health research and practice. Attention should also be paid to issues around authorships in global health, community participation, non-adversarial engagement, the importance of amplifying local or indigenous voices, and the critical roles of education, memorialization, and prevention in addressing historical injustices (Stahn, 2020).

Conclusion

Injustice and inequity in global health are recognized to be driven by the colonial legacies of the past. Because the colonization of global health is primarily driven by coloniality, which is vastly different from the agendas of political colonization, decolonizing global health requires a different approach to those employed to achieve political decolonization. Decoloniality seeks to root out what remains in culture, education, society, and so on from the colonial era. It thus entails removing "all forms of supremacy within all spaces of global health practice, within countries, between countries, and at the global level."

Therefore, decolonizing global health requires changing the ideologies and mindsets guiding global health practice and research. In this chapter, I propose the adoption of counter-hegemonic discourse, which entails decolonizing the mind, combating colonial amnesia, going beyond traditional mastery (global health expertise), establishing meaningful global health collaborations, valorizing local knowledge, and having a self-reliant mindset.

References

Abimbola, S. (2019). The foreign gaze: authorship in academic global health. *BMJ Global Health*, 4(5), 2068. https://doi.org/10.1136/BMJGH-2019-002068

Abimbola, S., & Pai, M. (2021). Undoing supremacy in global health will require more than decolonisation—Authors' reply. *The Lancet*, 397(10279), 1058–1059. https://doi.org/10.1016/S0140-6736(21)00373-1

Abimbola, S., Van De Kamp, J., Lariat, J., Rathod, L., Klipstein-Grobusch, K., Van Der Graaf, R., & Bhakuni, H. (2024). Unfair knowledge practices in global health: a realist synthesis. *Health Policy and Planning*, 39(6), 636–650. https://doi.org/10.1093/HEAPOL/CZAE030

Achieng, G. F., Kabasa, M., & Onyango, J. (2024, December 10). Decolonizing the mind to change the narrative. www.acts-net.org/blogs/challenging-the-narrative/decolonizing-the-mind-to-change-the-narrative.

Adeyi, O., & Nonvignon, J. (2024, February 19). Transition to sunset: The future of foreign aid for basic health services in Africa. *Development Today*. www.development-today.com/archive/2024/dt-2--2024/transition-to-sunset-the-future-of-foreign-aid-for-basic-health-services-in-africa.

Adkin, L. (2022). Hegemony & counter-hegemony. https://ecampusontario.pressbooks.pub/showingtheory/chapter/hegemony-and-counter-hegemony.

Affun-Adegbulu, C., Cosaert, T., Meudec, M., Michielsen, J., Van De Pas, R., Van Belle, S., Van De Put, W., Soors, W., Robertson, F., & Ddungu, C. (2023). Decolonisation initiatives at the Institute of Tropical Medicine, Antwerp, Belgium: Ready for change? *BMJ Global Health*, 8(5), e011748. https://doi.org/10.1136/BMJGH-2023-011748

Amster, E. J. (2022). The past, present and future of race and colonialism in medicine. CMAJ: *Canadian Medical Association Journal*, 194(20), E708. https://doi.org/10.1503/CMAJ.212103

Banerji, D. (2004). The people and health service development in India: A brief overview. *International Journal of Health Services*, 34(1), 123–142. https://doi.org/10.2190/9N5U-4NFK-FQDH-J46W

Beghin, N. (2022). Decoloniality as the only pathway to the right to development in Latin America. *Development*, 65(2–4), 178. https://doi.org/10.1057/S41301-022-00349-W

Betts, R. F., (2012). Decolonization: A brief history of the word. In E. Bogaerts, & R. Raben (Eds.), *Beyond empire and nation: The decolonization of African and Asian societies*, 1930s–1970s (pp. 23–37). Brill.

Bhakuni, H., & Abimbola, S. (2021). Epistemic injustice in academic global health. *The Lancet Global Health*, 9(10), e1465–e1470. https://doi.org/10.1016/S2214-109X(21)00301-6

Bharadwaj, L. (2014). A framework for building research partnerships with First Nations communities. *Environmental Health Insights*, 8. https://doi.org/10.4137/EHI.S10869

Bua, E., & Sahi, S. L. (2022). Decolonizing the decolonization movement in global health: A perspective from global surgery. *Frontiers in Education*, 7. https://doi.org/10.3389/feduc.2022.1033797

Byskov, M. F. (2021). What makes epistemic injustice an "injustice"? *Journal of Social Philosophy*, 52(1), 114–131. https://doi.org/10.1111/JOSP.12348
Charani, E., Abimbola, S., Pai, M., Adeyi, O., Mendelson, M., Laxminarayan, R., & Rasheed, M. A. (2022). Funders: The missing link in equitable global health research? *PLOS Global Public Health*, 2(6), e0000583. https://doi.org/10.1371/JOURNAL.PGPH.0000583
Chaturvedi, S., Porter, J., Gopalakrishna Pillai, G. K., Abraham, L., Shankar, D., & Patwardhan, B. (2023). India and its pluralistic health system—a new philosophy for Universal Health Coverage. *The Lancet Regional Health—Southeast Asia*, 10, 100136. https://doi.org/10.1016/j.lansea.2022.100136
Connelly, J. (2001). Critical realism and health promotion: effective practice needs an effective theory. *Health Education Research*, 16(2), 115–120. https://doi.org/10.1093/her/16.2.115
de Campos-Rudinsky, T. C., Bosha, S. L., Wainstock, D., Sekalala, S., Venkatapuram, S., & Atuire, C. A. (2024). Decolonising global health: why the new Pandemic Agreement should have included the principle of subsidiarity. *The Lancet Global Health*, 0(0). https://doi.org/10.1016/S2214-109X(24)00186-4
Dunham, A., & Shinard, V. (2022). The question of reparations to postcolonial states. https://abcnews.go.com/US/wireStory/reparations-draw-scrutiny-whod-pay-80273817
Eichbaum, Q. G., Adams, L. V., Evert, J., Ho, M.-J., Semali, I. A., & Van Schalkwyk, S. C. (2021). Decolonizing global health education: Rethinking institutional partnerships and approaches. *Academic Medicine*, 96(3), 329–335. https://doi.org/10.1097/ACM.0000000000003473
Ejdus, F. (2022). Anxiety, dissonance and imperial amnesia of the European Union. *International Relations*, 19(73), 45–60.
Elder-Vass, D. (2019). Realism, values and critique. *Journal of Critical Realism*, 18(3), 314–318. https://doi.org/10.1080/14767430.2019.1614744
Elder-Vass, D. (2022). Pragmatism, critical realism and the study of value. *Journal of Critical Realism*, 21(3), 261–287. https://doi.org/10.1080/14767430.2022.2049088
Erondu, N. A., Dhar Sharma, V., Mulumba, M., & na Haki, A. (2025). Decolonial framings in global health law: Redressing colonial legacies for a just and equitable future. *Journal of Law, Medicine & Ethics*, 1–3. https://doi.org/10.1017/JME.2025.25
Fletcher, R. (2012). The art of forgetting: imperialist amnesia and public secrecy. In Source: *Third World Quarterly*, 33(3).
Fonchingong, C. C., & Fonjong, L. N. (2002). The concept of self-reliance in community development initiatives in the Cameroon grassfields. *GeoJournal*, 57(1), 83–94. https://doi.org/10.1023/A:1026042718043
Fricker, M. (2007). *Epistemic injustice: Power and the ethics of knowing*. Oxford University Press.
Galtung, J. (1967). Scientific colonialism. *Transition*, 30, 10–15.
Goldstone, Z. (2024). Migration as reparation for colonialism. *Res Publica*, 30(4), 763–781.
Gopal, P. (2016). Redressing anti-imperial amnesia. *Race & Class*, 57(3), 18–30. https://doi.org/10.1177/0306396815608127
Greenwood, A. (2022). Diagnosing the medical history of British imperialism. *The Lancet*, 400(10354), 726–727. https://doi.org/10.1016/S0140-6736(22)01648-8
Grosfoguel, R. (2007). The epistemic decolonial turn: Beyond political-economy paradigms. *Cultural Studies*, 21(2–3), 211–223. https://doi.org/10.1080/09502380601162514
Hirsch, L. A. (2021). Is it possible to decolonise global health institutions? *The Lancet*, 397(10270), 189–190. https://doi.org/10.1016/S0140-6736(20)32763-X
Hoan Tram, K., Ratevosian, J., & Beyrer, C. (2025). By executive order: The likely deadly consequences associated with a 90-day pause in PEPFAR funding. *Journal of the International AIDS Society*, 28, 26431.

Hope, K. R. (1983). Self-reliance and participation of the poor in the development process in the Third World. *Futures*, 15(6), 455–462. https://doi.org/10.1016/0016-3287(83)90083-6
Houston, S., & Montgomery, L. (2018). Learning to absent the absent: Critical realism and social work education. In M. Kjørstad & M.-B. Solem (Eds.), *Critical realism for welfare professions* (1st edition, pp. 57–74). Routledge. https://doi.org/10.4324/9781315517537
Johnson, R. (2010). "An all-white institution": Defending private practice and the formation of the West African medical staff. *Medical History*, 54(2), 237–254. https://doi.org/10.1017/S0025727300006736
Jones, P. (2013). History matters: New evidence on the long run impact of colonial rule on institutions. *Journal of Comparative Economics*, 41(1), 181–200. https://doi.org/10.1016/J.JCE.2012.04.002
Kalbarczyk, A., Perkins, S., Robinson, S. N., & Ahmed, M. K. (2023). Decolonizing global health curriculum: from fad to foundation. *Frontiers in Education*, 8. https://doi.org/10.3389/feduc.2023.1217756
Katumba, A. (2025, March 21). Beyond dependency: Rethinking Africa's relationship with foreign aid Health. PLoS Blogs. https://speakingofmedicine.plos.org/2025/03/21/beyond-dependency-rethinking-africas-relationship-with-foreign-aid/
Kaufman, R., Fair, E., Reid, M., & Mirzazadeh, A. (2023). Authorship equity in global health research: who gets the credit at University of California, San Francisco? *BMJ Global Health*, 8(10), 13713. https://doi.org/10.1136/BMJGH-2023-013713
Keshri, V. R., & Bhaumik, S. (2022). The feudal structure of global health and its implications for decolonisation. *BMJ Global Health*, 7(9), 10603. https://doi.org/10.1136/BMJGH-2022-010603
King, N. B., & Koski, A. (2020). Defining global health as public health somewhere else. *BMJ Global Health*, 5(1), 2172. https://doi.org/10.1136/BMJGH-2019-002172
Kolawole, O. D. (2019). Science, social scientisation and hybridisation of knowledges. *Science as Culture*, 28(3), 391–401. https://doi.org/10.1080/09505431.2019.1645825
Kolawole, O. D. (2022). Is local knowledge peripheral? The future of Indigenous knowledge in research and development. *AlterNative: An International Journal of Indigenous Peoples*, 18(1), 132–140. https://doi.org/10.1177/11771801221088667
Koum Besson, E. S. (2022). How to identify epistemic injustice in global health research funding practices: a decolonial guide. *BMJ Global Health*, 7(4), 8950. https://doi.org/10.1136/BMJGH-2022-008950
Kwete, X., Tang, K., Chen, L., Ren, R., Chen, Q., Wu, Z., Cai, Y., & Li, H. (2022). Decolonizing global health: what should be the target of this movement and where does it lead us? *Global Health Research and Policy*, 7(1). https://doi.org/10.1186/s41256-022-00237-3
Kyobutungi, C., Okereke, E., & Abimbola, S. (2025). After USAID: what now for aid and Africa? *BMJ*, 388, r479. https://doi.org/10.1136/BMJ.R479
Lancet. (2025). The demise of USAID: time to rethink foreign aid? *The Lancet*, 405(10483), 951. https://doi.org/10.1016/S0140-6736(25)00556-2
Lankiewicz, E., Sharp, A., Drake, P., Sherwood, J., Macharia, B., Ighodaro, M., Honermann, B., & Russell, A. (2025). Early impacts of the PEPFAR stop-work order: A rapid assessment. *Journal of the International AIDS Society*, 28, 26423.
Lassa, S., Saddiq, M., Owen, J., Burton, C., & Balen, J. (2022). Power dynamics among health professionals in Nigeria: A case study of the global fund policy process. *International Journal of Health Policy and Management*, 11(12), 2876. https://doi.org/10.34172/IJHPM.2022.6097
Lawrence, D. S., & Hirsch, L. A. (2020). Decolonising global health: transnational research partnerships under the spotlight. *International Health*, 12(6), 518. https://doi.org/10.1093/INTHEALTH/IHAA073
Loomba, A. (2015). *Colonialism/postcolonialism* (3rd edition). Routledge.

Maldonado-Torres, N., Vizcaíno, R., Wallace, J., & We, J. E. A. (2018). Decolonising philosophy. https://philarchive.org/rec/MALDP-3.
McCoy, D. (2024, October 25). An anti-colonial agenda for the decolonisation of global health. www.miamisocialsciences.org/home/kfcz2ou06zszpv4bhcr4yw4fvx5y6g
McIntosh, K., Messin, L., Jin, P., & Mullan, Z. (2023). Countering helicopter research with equitable partnerships. *The Lancet Global Health*, 11(7), e1007–e1008. https://doi.org/10.1016/S2214-109X(23)00278-4
McKinnon, R. (2016). Epistemic injustice. *Philosophy Compass*, 11(8), 437–446. https://doi.org/10.1111/PHC3.12336
Mignolo, W. D., & Walsh, C. E. (2018). On decoloniality: Concepts, analytics, praxis. In *On decoloniality*. Duke University Press. https://doi.org/10.1215/9780822371779
Muyebe, F. S. (2025, March 11). How Africa can recover from the disease of aid dependency. *The Mail & Guardian*. https://mg.co.za/thought-leader/2025-03-11-how-africa-can-recover-from-the-disease-of-aid-dependency/
Naidu, T., Gingell, G., & Zaidi, Z. (2024). Decolonial framework for applying reflexivity and positionality in global health research. *Global Health Promotion*, 31(2), 52–58. https://doi.org/10.1177/17579759241238016
Nayar, K. R., Kyobutungi, C., & Razum, O. (2004). Self-help: What future role in health care for low and middle-income countries? www.equityhealthj.com/content/3/1/1.
Ndlovu-Gatsheni, S. J. (2013). *Coloniality of Power in Postcolonial Africa* (1st ed.). CODESRIA. https://muse.jhu.edu/book/25053
Neill, R., Shawar, Y. R., Kunnuji, M., Manoj, M., & Shiffman, J. (2023). Frames of self-reliance: an analysis of evolving international development discourse. *Third World Quarterly*, 44(3), 532–553. https://doi.org/10.1080/01436597.2022.2149484
Nonvignon, J., Soucat, A., Ofori-Adu, P., & Adeyi, O. (2024). Making development assistance work for Africa: from aid-dependent disease control to the new public health order. *Health Policy and Planning*, 39, I79–I92. https://doi.org/10.1093/HEAPOL/CZAD092
Ojiako, C. P. (2022, August 2). How not to become a global health expert. https://speakingofmedicine.plos.org/2022/08/02/how-not-to-be-a-global-health-expert/
Ojiako, C. P., Weekes-Richemond, L., Dubula-Majola, V., & Wangari, M. C. (2023). Who is a global health expert? *PLOS Global Public Health*, 3(8), e0002269. https://doi.org/10.1371/JOURNAL.PGPH.0002269
Opara, I. N. (2021). It's time to decolonize the decolonization movement. https://speakingofmedicine.plos.org/2021/07/29/its-time-to-decolonize-the-decolonization-movement/
Pace, M., & Roccu, R. (2020). Imperial pasts in the EU's approach to the Mediterranean. *Interventions*, 22(6), 671–685. https://doi.org/10.1080/1369801X.2020.1749702
Pant, I., Khosla, S., Lama, J. T., Shanker, V., AlKhaldi, M., El-Basuoni, A., Michel, B., Bitar, K., & Nsofor, I. M. W. (2022). Decolonising global health evaluation: Synthesis from a scoping review. *PLOS Global Public Health*, 2(11), e0000306. https://doi.org/10.1371/JOURNAL.PGPH.0000306
Parashar, S., & Schulz, M. (2021). Colonial legacies, postcolonial "selfhood" and the (un)doing of Africa. *Third World Quarterly*, 42(5), 867–881. https://doi.org/10.1080/01436597.2021.1903313
Puri, S. (2020). *The great imperial hangover: How empires have shaped the world*. Atlantic Books.
Rabin, T. L., Mayanja-Kizza, H., & Barry, M. (2021). Global health education in the time of COVID-19: An opportunity to restructure relationships and address supremacy. *Academic Medicine*, 96(6), 795. https://doi.org/10.1097/ACM.0000000000003911
Rahman, F. A., Djoudalbaye, B., Gomes, J. C., Karhili, N., Lara, J. C., & Mustaffa, M. (2025, March 18). A roadmap for South–South cooperation. *The Diplomat*. https://thediplomat.com/2025/03/a-roadmap-for-south-south-cooperation/

Sarmiento, I., Zuluaga, G., Paredes-Solís, S., Chomat, A. M., Loutfi, D., Cockcroft, A., & Andersson, N. (2020). Bridging Western and Indigenous knowledge through intercultural dialogue: Lessons from participatory research in Mexico. *BMJ Global Health*, 5(9). https://doi.org/10.1136/BMJGH-2020-002488

Scheiner, A., Rickard, J. L., Nwomeh, B., Jawa, R. S., Ginzburg, E., Fitzgerald, T. N., Charles, A., & Bekele, A. (2020). Global surgery pro-con debate: A pathway to bilateral academic success or the bold new face of colonialism? *The Journal of Surgical Research*, 252, 272–280. https://doi.org/10.1016/J.JSS.2020.01.032

Schenberg, E. E., & Gerber, K. (2022a). Epistemic losses, cultural exclusions, and the risk of biopiracy in the globalization of ayahuasca: A reply to Labate et al. *Transcultural Psychiatry*, 59(5), 714–717. https://doi.org/10.1177/13634615221131597

Schenberg, E. E., & Gerber, K. (2022b). Overcoming epistemic injustices in the biomedical study of ayahuasca: Towards ethical and sustainable regulation. *Transcultural Psychiatry*, 59(5), 610–624. https://doi.org/10.1177/13634615211062962

Shawar, Y. R., Neill, R., Kunnuji, M., Manoj, M., & Shiffman, J. (2023). Understanding resilience, self-reliance and increasing country voice: A clash of ideologies in global health. *BMJ Global Health*, 8(1), e010895. https://doi.org/10.1136/BMJGH-2022-010895

South Commission. (1990). *The challenge to the South: The report of the South Commission*. Oxford University Press.

Stahn, C. (2020). Confronting colonial amnesia. *Journal of International Criminal Justice*, 18(4), 793–824. https://doi.org/10.1093/jicj/mqaa052

Stark, A. (2019). Institutional amnesia and crisis management analysis. *Oxford Research Encyclopedia of Politics*. https://doi.org/10.1093/ACREFORE/9780190228637.013.1526

Tobi, A. T. (2020). Towards a plausible account of epistemic decolonisation. *Philosophical Papers*, 49(2), 253–278. https://doi.org/10.1080/05568641.2020.1779602

Tupper, K. W. (2008). The globalization of ayahuasca: Harm reduction or benefit maximization? *The International Journal on Drug Policy*, 19(4), 297–303. https://doi.org/10.1016/J.DRUGPO.2006.11.001

Turner, S. P. (2015). *The politics of expertise*. Routledge.

Wa Thiong'o, N. (1986). *Decolonising the mind: The politics of language in African literature, vol. 1*. James Currey.

Weekes-Richemond, L. (2022, March 29). Why I left my career in global health. https://speakingofmedicine.plos.org/2022/03/29/why-i-left-my-career-in-global-health/

Wong, B. (2019). On relational injustice: Could colonialism have been wrong even if it had introduced more benefits than harms? *Journal of Practical Ethics*, 7(1). https://ssrn.com/abstract=3474950

Wright, E. O. (2010). *Envisioning real utopias*. Verso

Zaman, M., Afridi, G., Ohly, H., McArdle, H. J., & Lowe, N. M. (2020). Equitable partnerships in global health research. *Nature Food*, 1(12), 760–761. https://doi.org/10.1038/s43016-020-00201-9

6 Dialectic of Freedom

A Framework for Decolonizing Global Health

Introduction

The previous chapters integrated postcolonial and decolonial discourses and the principles of critical realism to establish postcolonial critical realism as a philosophical foundation for understanding the decolonization of global health following Tinsley's (2021) lead. I started by reflecting on the dominance of postcolonial discourses, which focus on how colonialism's legacies continue to shape identities and power dynamics, and decolonial discourses, which seek to understand and dismantle the colonial matrix of power and continue to shape contemporary societies. Postcolonial and decolonial discourses have provided academic and practical arguments to decolonize every aspect of society and strive toward equity and justice in modernity. I acknowledged that these discourses have provided a valuable foundation for understanding the historical events and operations of the colonizers on the colonized. I then argued that integrating the tenets of basic critical realism into postcolonial and decolonial discourses would offer a more robust philosophical paradigm—postcolonial critical realism—to unpack global health's decolonization. The explanatory nature of critical realism, which offers a transcendental approach focusing on the interactions between structures, mechanisms, and contexts and how they generate observations, informs this understanding. Thus, the postcolonial critical realist approach can provide a deep explanation of how (de)colonization occurred and how it continues to influence the practice of global health today by unearthing the causal mechanisms and structures involved in orchestrating and maintaining coloniality in global health.

In this chapter, I explored Bhaskar's dialectical critical realism as a framework to inform the decolonization agenda as they are imbricated in the logic of human emancipation. Bhaskar developed dialectical critical realism as an extension of basic critical realism to address the dualism of human freedom and well-being. Therefore, the goal of dialectical critical realism was not to alter basic critical realism but to incorporate the notion of dialectic, which was achieved in at least two ways (Norrie, 2024). The first is to take the idea of

DOI: 10.4324/9781032700786-6

dialectic as logical negation (from Hegel) and to relocate it to the idea of change and movement in history (in line with Marx)—real movements in the spatio-temporal do not ultimately reduce to movements of underlying ideas. The second emphasized the nature of real things as always existing vis-à-vis other things—when is a thing itself and when it becomes something else (Norrie, 2024).

Bhaskar's development of dialectical critical realism was meant to serve three aims: (1) to dialecticize basic critical realism, (2) to introduce a critical realist understanding of ontology and deep structure to existing, especially Hegelian dialectical theory, and (3) to develop a metacritique of western philosophy (Norrie, 2010, 2024). All three aims are related to how social theory should best handle the complex nature of social phenomena, especially regarding tackling social ills with the notions of oppression and freedom and their corresponding synonymous variants, which are taking center stage in the dialectical argument. The first two objectives of dialectical critical realism align more with my goals of providing a mechanism-based explanation of the impact and influence of colonialism in global health practice and research, as well as how global health can be decolonized.

Adopting an ethical view of things and arguing for redressing social ills, Bhaskar's intention for developing dialectical critical realism was to improve our efforts to understand "how we could do things differently to achieve better circumstances that are conducive to human well-being" (Bhaskar, 2020, p. 113). Bhaskar then developed dialectical critical realism as the dialectic of freedom (Bhaskar, 2008, 2020), which more conspicuously accentuates his intention to contribute to addressing social ills through his philosophical thinking. In the previous chapters, I have established how coloniality and its effects constitute a social ill as it perpetuates health and social inequities and injustice. It is, therefore, on this premise that I considered dialectical critical realism as a helpful ontological framework for understanding and reflecting on a vision, objective, and process of decolonizing global health.

The Logic of Dialectics

"Dialectics" is a philosophical argument approach involving contradictory processes between opposing sides (Maybee, 2016). In philosophy, dialectic arguments describe situations, theories, and methods that depend on resolving opposing arguments. In the early conceptualization of "dialectics," the ancient Greek philosopher Plato (429–347 BCE) considered dialectics as a conversation between individuals with differing perspectives on a topic, intending to reach the "truth" through thoughtful discussions. Immanuel Kant (1724–1804) adopted the term "transcendental dialectic" to describe efforts to uncover the illusions that arise when applying categories and principles of understanding beyond the boundaries of phenomena and possible experience (Kant, 1933). German philosopher Georg Wilhelm Friedrich Hegel (1770–1831) acknowledged Immanuel

Kant as pivotal in developing the dialectic concept's modern philosophical revival. In its later development, Hegel proposed "dialectical" methods as a contradictory process between opposing sides.

While Plato's "opposing sides" were people (Socrates and his interlocutors), Hegel's "opposing sides" referred to a subject matter under deliberation (Maybee, 2016). Like Plato's dialectics, a contradictory process between "opposing sides" in Hegel's dialectics leads to a linear evolution or development from less sophisticated definitions or views to more sophisticated ones later. Kant (1933) developed his dialectics, suggesting that the two arguments he called the thesis and the antithesis were not necessarily contradictory opposites. Kant was of the view that dialectics, as a form of "opposition" between thesis and antithesis, is not necessarily a contradiction because "two dialectically opposed judgments both may be false; for the one is not mere contradictory of the other but says something more than is required for a simple contradiction" (Kant, 1933).

Bhaskar builds his dialectical critical realism from the foundations of the previous philosophers, especially Hegel and Kant. To this end, I begin with a synopsis of how Hegel and Kant conceptualized their dialectical logic and process. Hegel introduced his logic of dialectics through his book *Science of Logic*. According to Maybee (2016), Hegel's logic of dialectics begins with the simple, immediate, and abstract concept of pure "being," or "bare existence," which is used to illustrate the moment of understanding. Pure being, he says, is pure indeterminateness and has in it no object for thought to grasp, suggesting that it is empty and Nothing (Panovski, 2024). The "being" and "nothing" analogy formed the basis of Hegel's dialectical process; the first thesis, "being," turned into its antithesis, "nothing." Hegel illustrated his logic through his explanation of how Greek society functioned. He explained that Greece was a society rooted in customary morality, where citizens identified closely with their community and rarely considered acting against it. This customary community typifies the foundation for the dialectical movement known as the thesis—the state of pure being. The dialectical opposition of the thesis is to show itself to be inadequate or inconsistent (Panovski, 2024). In ancient Greece, the inadequacy of traditional thought was exemplified by the life and death of Socrates. He encouraged the citizens to think independently, giving them independent intellectual thought. Consequently, the community grounded in customs began to crumble in favor of the principle of intellectual thought and not just going along with the customary morality.

The transition from a customary community to an emphasis on intellectual thought allowed the acceptance of individual conscience as a guiding principle for a new way of life. The harmony of the Greek community was lost through the rise of the individual conscience ideology, and freedom prevailed (the process of becoming). This notion of "becoming" represents the second stage of dialectical logic, antithesis, which contrasts the first customary morality (Panovski, 2024). Nevertheless, having a society of absolute freedom is unsustainable, as illustrated by the terror of the French Revolution, which indicates that individuals' conscience now becomes a one-sided abstract freedom. Hegel then proposed that both sides could be united and unified to preserve them and avoid their different forms of one-sidedness (Panovski, 2024). Consolidating the two ends results in a third and more adequate stage, the synthesis. In Hegel's time, he considered German society to be the synthesis of the overall dialectic movement. He suggested that German society was harmonious because it preserved the organic community and embraced individual freedom because it was rationally organized.

The new state of freedom, which Hegel conceptualizes as a state of becoming, cancels, replaces, or negates the original state of being. This dialectic method culminates in the absolute idea. This absolute idea serves as the destination of the process, which moves from thesis to antithesis and then through synthesis. This progression aims to overcome one-sidedness until we arrive at the absolute idea. For Hegel, every dialectical movement follows a specific path: thesis, antithesis, and synthesis. In terms of logic, a concept is first introduced as a "thesis" or positive idea. This thesis then develops into an opposing concept, known as the "antithesis," which negates or contradicts the first. Ultimately, this process leads to a third concept, the "synthesis," which unifies both the thesis and antithesis (Maybee, 2016). Although the synthesis is intended to reconcile the thesis and antithesis, it is often not symmetrical or balanced when considering both sides. As a result, it tends to favor one aspect over the other. This synthesis becomes the thesis for a new dialectical movement, allowing the process to continue.

Hegel also shifted his idea of dialectical logic by further dissecting the notion of being or bare existence. He then argued that pure being is indeterminate (Panovski, 2024). Being's lack of determination leads it to sublate itself, transitioning into the concept of nothing. This illustrates the dialectical moment (Maybee, 2016). He argued that the opposite of being is nothing and described being as undefined content, taken as or meant to be present, while nothing is undefined content, taken as or meant to be absent. He suggested that the notion of being is not different from the assertion of pure negation or the negative, which he views as bare existence equal to nothing. Becoming negates or cancels being and nothing, as it emerges as a new concept that supersedes these earlier ideas; however, it simultaneously preserves both being and nothing, as it depends on these foundational concepts for its definition (Maybee, 2016). Indeed, becoming represents the first concrete concept within this logical framework.

In contrast to being and nothing, which lacks definitive characteristics and thus remains purely abstract, becoming constitutes a determinate unity in which there is both being and nothing. The logic of being-nothing-becoming is closely related to the traditional view that Hegel's dialectics follows: a thesis-antithesis-synthesis pattern. A thesis that leads to its reaction, an antithesis that contradicts or negates the thesis. A synthesis resolves the tension between the two. Applying the thesis-antithesis-synthesis pattern to understand the decolonization of global health should start with unpacking the thesis of how the Global North, with political and economic domination over the Global South, established and maintained coloniality, which dictates the practice, knowledge ecosystem, and agenda setting in global health. This thesis would progress to its antithesis, where the Global South focuses on sourcing resources and addressing the health challenges plaguing the nations in the Global South with little or no reliance on the Global North—self-determination. A synthesis would then be the practice of global health achieved through shared decision-making, mutual respect, epistemic justice, and equitable resource distribution with both sides' political power. Some authors have deemed this synthesis an unattainable utopia, arguing that it will require the Global North to cede its power and privilege and make major compromises. To this end, other authors have argued for allyship—leadership by the Global South with support from the formal colonizers (Oti, 2024; Pai et al., 2024; Anti-Oppression Network, 2015).

One of the drawbacks of Hegel's thesis–antithesis–synthesis dialectical logic is that antinomies—the thesis and antithesis (such as infinite space, eternal time, and first cause)—are challenging to operationalize, and these antinomies cannot be resolved through a synthesis. For instance, if a thesis contends that "the world has a beginning in time and is limited in space" (Overend, 2020), the antithesis to this thesis contends that the world has no beginning and end. There is no synthesis to address these antinomies appropriately. According to Kant, space, time, and causality are modes of perception and conception that shape all our experiences; they are not external entities that exist independently of our perception. Also, there is the opposition between parts and the whole. The thesis contends that everything is divisible by simple parts. The antithesis contends that the "composite thing" is the whole and not divisible into parts (Overend, 2020).

Kant argued that antitheses can be addressed through the epistemological distinction between pure reason and understanding (Gasparyan, 2023). To this end, he introduced the notion of Transcendentalism, adopting a negative connotation of dialectics, and described it as the "logic of Schein" (appearance). However, Hegel rejected the concept of a fixed and unknowable realm of things in themselves, proposing instead that reality is fundamentally a dynamic and interconnected process (Panovski, 2024). For Kant, while reason has a structural tendency, as seen in the thesis—antithesis—synthesis model, it should move beyond the realm of experience into the unknowable. This argument lends itself to the "dialectical battlefield" between the Transcendentalism thesis and Empiricism's antithesis. Kant describes the "transcendental dialectic" as a "logic of illusion," which seeks to reveal the misconceptions that occur when reason is used beyond the boundaries of experience. He contends that reason is only valid when applied to things as they appear in experience; thus, our understanding of what things are in themselves is constrained by our experiential knowledge (Gasparyan, 2023).

With the offering of unpacking arguments from the initial state of being to a state of nothing and arriving at the state of Becoming, dialectics offers a starting point of reflections on the nature of what a decolonized global health would look like—a merge of elements of Global North–South collaborations and self-determination of the Global South. To this end, I found the dialectical logic of understanding a valuable philosophical framework for unpacking the implications of colonization and coloniality against the notions of decolonization and decoloniality. Dialectics is a useful framework for questioning the power dynamics of colonialism and how it has shaped societies, thus fostering a nuanced understanding of the impact of colonialism by considering opposing viewpoints and contradictions.

Dialectical Critical Realism

Scaffolded by the above philosophical discourse on dialectical engagements, Bhaskar (2008) builds on the tenets of basic critical realism to develop dialectical critical realism. He proposed this as being, negation, and becoming, then agency, and developed a MELD system, his dialectic form. His thoughts were that original critical realism was the "first moment" (1M), from which the dialectical work developed a "second edge" (2E) based on negation, which was followed by a further "third level" (3L) of totality (representing synthesis), before finding a "fourth dimension" (4D) around agency (Norrie & Morgan, 2021). So, MELD described Bhaskar's overall dialectical movement, starting from what he had done in basic critical realism (1M); he then added to it the importance of understanding what material change meant (2E)—the real determinate negation of what was presently there. He then argued for a world in which material change related to structure and mechanism entailed an understanding of how a material totality or whole operated (3L)—with holistic causality and concepts like the constellation and four planar social being; before circling to understand how real agency and moral commitment were possible in this material world (4D)—the possibility of a world of human flourishing and praxis (Norrie & Morgan, 2021).

According to Creaven (2001), critical realism must be more explicitly dialectical to realize its rich potential for capturing sociocultural dynamics. As seen above, dialectical critical realism goes beyond the traditional thesis-antithesis-synthesis model, proposing a fourth level to the dialectical process leading to action for or advocating change (Bagley et al., 2016). In the most general of terms, Bhaskar views dialectic as both a structure-in-process and a process-in-structure, highlighting the interconnections and oppositions that lead to the elaboration or transformation of a particular system, its totality, or some of its elements (Creaven, 2009). For structure-in-process, social structures (e.g., economic systems, cultural norms) are not static but exist through ongoing human agency and activity processes. Structures emerge, persist, and transform via these processes. For example, coloniality as a structure is maintained or altered through daily practices like funding operations and mechanisms and the adoption of participatory research methods. Process-in-structure processes (global health practice and research activities) are always embedded within and conditioned by pre-existing structures such as the guiding principles of the funding agencies. Structures provide the material and relational constraints/enablers that shape agency. For instance, the distribution of funds between the Global North–South institutions is based on the specifications of the funding bodies.

As discussed earlier, for Hegel, the dialectical process is the logic of negation (contradictory process between opposing sides), but Bhaskar explained "negative dialectics" as (generally) the absenting of absence and (specifically) the absenting of constraints or ills. According to Bhaskar (2008), dialectical engagements should not start with "Being"—what was there or present, as Hegel had done, but rather from "absence" (what was not present). For instance, decolonization should start from the "absence" (what is missing), such as the absence of equity in global health practice, especially concerning the Global South, women, persons with disabilities, and migrants (Tangcharoensathien et al., 2023). Bhaskar (2008) sees dialectics as removing absences (a process he called "absenting absences"). Alderson (2016a) also considers aporia (contradictions and constraints, ills and untruths) absences. Therefore, interventions to address health inequalities should address the maldistribution of power ubiquitous in global health. In dialectical critical realism, dialectics is the identification and transformative elimination of absences, crucial to the logic of change, freedom, and human flourishing. Concerning the decolonization of global health, the role of dialectical critical realism would be to undo the colonial matrix of power to achieve equity and justice in global health.

While dialectical realism has not gained traction in health care, some authors have successfully applied it to explore the possibility of freedom or emancipation among selected populations. For example, her two volumes (Alderson, 2016b, 2013) provided accounts of how to successfully liberate children (especially those in contact with healthcare systems) so that their rights are fully realized. Scambler and Scambler (2015) also applied Bhaskar's dialectical critical realism model to explain health inequalities and interventions to reduce health inequalities. They found it useful to unpack the underlying causal mechanisms informing health inequities and how these mechanisms can be neutralized through interventions to address health inequities. Following the stellar examples provided by these scholars, I believe that Bhaskar's political-moral theory offers a useful emergent epistemic framework for understanding the process of decolonizing global health.

I found dialectical critical realism's focus on eliminating constraints to achieve "freedom" attractive to unpack decolonization through decoloniality. This consideration is enhanced by process/product bipolarity of dialectical critical realism: it can refer to the process and outcome of the transformative elimination of "absences." In Chapter 4, I argued that inequities and injustice in global health (absences) are underpinned by the mechanisms of racism, hegemony, religious paternalism, white saviorism, and white supremacy, and decolonizing global health requires eliminating the colonial matrix of power guiding global health practice and research—coloniality. It is my argument that the transformative elimination of "absences" requires a change of mindset or epistemic re-orientation, which entails decolonizing the mind of the formerly colonized, combating colonial amnesia among the former colonizers, going beyond traditional mastery to identify global health expertise, establishing meaningful global health Global North–South collaborations, valorizing local or indigenous knowledge and for the Global South to develop a self-reliant mindset—decoloniality.

Agents possess various capacities, including mind, self, intentionality, and rationality. They express their needs and interests with these capabilities and consciously act on them (Hartwig, 2001). When agents find themselves in social relations rooted in economic exploitation and political domination, such as in the case of colonialism and imperialism, they are denied the same freedom and life chances as others in more privileged positions. They may also be deprived of the consumption of their labor, as was the experience of the colonized nations. In such situations, agents perceive these social relations as unjust and oppressive and strive to resist reform to overturn them (Hartwig, 2001). However, they face opposition from elite groups who benefit from the status quo due to their control over resources and authority. This "dialectic of control" between collectives who seek to maintain the current societal order and those who pursue societal change is a significant driving force in history, as Marx aptly noted (all history is the history of class struggle). The "dialectic of control" illustration introduces the notion of power (the ability to control others and change situations inherent to agency). Sayer (2012) argues that power aligns with causation or power as derived from agents' capacities and concludes that dispersed power presupposes causality and causal powers.

In a revised version of dialectical critical realism, Bhaskar (2020) considered individuals or agents as central to the transformational model of social action. The transformational properties of agents are related to their human nature and their emergent properties. Agents are considered stratified and relational entities defined by their historical context, rhythms of change, and the complex web of relationships they have with everything else around them. Essentially, agents cannot be understood in isolation but must be analyzed within the totality of their connections and historical development. Power is the transformative capacity intrinsic to agency; $Power_1$ and $Power_2$ in colonial relations were expressed in domination, exploitation, subjugation, and control structures. Bhaskar (2020) describes $Power_1$ as the implicit potentialities of persons, which they can use to achieve their potentialities (human emancipation). $Power_1$ is the reflexivity and voice that can be used to seek unity through diversity and reestablish transformative action, challenging the status quo and creating a deadlock against oppressors. $Power_1$ is a group of dialectics aimed at restoring agency to the marginalized, promoting mutual recognition and respect for diverse identities.

Power$_2$, conversely, encompasses a more sociological understanding of power. It relates to the social relationships that regulate the distribution of material goods, political and military power, and social and cultural hierarchies determined by class, gender, ethnicity, and age. Power$_2$ relations allow individuals to overcome others or protect their advantages by going against the hidden desires and/or genuine interests of others. Bhaskar emphasizes that power can be enabling and repressive (Scambler & Scambler, 2015). Bhaskar argues that the significance of the second power source is not that it grants agents the capacity to exercise control over the social and natural environments but to intervene causally in the world (Creaven, 2009). Power$_2$ can be used to organize and control the uneven distribution of power among human agents, limiting their autonomy and hindering their ability to thrive. The manifestations of Power$_2$ are evident in situations like colonialism, where people are subjected to governance that restricts their freedom.

As seen in Chapter 2, the workings of coloniality driven by the colonial matrix of power underscore the role of Power$_2$. The colonial matrix of power represents the nature of Power$_2$ in contemporary global health research and practice, with clear marginalization observed in practices such as helicopter research and inequitable global health publication landscape. The ongoing struggle between agents with Power$_1$ and those with Power$_2$ leads to a constant redefinition of needs and desires, shaping cultural definitions of what is necessary and consequently redefining and reshaping social structures (Scambler & Scambler, 2015). Applied to the decolonization agenda, the Global North (Power$_1$) often resists decoloniality because it challenges their historical dominance and the power structures and privileges constructed during colonialism. This resistance results in a reluctance to relinquish the control and advantages gained through colonial legacies in politics, economics, and culture. It can manifest in overt actions and subtle ideological pushback against critiques of Western-centric perspectives. On the other hand, the decolonization movement represents Power$_1$ and advocates that the formerly colonized nations break free from the colonial matrix of power and create more just and equitable societies. This power imbalance or opposing agendas perpetuates a system that prioritizes broader notions of freedom, disregarding the needs of vulnerable and marginalized individuals (including basic survival needs and those influenced by cultural perspectives). As a result, there is a yearning for freedom from these oppressive forces.

Bhaskar (2008) sought to connect his earlier conceptualization of critical realism with dialectical methods, thereby providing an ontological foundation for the dialectic concept. From the above writings, we see how Bhaskar attempts to merge his dialectical arguments with the transcendental principles that he had developed in his earlier work on basic critical realism to formulate the dialectical critical realist position (Figure 6.1).

Figure 6.1 represents Bhaskar's onto-axiological schema for absenting absences or removing ills from society to achieve justice and equity. He started by elaborating on the nature of the absence or the identified ills, such as

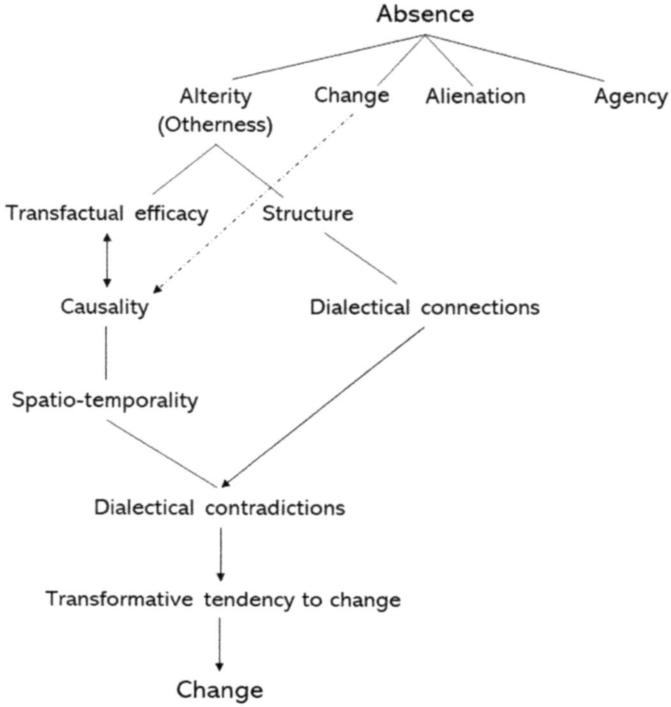

Figure 6.1 Bhaskar's proposed onto-axiological process of absenting absences.

inequities in global health practices. The agency highlights the mutual recognition and respect for identity differences that seek unity through diversity and recentralize transformative praxis, regressing against the status quo to create a stalemate against oppressors. He suggested that the absence is agentic (perpetuated and redressed through social interactions or individuals through their thoughts and actions).

By *alienation*, he suggested that absences involve some form of alienation of a group of persons based on the operations of $Power_1$ and $Power_2$. Hartwig (2007) conceptualized alienation as "separation from self," stating that it encapsulates the erosion of authentic agency and identity within a capitalist system. Alienation, according to Bhaskar (2008), is the unfair treatment of one group by another. As I understand it, Bhaskar's operationalization of alienation aligns with the agenda of decolonizing global health as it gives meaning to the marginalization of the people on the periphery by those in the center. Grounding this argument is global health decolonization would imply that alienation can be expressed through epistemic injustice whereby the knowledge of researchers from the Global South and indigenous persons are considered inferior to those of their Global North counterparts, who are most often considered the experts even in issues affecting predominantly the Global South.

By *change*, Bhaskar suggested that what is ignored matters when things change, transition, or transform; the state of absence is not static (it can be changed through actors' actions). In other words, it is possible to achieve equity, although global health practice is inequitable, and equity will be relevant in the absence of inequity. His emphasis on *alterity* as one of the ontological nature of absences illustrates that absences are a reality. By understanding the causal pathway and structures of how epistemic injustice manifests, one can start formulating dialectical contradictions (how to counter epistemic injustice) or find a better way to consider and appreciate knowledge in global health.

After establishing the ontological nature of absences, Bhaskar (2008) presented a transcendental process through which undoing these social ills or injustices (absenting these absences) can be achieved. Focused on the nature of the absences, Bhaskar suggested that one must understand their transfactual efficacy and the structures implicated in developing and sustaining the absence. He also proposes unpacking the causal processes of generating and sustaining these absences through space and time. Understanding these absences' causal processes and dialectical connections can inform the development of dialectical contradictions, a precursor for formulating a transformative pathway to change and achieving the change. For instance, considering epistemic injustice as the absence that requires absenting, Bhaskar suggests that one should start by unpacking the causal processes (underlying mechanisms), including highlighting the structures of how epistemic injustice occurs and is maintained in global health.

In grounding the arguments for merging the dialectical arguments and the critical realist philosophical position, Bhaskar (2008, p. 12) stated that "the moments of critical realism are affected by its dialectical deepening, which is also a cross-fertilization" because "they are co-present and systematically 'intermingle' in reality." Based on this premise, he formed dialectical critical realism as a way of critical realism extending its realism to cover an aspect of the concept of truth, morality, and spatio-temporality—a phenomenon in a specific location and time (Bhaskar, 2008). He captured these three constructs of dialectical critical realism in the following excerpt:

> By alethic realism [otherness], I mean to connote the reason for or truth of things as distinct from propositions (in the intransitive dimension). Moral realism specifies a first-person action-guiding relation to, in the social world, typically a set of relations that includes, but is not reducible to, actually existing moralities which may be described, redescribed, critically explained (in descriptive, re-descriptive, and explanatory critical morality), accepted or changed (reproduced or transformed). What is most distinctive about the spatio-temporal realism I will be advancing is its insistence on the reality of tense (as a spatializing process) and becoming—in the intransitive and transitive dimensions alike.
>
> (Bhaskar, 2008, p. 81)

In the above excerpt, Bhaskar synthesizes ontology and ethics, arguing that objective structures (e.g., social inequalities) and temporal processes (e.g., historical change) are real, yet humans retain agency to engage and transform them critically. This framework underpins his dialectical critical realism, aiming to bridge positivism and postmodernism.

By alethic realism (truth/otherness), Bhaskar reveals truth as the intransitive dimension (objective reality existing independently of human cognition), and "otherness" signifies the irreducible reality of entities/structures beyond our propositions (e.g., social structures, natural laws), which constrain or enable human agency. He thus meant that moral facts exist objectively in the social world but are not reducible to existing moral codes ("actually existing moralities"). In this way, moral agents can describe, critique, explain, and transform moral systems through dialectical praxis (combining theory and action).

Although Bhaskar characterizes the dialectic of freedom as a process of acting to absent constraining ills, such as inequities in global health, I think it can be extended to embrace communicative action more generally, including moral or ethical judgment. Bhaskar's statement below outlines the dialectical logic of emancipation in his critical realism philosophy, arguing that every moral judgment inherently points toward universal human flourishing:

> Insofar as an ill is unwanted, unneeded and remedial, the spatio-temporal-causal-absenting or real transformative negation of the ill presupposes universalizability to absenting agency in all dialectically similar circumstances. This presupposes, in turn, the "absenting" of all similar constraints. Moreover, by the inexorable logic of dialectical universalizability, insofar as all constraints are similar in virtue of "their being constraints", i.e., qua constraints, this presupposes the absenting of all constraints as such ... And this presupposes in its wake a society-oriented to the free development and flourishing of each and all, and of each as a condition for all, that is to say, universal autonomy as flourishing ... So, the goal of universal human autonomy is implicit in every moral judgement.
>
> (Bhaskar, 2008, p. 79)

Although Bhaskar avidly defends the need for human emancipation, which is seen through his arguments in dialectical critical realism, Norrie and Morgan noted that "For some critical theorists, it seems to be very dangerous even to talk about emancipation because, I think, this is associated with past promises that have become a part of the social process of domination under modern conditions" (Norrie & Morgan, 2021, p. 108). This expression accurately describes the situation of (de)colonization. When political decolonization was offered to the formerly colonized countries, they were promised complete independence and control over their political, economic, and religious affairs. Nevertheless, treaties and agreements were made between the formerly colonizers and their formal colonies, which continue to hold them in a state of colonization: neo-colonization (the control of less-developed countries by developed countries through indirect means). This scenario fulfills the conditions described by Norrie and Morgan; the promise of emancipation was not delivered. They insisted, nevertheless, that although there was a failure to deliver emancipation as expected, "it ought not to be allowed to stop us talking about what emancipation would mean today, and in a way that links the past struggles to ones in the present" (Norrie & Morgan, 2021, p. 108). This assertion gives credence and impetus to the decolonization movement observed in many fields, including global health. Given Bhaskar's emphasis on the enduring relevance of power dynamics—or generalized master-slave relations—in contemporary society, he could not sidestep the imperative of emancipation, and critical analysis is scarcely conceivable without this emancipatory aim at its core.

Bhaskar (2008) went further in his writing to explore within the dialectical critical realism what he noted as dialectics of master-slave, and he suggested that this relationship should be considered with a much richer and deeper conception of freedom, democracy, rights, education, health, and well-being. This position, in my opinion, sits right down the alley of coloniality, considering that, as we have seen in Chapter 4, it is scaffolded by colonialism-led power patterns. The absence at the heart of Western societies, which drives them forward through successive forms of master-slave and colonized-colonial type relations, is precisely what philosophy finds the hardest to comprehend. Indeed, it is precisely the thing, absence, in its very concept, that philosophy seeks to suppress. Bhaskar's analysis of absence is an idea of "philosophy operating in a geo-historical context that fundamentally lacks emancipation, which leads to the denial of absence—emancipation from specific constraints such as exploitation, domination, subjugation, oppression, repression, and control" (Bhaskar, 2008, p. 176). To this end, I found Bhaskar's political-moral theory a useful framework to unpack the idea of decolonizing global health.

Bhaskar's Political-Moral Theory

The desire to absent the absences is described as negation—the transformative tendency to change. Bhaskar distinguishes between three types of negation: real, transformative, and radical negation. Real negation, which signifies the absence of consciousness (the unknown), is the foundation for dialectic. Transformative and radical negation are derived from or a part of this foundation. Transformative negation involves changing something, a quality, or a situation, which entails the cessation or removal of something that already existed (Scambler & Scambler, 2015). Radical negation, on the other hand, is a specific form of transformative negation. It pertains to the self-subversion, transformation, or overcoming of a being or a state (in other words, negation as self-transformation). Bhaskar's transformational model of social action, which holds that agents do not create or produce structures from scratch but rather recreate, reproduce, and/or transform a set of pre-existing structures, places transformational negation at the center of addressing societal ills. I argue that the agenda of decolonizing global health entails understanding the sets of pre-existing structures (political and economic systems) and generative mechanisms (racism, hegemony, white supremacy saviorism, and religious propaganda) constitutes what Bhaskar will describe as transformational negation, to negate the enduring effects of colonialism in global health. In Chapter 5, I propose that these pre-existing structures can be transformed by decolonizing the mind, combating colonial amnesia, going beyond traditional mastery (global health expertise), establishing meaningful global health collaborations, valorizing local knowledge, and having a self-reliant mindset.

In critical realism, ontology is stratified and transformational (Scambler & Scambler, 2015). The stratified and transformational ontology of critical realism switches the emphasis from the levels of the empirical and actual and "event patterns" to the level of the real and the mechanisms that govern events. In this way, the characteristics of transformative negation align with Bhaskar's conceptualization of entities as existing in the realm of the "real," "actual," and "empirical" (Bhaskar, 1975). Ontologically, the process of transformative negation is synonymous with social and natural geo-history. Epistemologically, transformative negation equates to progress in philosophical and theoretical thought, particularly concerning the logic of scientific discovery. From a normative and practical perspective, this process embodies "the axiology of freedom" (Creaven, 2009). To this end, Bhaskar (2008) posits that social structure is both a necessary condition and a medium for intentional agency, essential for the reproduction or transformation of social forms.

Based on the above premise, he proposed a practical approach to transformative negation as a contribution to the traditional dialectical search for truth. To this end, from the triadic process of negation generally associated with Hegel (thesis–antithesis–synthesis), Bhaskar developed a political-moral theory using an open-ended four-stage model—prime moment (1M), second edge (2E), third level (3L), and fourth dimension (4D)—to conceptualize and generalize the transformational model of social action based on his dialectic principles (Bhaskar, 2020). MELD is a process of identifying ills and developing theories of transformations to work towards change (towards concrete utopias). So there is a movement from investigation to identify structures and mechanisms—why the thing is how it is (1M); then looking wider at interactions and what things could be like instead (to absent the absences) at a micro/meso-level (2E); then wider again to larger contexts and effects, totality, theories for change with Bhaskar's transformational model of social action, etc. to guide "completeness" (3L); then action at 4D (with critical and reflexive processing).

Dialectical critical realism involves its extension from the understanding of being as such and as structured (1M) to being as a process (2E), being as a whole (3L), and being as incorporating transformative practice through human agency (4D). He elaborated on these stages as below:

1M: We think of being as such, non-identity and structured.
2E: We think of being a process; involving absence, negativity, and change.
3L: We think of being as together, as a whole or as a totality.
4D: We think of being as incorporating transformative praxis.

Bhaskar's MELD model was a way to incorporate the complexities of power and conflict, representing dialectical critical realism as sociology, politics, and ethics. The notion of decolonizing global health is sociological, political, and ethical. Therefore, the interdisciplinarity that dialectical critical realism offers by integrating these three fields suits my agenda of exploring an approach to decolonizing global health.

Prime Moment: Knowledge of "What Is and What Is Not"

Prime moment (1M) represents the first step of Bhaskar's four-stage of transformative negation and deals with the knowledge of being—knowledge of what is and is not (Schudel, 2017). The prime moment represents the "first moment" of recognition of ontology (the state of being). It is, therefore, focused on describing the situation, usually something that must be changed (negated). 1M describes how things are, viewing them primarily ontologically by looking backward in time and "down" in terms of ontological depth to the real to describe what is. Bhaskar (2008) used "Non-identity" based on Marx's materialist dialectics and replaced the Hegelian notion of identity to describe the world into which we are "thrown"—a world into which we come to be. Non-identity is about understanding the nature of the world we find ourselves in. Non-identity, as relates to decolonizing global health, would mean understanding the colonized nature of global health, the forces undergirding the inequitable and unjust nature of global health practice, leading to the understanding that the way global health is practiced in contemporary times is informed by the relics of colonialism. Indeed, it is about acknowledging the epistemic and social injustices and health inequities pervasive in global health and what perpetuates them.

1M is about understanding "thrownness,"—the existential condition of being "thrown" into the world, meaning we are born into specific circumstances and inherit a pre-existing reality without having a choice in the matter—or "what is and what is not." 1M relates to understanding what is missing in the world in which we are, highlighting the ills that befall the world (Bhaskar, 2008). Considering global health, what is missing is equity and justice (social and epistemic) in the different aspects of global health practice, from knowledge generation to informed evidence-based practice to the distribution of human and other resources for health. Inequity and injustice are pervasive in most global health partnerships and are fueled by a lack of transparency. Asymmetry in power and funding pervades global health (Bain et al., 2024). Health inequity and social and epistemic injustice have been captured using various epidemiological studies and trace conditions. Empirical evidence shows that compared to the Global North, the Global South experiences significantly higher rates of infant mortality and poorer outcomes in life expectancy at birth, maternal health, and child health (Aginam, 2000). Global institutions such as the World Bank, World Trade Organization, and International Monetary Fund also systematically institutionalize these global health inequalities, leading to the maldistribution of power, money, and resources, establishing global coloniality (Deacon, 2015; Nare et al., 2024). This systemic critique underpins calls for decolonizing global governance and redistributing power/resources to achieve health justice (e.g., via a Global Health Equity Fund).

Bhaskar's philosophical groundwork in his critical realism suggests that to understand "what is and what is not," one is working at the level of the empirical. The understanding here is that our knowledge of "what is and what is not" is based on observations. From the multiple statistical associations emanating from quantitative and qualitative research, one can infer the existence and causal and explanatory force of mechanisms like class and command (Scambler & Scambler, 2015). For instance, qualitative studies have shown evidence of residual socio-politico-cultural effects of colonialism in postcolonial nations (Kim et al., 2017). The disparities between the Global North and Global South—adversely affect the health conditions of the world's poorer populations (Aginam, 2000). This disparity is the current nature of global health. It is NOT equitable! Figure 6.2 illustrates the nature of prime moment (1M) in decolonizing global health.

1M is about applying critical realist principles such as the layered ontology of reality, emergence, openness, and transitive/intransitive notions, retroduction, among others, meshed within the ideas of negation with fundamental values, which are often unseen or unrecognized but which inform or control action (e.g., covert power systems and alienation) to explain the change process. For instance, applying the principles of layered ontology to 1M means that absence is present not only in the "empirical" and "actual" (experiences and events) but also in the structures and mechanisms that exert power in society (Schudel, 2017). At the "actual" level, we observe limited participation of Global South experts and community representatives in the governance structures, global health journal editorial boards, and advisory bodies of organizations focusing on improving health in the Global South. At the level of the "real," these observations and events are perpetuated by the agents' struggle ($Power_1$) against successive forms of $Power_2$ relations like hegemony, racism,

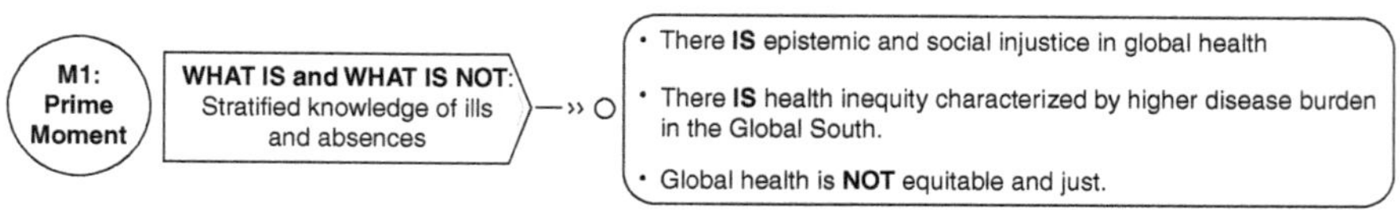

Figure 6.2 Pime moment in decolonizing global health.

white supremacy, religious paternalism, and white saviorism designed to maintain the status quo. Other conditions that could be relevant to the poor representation of experts from the Global South include greater value being attributed to the skill sets of Global North partners and little value being attached to the skill sets of Global South partners unless educated in the Global North.

Using the principles of the critical realist philosophy of science to unpack how and why an event occurs means that 1M entails knowledge of absence as a product. 1M represents knowledge of ills and power relations and the structures and mechanisms from which world events and experiences like a colonized global health emerge (Schudel, 2017). Consequently, the 1M stage is about searching for the original problems and causes that must be redressed at 2E (Alderson, 2016a). Absence also teaches us about diversity and uniqueness and allows us to explore alternative perspectives and possibilities. Recognizing the vastness of absence or non-existence reveals that our reality is a dynamic system capable of transformation. Dwelling on the challenge of colonialism, 1M focuses on uncovering coloniality and explaining, using causal principles, how decolonization occurs through time (historically) and space (geographically). 1M focuses on what is absent (equity and social justice in global health), and the awareness and explication of ills and absences move to the second edge—2E (Alderson, 2016a).

Second Edge: Knowledge of "What Could Be"

Bhaskar uses 2E as an abbreviation of the *second edge* of development. 2E stands for the absence of what is missing in our understanding to move to a new level (becoming). It, therefore, focuses on the knowledge of what could be done differently—knowledge of what could be (Schudel, 2017). 2E focused on "negativity," whereby Bhaskar radically changed Hegel's notion of negativity from a negative critique of identity to a notion highlighting a process of absenting absences in which multiple unrealized possibilities might become possible (Bhaskar, 2008). Understanding the nature of ills or absence at 1M, such as the nature of colonialism in global health, drives agents with $Power_1$ to desire to address the ill or absence, a process known as absenting. Therefore, 1M absence (event or observation) instigates the absenting process at 2E. Absenting absences requires formulating alternatives to mitigate the ills, absences, or harms and to propose transformative strategies for realizing those alternatives.

2E is the moment to propose different/alternative ways of being based on the knowledge of "what is and what is not" obtained from 1M. It is the narrowly dialectical moment in the four-staged dialectic and focuses on the very principles of indifference. It is the stage where the absence or lack of fulfillment is brought to the fore, and the yearning for change. In other words, the sources of failures (coloniality) to meet human needs should be removed to achieve equity. Dialectic equity requires that there must be grounds for difference, and if there is no such ground, then "we are rationally impelled to remove them" (Bhaskar, 2014, p. 12).

For Bhaskar, "to act is to absent," presupposing universal human emancipation. In recognizing and acting to negate the constraining ills that threaten their own "concrete singularity," actors are committed to recognizing and acting to negate the constraining ills that threaten others who share common situations and a common human-social-being-in-nature—"concrete universality" (Creaven, 2009). Regarding the decolonization of global health, 2E is concerned with the active intervention to negate coloniality that perpetuates colonial practices in global health. It entails considering decolonial measures even at a narrower level, such as engaging with indigenous groups and prioritizing local knowledge over Western theories and frameworks to conduct research in the Global South. It can also entail practical steps to pursue justice, equity, and dignity for all in global health (Prasad, 2024). Figure 6.3 displays the nature of the second edge (2E) in decolonizing global health.

In Chapter 5, I identified six counter-hegemonic processes that should be in place for global health decolonization to be achieved: which entails decolonizing the mind, combating colonial amnesia, going beyond traditional mastery (global health expertise), establishing meaningful global health collaborations, valorizing local knowledge and having a self-reliant mindset. Interventions and opportunities must be created to achieve these decolonial mindsets. These considerations require cooperative reflexivity and represent what Bhaskar describes as structure-in-process and process-in-structure.

Third Level: Knowledge of "What Should Be"

A reflective stage follows the practical 2E, the third level (3L). 3L stands for the totality—the completion of emergence into the new level. It speaks to knowledge of the implications of our choices for ourselves and others—knowledge of "what should be" (Schudel, 2017). Bhaskar adapted Hegel's concept of totality from an idealized completeness reached by rationally negating contradictions to a viewpoint that perceives totality as a complex of intra- and inter-relationships (Bhaskar, 2008). This understanding of the relationships between ourselves and others and the interacting mechanisms within society represents the core aspect of this connection in the chain, which is "totality" (Schudel, 2017). 3L, therefore, considers larger structures and totalities and entails understanding how social structures such as socio-economic, political, and international relations contribute to perpetuating neo-colonialism, for

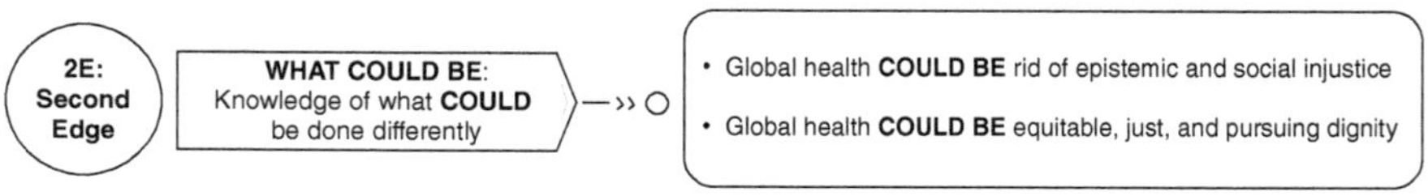

Figure 6.3 The expression of the second edge (2E) in the decolonization of global health.

example. At 3L, values and sentiments are deliberated through reflexivity to refine further the desirable absenting processes (what "should be") and reach a morally justifiable way forward. In this way, Bhaskar naturalistically grounds his moral realism and ethical naturalism, under human interactions, objectively presuppose trust, solidarity, and mutual aid (Creaven, 2009).

3L is also the level where concrete goals and visions (practical utopias) are put in place through practical wisdom *in tandem* with theory and practice to address unfairness or injustice. The role of 3L is not simply to justify the decolonization of global health but also to understand its more profound and prominent causes (entities existing in the "Real") to plan effective reforms at the global, international, and political levels and not only at the personal levels. The understanding is that there are "relationships of dependency and interdependency and their characteristic patterns of interaction and intra-action" (Schudel, 2017). This understanding lends itself to considering interventions or absences that cut across multiple socio-ecological model levels—individual, relationship, community, and societal. Decolonizing interventions to be considered at 3L include redressing political and economic reforms that negate the continuing practices and policies designed to exploit and extract from the Global South. Figure 6.4 illustrates the nature of 3L in the decolonization of global health.

Achieving emergence into the new level requires reflexivity as a corporate agency to formulate and make those choices for ourselves and others to address the "absence." Using a corporate agency to drive, command, and effect social change requires challenging higher powers (Power$_2$) and tapping into Power$_1$—the transformative capacity inherent in an agency. This level of reflexivity aligns with Archer's conceptualization of reflexivity. Archer (2007) defines "reflexivity" as the ability for creative self-mastery, which allows individuals (and indeed corporate agency) to assess their social circumstances and act purposefully within them. She thus thought of reflexivity as regular mental exercise shared by all normal people, to consider themselves concerning their (social) context and vice versa" (Archer, 2007, p. 4). She outlined four types of reflexivity that can inform the actions of individuals and groups (reflexivity as a corporate agency) to address their situation:

1) Communicative reflexives seek confirmation and approval from others before acting. This confirmation can be sought from other individuals or groups who are more experienced or knowledgeable about what the individual is reflecting on. In the case of decolonizing global health, this reflection

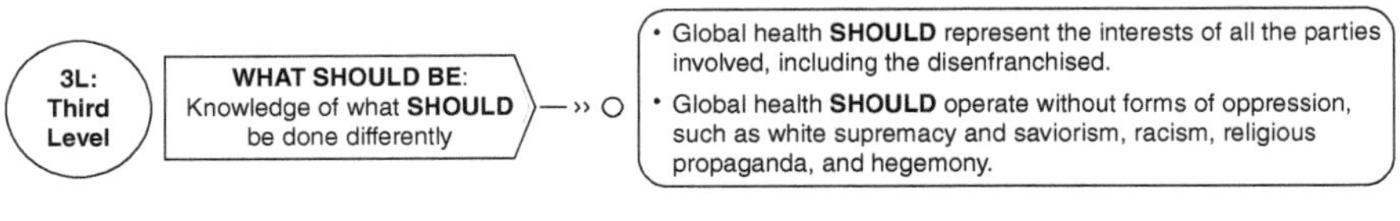

Figure 6.4 The nature of third level (3L) in the decolonization of global health.

can be with other Global South researchers or global health practitioners from the Global South.

2) Autonomous reflexives entail using internal conversations, and the individual is less inclined to seek advice from others before acting.
3) Meta-reflexives are critically reflexive about their internal conversations, the advice of others, and the value of potential actions. Meta-reflexives go beyond conforming to the norms to adopt a broader set of ideas and lifestyles—thinking outside the box.
4) Fractured reflexives are about having internal conversations that generate dissonance and distress rather than leading to purposive courses of action that benefit them. The case of internalized racism that I discussed in Chapter 4 is a great example of fractured reflexivity.

Researchers from the Global South and other stakeholders whose operations are relevant to the global health space can use these forms of reflexives to formulate concrete or practical solutions to addressing epistemic and social injustice and inequities pervasive in global health. I have discussed the role of reflexives in the process of absenting absences in global health (decolonial reflexivity) in Chapter 7 using Archer's morphogenetic approach to social change.

Fourth Dimension: Knowing "What Can Be"

The fourth dimension (4D) is the transformative agency, which focuses on the human agency to change the world practically (Bhaskar, 2008). It entails critically reflecting on achieving the desired social change and knowing what real change can be achieved in context (Schudel, 2017). Bhaskar (2008) suggests that 4D requires "active and reflexive engagement within the world in which we seek to achieve the unity of theory and practice in practice" (p. 234). With these words, Bhaskar suggests that practical actions should be taken to address the issue that needs corrective action. 4D, therefore, focuses on executing the plans formulated in 2E (micro to meso level) and 3L (macro level). Therefore, achieving 4D depends on the nature of the solutions or changes proposed in 2E and 3L. 4D is the moment to consider a context-sensitive transformative approach where the proposed change is specific to a particular individual or group and context (Hartwig, 2007). Wright (2010) calls this process a transformative strategy, which entails developing concrete or practical utopias. According to Bhaskar:

> Concrete utopianism marks out a legitimate role for visionary intellectuals, and of course for visionary funding agencies. Thinking alternatives in detail must be an important part of any vibrant democracy. Also important here would be collective concrete utopian projects, the working through together of alternative ways of satisfying the constraints (or objectives) of a household, school, medical practice, enterprise or borough.
> (Bhaskar, 2020, p. 117)

Concrete or practical utopias are more likely to be implemented than real utopias (Wright, 2010). Archer (2019) distinguishes concrete utopias from real utopias: while the latter are theoretical constructs that, despite being preferable to current social systems, remain unrealized, concrete utopias generate actionable alternatives (e.g., addressing epistemic injustice in global health by fostering Global South-led research investigations) and establish frameworks for reimagining global societal restructuring. An example of real utopia in the global health decolonization agenda would be for the Global South to strive for self-sufficiency. This real utopia has especially gained traction with the stopping aid for global health programs by the United States of America in January 2025. Self-sufficiency in global health seeks to dismantle colonial dependencies by empowering nations and communities to control their health systems. Self-sufficiency is not isolation but sovereignty—a decolonial shift from dependency to equitable partnerships. It demands dismantling extractive global systems (e.g., debt, patents) while fostering South–South collaboration and local innovation. My argument is that implementing local innovation and fostering South–South collaborations are achievable. Systemic issues such as dependency would be more challenging to address. For instance, after stopping the United States Agency for International Development funding, African countries are advancing innovative frameworks to reform health financing. For example, the Lusaka Agenda launched in 2023 emphasizes increased domestic investment in healthcare, a greater focus on health system strengthening, and improved coherence and coordination among donors (Demeshko et al., 2025). The goal is to ensure that countries take charge of their financing while maintaining continuous international support. While taking charge of financing their healthcare systems and needs is possible, what qualifies self-sufficiency as a real utopia is how challenging it would be, in practice, to dismantle the exploitative capitalistic systems enforcing dependency in the Global South.

Practical utopias at the micro–meso level will have better chances of being implemented than the macro-level interventions required to neutralize coloniality at 3L. For instance, it could be easier to improve the representation of members from the Global South on global health research committees of global health journal boards than to review economic and political reforms that dismantle the neocolonial puppet-master systems that use so-called indigenous political leaders to manipulate internal sociocultural and economic dynamics to plunder the resources of nations in the Global South continuously. Nevertheless, difficult is not impossible. The goal should be to dismantle the hegemonic and colonial foundations of international law and international relations that are currently in place through counter-hegemonic discourse. Figure 6.5 illustrates my conceptualization of 4D in the decolonization of global health. For Bhaskar, this is an essential aspect of an emancipatory project that aims to challenge the Power_2 relations that create obstacles and limit the ability of most people in the Global South to fulfill their basic needs and desires. Bhaskar's 4D can be likened to what Creaven calls the "practical agency energized by material interests." However, Bhaskar characterizes the dialectic of freedom as a process of acting to absent constraining ills.

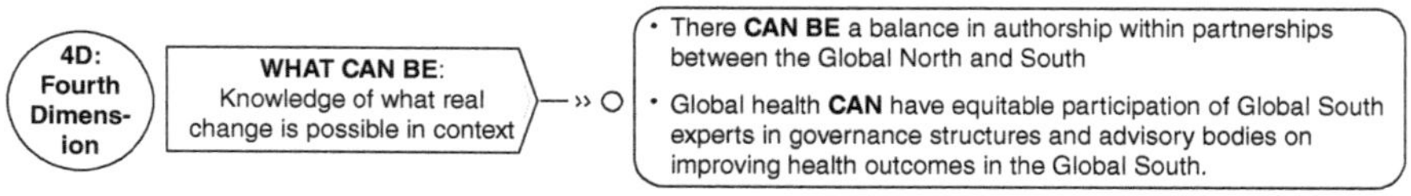

Figure 6.5 Fourth dimension (4D) in the decolonization of global health.

Political-Moral Theory of Transformative Decolonization of Global Health

In his conceptualization, Bhaskar would consider the absence of equity and justice in global health or the dominance of inequity and injustice between the Global North and the Global South an absence. I believe the notion of absenting absences also applies to correcting injustice and introducing equity in global health, for which I find the MELD model applicable. Figure 6.5 illustrates how the entire MELD model is applied to understanding the process of decolonizing global health.

The model presented in Figure 6.6 illustrates how 1M's knowledge and understanding of the global health context, including knowledge of "what is" and "what is not," provides insight into the ills that befall a system. Decolonization is an implicit process that requires challenging the socio-political status quo, moving from "what is" (1M) to "what ought to be" or "what should be" (3L). According to Bhaskar, addressing the unfairness, inequity, ills, and slavery should take an ethical/moral direction, which engages with the notion of fact (what is described based on empirical findings at 1M) and value (real possible change in the context) at 3L. I have argued earlier that the agenda of decolonizing global health is based on morality rather than responsibility, especially concerning those global health institutions that advocate for the decolonization of global health. Simply put, they are not obliged

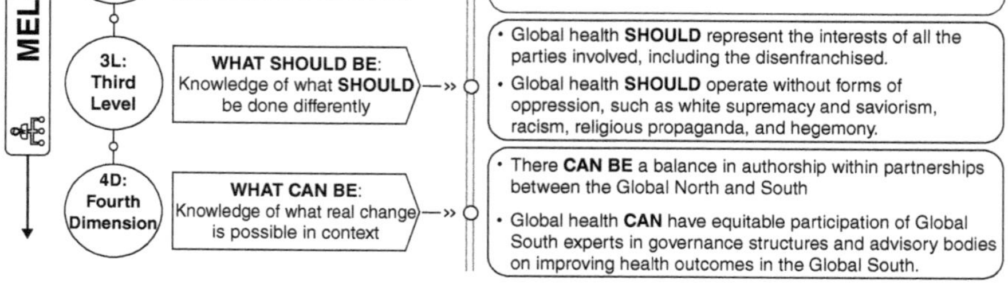

Figure 6.6 Dialectical process model of transformative decolonization of global health.

to engage in the decolonization agenda. However, they may be driven by morality, underscored by the principles of equity, the feeling of historical responsibility, and the goal of mutual benefit. While the effects of colonization on global health are factual — inequities in health outcomes—the call to decolonize global health is more on the moral/ethical side driven by decolonization moments (Opara, 2021; Pai, 2021). A moral/ethical approach to decolonizing global health is warranted because no legally enforceable mandates are compelling the Global North to support the Global South in achieving health equity. The United Nations Charter of 1945 laid the foundation for international cooperation to address economic, social, and humanitarian challenges worldwide, which drives most of the humanitarian efforts of the Global North carried out in the Global South. This framework explicitly acknowledges that the Global North assists the Global South in fostering global stability, peace, and prosperity, encompassing health concerns.

I argue that dialectical critical realism has the potential to identify the foundational history of the generative mechanisms of social phenomena such as colonization and decolonization and asks questions about how they came to be (1M). To this end, I dedicated Chapter 4 of this book to unpacking the social mechanism constituting coloniality, which continues to orchestrate inequities and injustice in global health. The chapter accentuated five social mechanisms—hegemony, (internalized) racism, religious paternalism, white saviorism, and white supremacy—as a bundle of social mechanisms perpetuating inequities and injustice in global health. Of course, these mechanisms operate in the context of larger political and economic contexts and structures. Focusing on what things could be like instead (absenting the absences) at a micro/meso level, dialectical critical realism can inform value and valuation through a continuous process in a social system with continuous feedback (inter-relational reflexivity) between "agents" (the actors or advocacy groups and decolonization movements) or between various individuals (2E and 3L). To this end, in Chapter 7 I make a case for decolonial reflexivity through Archer's morphogenetic approach. Through these reflexive ideas, exchanges, and actions, global health institutions and organizations from the Global North and South engage in continuous change and adjustment to obtain new feedback toward changing the prevalent social structures and social mechanisms (mindsets and ideologies) for achieving decolonization (4D). Considering that we unveil oppressive mechanisms operating at the causal level of reality, the social scientist is morally obligated to apply measures to negate their effects and expose them for what they are (Houston & Montgomery, 2018).

In addition to supporting efforts to unearth generative mechanisms, specifically in adopting Bhaskar's transformational model of social action, dialectical critical realism offers an explanatory framework to explore a possible transformative negation of a colonized global health practice. The transformational model of social action is a sociological framework that explains the dynamic interplay between social structures and human agency. To explore the dynamic interaction between human agency and social structures, it asserts that society shapes individuals, who, in turn, reproduce or transform societal structures through their actions over time. The premise of the transformational model of social action suggests that one can explain how colonialism through social structures such as imperialism and capitalism shaped the colonizers and colonized. This influence continued through coloniality after political decolonization. Decoloniality to achieve global health decolonization would require the reflexivity and actions of the different actors in global health. The transformational model of social action posits that social structures such as capitalism and imperialism are not merely static frameworks but are constantly being shaped and reshaped by the actions of individuals while simultaneously influencing those individuals' actions. It offers a process by which one starts by appreciating the role of the different agents with their structures ($Power_1$ or $Power_2$) and their roles in maintaining the status quo or addressing the injustices and inequities in their society.

Agents as Social Beings: Implications of the Four Planes of Social Being within MELD

Global health involves various actors, including traditional players like national health ministries and the World Health Organization (WHO), alongside newer actors such as civil society organizations, private firms, and philanthropists. Collaboration between these global health actors is fundamental to effective global health practice, requiring partnerships across various sectors and disciplines to address complex health challenges and achieve better outcomes for vulnerable populations. International collaborations are essentially the standard model for global health practice and research but continue to be underpinned by coloniality. Táíwò (2022) confirms that the main issue with decolonization discourse is its frequent failure to recognize the complexity of (Global South) agency and the diverse ways it has interacted with colonialism and its aftermath. In Bhaskar's dialectics, 4D was based on understanding how real agency and moral commitment were possible in this material world. In addition, Bhaskar and Archer put agency or the role of agents at the center of their conceptualization of social transformation. Thus, it stands to reason that the role of agents and actors should be considered in any decolonization agenda, as noted by Creaven:

> For Bhaskar, it is the dialectical interaction of agents with structural properties and/or practices on these analytically distinct planes (material transactions with nature, i.e., cooperative labor to produce subsistence; social relations between agents, i.e., as incumbents of structured "positions" and "practices" of the social system; interpersonal relations, i.e., interactions between individuals as subjects rather than as agents of positions or institutional roles; and intra-subjective relations, i.e., internal relations of the subject, such as the self-construction of personal and cultural identities), which constitute the social cube.
>
> (Creaven, 2009)

In unpacking the agency's role in decoloniality and decolonization, two agential positions are identified: that of the colonizer with coercive $Power_2$ and that of the colonized with $Power_1$. The colonized are more likely to appreciate the unfairness and injustices that they face in the hands of the colonizers than the colonized are willing to acknowledge that a colonial matrix of power underpins the injustices and inequities experienced by the colonized. Of course, my position is that of the colonized, which is the perspective Bhaskar used to develop the MELD framework, the position of the enslaved, and the position of the unjustly treated. First, in the context of decolonizing global health, all four planes of the four-planar social being can be understood through the coloniality of global health orchestrating sustained health inequities and injustices on certain groups of individuals. According to Hartwig (2015), explanations of geohistorical events (such as colonialism) can be robustly understood by prioritizing the role of the social context and the creativity that comes from agents, from people, from "below," and in a major crisis the context cracks. Therefore, the centrality of decoloniality (absenting of absences in global health) is for the benefit and emancipation of these disenfranchised individuals and groups.

Bhaskar also suggested that while his philosophy of meta-reality begins to mark out ways in which we can approach the resolution of these crises, such as the injustices and inequities that exist in global health, one should also be cognizant of the fact that human beings are concretely singularized (having individual agency), which makes them replete with differences of various sorts, but require collective action which is *necessary* to address absences of a global nature such as decolonizing global health. For instance, oppressive neoliberal global institutions are sometimes led by people originally from the Global South, while some individuals from the Global North are strong advocates for real justice in global health. For instance, I have argued that individuals from the Global South who are trained in Global North institutions and philosophies can also practice white saviorism when engaged in global health practice. To this end, Bhaskar proposes adopting a universal solidarity approach, which he defines as "the capacity that everyone has to identify or empathize with anyone else" (Bhaskar, 2020, p.119). He further explains that universal solidarity involves the notion that the other is not just something I could have been but rather that the other is indeed a part of oneself. This perspective calls for other stakeholders in the Global North to consider the goal of decolonizing global health by identifying with the Global South more radically through copresence.

Of course, copresence should be a key element in the global health decolonizing agenda as the nature of global health practice and research is collaborative, predominantly between the Global North and South. Within the social theory, copresence is the central mechanism through which micro-macro dynamics are mediated: mutual attention, emotion, and behavior (Campos-Castillo & Hitlin, 2013). Cooperations of the different identity groups in the copresence dynamic also compete for resources and power (Tverskoi et al., 2021). In decolonizing global health, copresence possesses the dynamics of cooperation and competition between the different identity groups (Global North with $Power_2$ and Global South with $Power_1$). However, when each side exercises power, they infiltrate the other side. There is not a whole division. Therefore, class positions within emergent relations between the Global North and the Global South play a crucial role in determining access to authoritative and allocative resources for researchers and other stakeholders in the Global South. One party possesses $Power_1$ while the other possesses $Power_2$ due to the power differentials established. Copresence should include making the atmosphere conducive for the disenfranchised to address the absence (in the case of global health inequalities and injustices). One form of copresence relationship that can be helpful in the decolonization of global health is allyship, which is based on the awareness of the power difference between the Global North and South. The Anti-Oppression Network (2015) defines allyship as "an active, consistent, and arduous practice of unlearning and re-evaluating, in which a person in a position of privilege and power seeks to operate in solidarity with a marginalized group." Pai et al. (2024) argue that shifting power in global health to achieve health equity and justice will require leadership by the Global South and allyship by the Global North.

Following the calls for a transformative praxis to address the absence of systemic injustice in global health practice, for example, the Global South should not only take leadership and expect allyship from the Global North but strive for self-determination to underpin their action and practice of global health. Although the call for Global South-led leadership in global health is timely, it overlooks a crucial element: the critical need for capacity building in the governance, business, politics, and economics of global health (Wiyeh & Mukumbang, 2025). In a recent publication in the Lancet, we argued against the Global South remaining at the level of allyship with the Global North as an approach to transform the inequitable and unjust situation that pervades global health practice. We argued that sustainable decolonization extends beyond technical public and global health skills but requires empowered Global South leaders who can effectively navigate the interdisciplinary complexities of the global health landscape (Wiyeh & Mukumbang, 2025). These leaders should be able to leverage available local governance tools to protect national autonomy and advance prioritized health outcomes for their nations. Strengthening these leaders' capacities enables them to negotiate favorable terms with external partners and allows for the prioritization of local development goals. Unfortunately, current Global Health training programs often fall short, leaving future leaders ill-equipped to confront entrenched power structures.

Conclusion

Epistemic relations are informed by critical realist thinking tools such as concrete utopianism transformative praxis. The facts of colonization's broader social, economic, cultural, political, and global health effects have been established. Redressing the social situation of colonial relics still operating in global health provides grounds for a critique of colonialism and exploring an ethical and political case for decolonizing Global Health. According to Connelly (2001), "The ethical and political aspects of the analysis of a social situation [colonization and decolonization] are also seen as centrally relevant in understanding generative mechanisms, and in any subsequent planning, implementation, and interpretation of interventions for change." Bhaskar's MELD model was a practical philosophical proposition to unpack the transformative process of moving from global health colonization to decolonization of global health.

Dialectical critical realism provides a robust framework for sustainable social inequity problem solving and not just to offer practical solutions. Of course, some suggested actions achieved through the MELD model might not be easy to implement in every situation because we live in an open and complex social world. As illustrated using the MELD model, unpacking the root cause of the problem, and engaging in discussion on what should be provided a robust approach to consider utopias that could lead to better decolonization outcomes. For real decolonization of global health, besides concrete utopianism, we need a transition theory and its conditions to be satisfied, which will often include (at the political level) a movement or party that will embrace it. In Chapter 7, I explore Margaret Archer's social morphogenesis as the theory of the transition from a global health underpinned by colonial relics to an equitable and just global health.

References

Aginam, O. (2000). Global village, divided world: South-North gap and global health global village. *Indiana Journal of Global Legal Studies*, 7(2), 10.

Alderson, P. (2013). *Childhoods real and imagined, vol. 1*. Routledge.

Alderson, P. (2016a). The philosophy of critical realism and childhood studies. *Global Studies of Childhood*, 6(2), 199–210. https://doi.org/10.1177/2043610616647640

Alderson, P. (2016b). *The politics of childhoods real and imagined: Practical application of critical realism and childhood studies*. Routledge.

Anti-Oppression Network. (2015). Allyship. https://theantioppressionnetwork.com/allyship.

Archer, M. S. (2007). *Making our way through the world*. Cambridge University Press.

Archer, M. S. (2019). Critical realism and concrete utopias. *Journal of Critical Realism*, 18(3), 239–257. https://doi.org/10.1080/14767430.2019.1619428

Bagley, C., Sawyerr, A., Abubaker, M., Bagley, C., Sawyerr, A., & Abubaker, M. (2016). Dialectic critical realism: Grounded values and reflexivity in social science research. *Advances in Applied Sociology*, 6(12), 400–419. https://doi.org/10.4236/AASOCI.2016.612030

Bain, L. E., Adeagbo, O. A., Avoka, C. K., Amu, H., Memiah, P., & Ebuenyi, I. D. (2024). Identifying the conundrums of "global health" in the Global North and Global South: a case for Sub-Saharan Africa. *Frontiers in Public Health*, 12, 1168505.

Bhaskar, R. (1975). Forms of realism. *Philosophica*, 15(1), 99–127.

Bhaskar, R. (2008). *Dialectic: The pulse of freedom*. Routledge. https://doi.org/10.4324/9780203892633

Bhaskar, R. (2014). *The possibility of naturalism: A philosophical critique of the contemporary human sciences* (4th ed.). Routledge.

Bhaskar, R. (2020). Critical realism and the ontology of persons. *Journal of Critical Realism*, 19(2), 113–120. https://doi.org/10.1080/14767430.2020.1734736
Campos-Castillo, C., & Hitlin, S. (2013). Copresence: Revisiting a building block for social interaction theories. *Sociological Theory*, 31(2), 168–192. https://doi.org/10.1177/0735275113489811
Connelly, J. (2001). Critical realism and health promotion: effective practice needs an effective theory. *Health Education Research*, 16(2), 115–120. https://doi.org/10.1093/her/16.2.115
Creaven, S. (2001). *Marxism and realism: A materialistic application of realism in the social sciences*. Routledge.
Creaven, S. (2009). *Emergentist Marxism: Dialectical philosophy and social theory*. Routledge.
Deacon, B. (2015). After "08": Social policy and the global financial crisis. In S. McBride & R. Mahon (Eds.), *The ILO and social protection policy after the global financial crisis* (pp. 101–120). University of British Colombia Press.
Demeshko, A., Drake, T., & Yakhelef, N. (2025). A new era for global health: Can African countries agree a new compact with external donors? www.cgdev.org/publication/new-era-global-health-can-african-countries-agree-new-compact-external-donors
Gasparyan, D. (2023). False contradiction: a critique of Immanuel Kant's transcendental dialectic in the Kantian thought of Valentin Asmus. *Studies in East European Thought*, 75(4), 613–628.
Hartwig, M. (2001). Creaven, Marxism, and realism. www.criticalrealism.com/archive/mhartwig_cmr.html
Hartwig, M. (2007). *Dictionary of critical realism*. Routledge.
Hartwig, M. (2015). From the anatomy of the global crisis to the ontology of human flourishing. *Journal of Critical Realism*, 14(3), 227–237. https://doi.org/10.1179/1476743015Z.00000000069
Houston, S., & Montgomery, L. (2018). Learning to absent the absent: Critical realism and social work education. In M. Kjørstad & M.-B. Solem (Eds.), *Critical realism for welfare professions* (pp. 57–74). Routledge. https://doi.org/10.4324/9781315517537
Kant, I. (1933). *Critique of pure reason* (N. K. Smith, Ed.). Macmillan and Co. https://archive.org/details/critickpurereas00haywgoog
Kim, J. U., Oleribe, O., Njie, R., & Taylor-Robinson, S. D. (2017). A time for new north–south relationships in global health. *International Journal of General Medicine*, 10, 401. https://doi.org/10.2147/IJGM.S146475
Maybee, J. E. (2016). Hegel's dialectics. Stanford Encyclopedia of Philosophy. https://plato.stanford.edu/ENTRIES/hegel-dialectics/
Nare, M., Moopi, P., & Nyambi, O. (2024). Global coloniality and ecological injustice in Imbolo Mbue's *How Beautiful We Were* (2021). *Journal of Black Studies*, 55(4), 349–372. https://doi.org/10.1177/00219347241238445
Norrie, A. (2010). *Dialectic and difference: Dialectical critical realism and the grounds of justice*. Routledge.
Norrie, A. (2024). Dialectical critical realism, complexity and the psychology of blame. *Journal for the Theory of Social Behaviour*. https://doi.org/10.1111/jtsb.12411
Norrie, A., & Morgan, J. (2021). Realism, dialectic, justice and law: an interview with Alan Norrie. *Journal of Critical Realism*, 20(1), 98–122. https://doi.org/10.1080/14767430.2021.1881274
Opara, I. N. (2021). It's time to decolonize the decolonization movement. https://speakingofmedicine.plos.org/2021/07/29/its-time-to-decolonize-the-decolonization-movement/
Oti, S. O. (2024). Towards authentic institutional allyship by global health funders. *PLOS Global Public Health*, 4(3), e0003024. https://doi.org/10.1371/JOURNAL.PGPH.0003024

Overend, T. (2020, November 20). Immanuel Kant and the origin of the dialectic. *The Fortnightly Review*. https://fortnightlyreview.co.uk/2020/11/immanuel-kant-origin-dialectic/

Pai, M. (2021). Decolonizing global health: A moment to reflect on a movement. www.forbes.com/sites/madhukarpai/2021/07/22/decolonizing-global-health-a-moment-to-reflect-on-a-movement/?sh=5887aaed5386

Pai, M., Bandara, S., & Kyobutungi, C. (2024). Shifting power in global health will require leadership by the Global South and allyship by the Global North. *The Lancet*, 404(10464), 1711–1713. https://doi.org/10.1016/S0140-6736(24)02323-7

Panovski, A. (2024). What is Hegel's dialectic method? www.thecollector.com/hegel-dialectic-method.

Prasad, A. (2024). Ngozi Erondu: pursuing justice, equity, and dignity in global health. *The Lancet*, 403(10429), 799. https://doi.org/10.1016/S0140-6736(24)00361-1

Sayer, A. (2012). Power, causality and normativity: A critical realist critique of Foucault. *Journal of Political Power*, 5(2), 179–194. https://doi.org/10.1080/2158379X.2012.698898

Scambler, G., & Scambler, S. (2015). Theorizing health inequalities: The untapped potential of dialectical critical realism. *Social Theory and Health*, 13(3–4), 340–354. https://doi.org/10.1057/sth.2015.14

Schudel, I. J. (2017). Modelling dialectical processes in environmental learning: An elaboration of Roy Bhaskar's onto-axiological chain. *Journal of Critical Realism*, 16(2), 163–183. https://doi.org/10.1080/14767430.2017.1288061

Táíwò, O. (2022). *Against decolonisation: Taking African agency seriously*. Hurst & Company.

Tangcharoensathien, V., Cetthakrikul, N., Lekagu, A., Ontong, S., Suphanchaimat, R., & Patcharanarumol, W. (2023). Global health inequities: a call for papers. *Bulletin of the World Health Organization*, 101(4), 230. https://doi.org/10.2471/BLT.23.289906

Tinsley, M. (2021). Towards a postcolonial critical realism. *Critical Sociology*, 48(2). https://doi.org/10.1177/08969205211003962

Tverskoi, D., Senthilnathan, A., & Gavrilets, S. (2021). The dynamics of cooperation, power, and inequality in a group-structured society. *Scientific Reports*, 11(1), 1–16. https://doi.org/10.1038/s41598-021-97863-7

Wiyeh, A. B., & Mukumbang, F. C. (2025). Global South leaders should strengthen strategic capacity. *The Lancet*, 405(10475), 297. https://doi.org/10.1016/S0140-6736(24)02637-0

Wright, E. O. (2010). *Envisioning real utopias*. Verso.

7 Social Morphogenesis and Decolonial Reflexivity

Introduction

In the preceding chapter, Bhaskar's dialectical critical realism was used to develop a transformational global health decolonization model. Dialectical critical realism offered an opportunity to explore how dialectics can be used to contemplate social action to achieve justice and equity in global health practice. Following Bhaskar's planar social being (MELD), I explored the possibility of moving beyond current practical and theoretical approaches to decolonizing global health under consideration. The abstract nature of dialectical critical realism is informed by its sophisticated causality based on its understanding of an in-depth ontology of structures and generative mechanisms, causal tendencies in open systems, and the reasoning of agents as causes in structures (Norrie, 2024). Consequently, dialectical critical realism was more useful in providing a framework and laying a theoretical foundation for the complexity of structural conditioning and social reproduction/transformation.

Thus far, I have focused on the transcendental component of understanding how colonization was achieved and maintained through coloniality (Chapter 4) and the decolonial process toward decolonizing global health practice and research (Chapter 5). Equally important but missing is unpacking how the decolonization of global health can be achieved through space and time—spatio-temporality—from colonization to decolonization through coloniality and decoloniality. Transcendentally, I considered Sayer's conceptualization of generative causality to identify five generative mechanisms hypothesized to underpin coloniality, thus maintaining the colonization of global health (Chapter 4). I also identified possible ideologies and mindsets (mechanisms) that can drive the decoloniality agenda towards a possible concrete utopia (goal) to decolonize global health (Chapter 5). I am not saying that Bhaskar did not consider temporality in his conceptualization of critical realism. Indeed, the spatio-temporality was important when Bhaskar developed dialectical critical realism. He engaged in truth, morality, and spatio-temporality to offer the notions of specific location and time through the MELD schema (Bhaskar, 2008). For temporality, nevertheless, I found that the social morphogenetic

DOI: 10.4324/9781032700786-7

framework proposed by Margaret S. Archer (1943–2023) provides a more robust metatheoretical underlaboring to develop a theoretical understanding and practical possibilities of the transition process from the current colonized status of global health currently to a decolonized global health (concrete utopia).

Social morphogenesis is Archer's most telling contribution to developing critical realism (Archer & Morgan, 2020), addressing key debates surrounding structure, agency, and culture and how they contribute to social change. She developed social morphogenesis to critique Giddens's (1979) structuration theory, which analytically conflates structure and agency. According to Archer (2010), Giddens' structuration theory is problematic because it overly emphasizes the "duality of structure," essentially claiming that social structures are constantly being created and reproduced through individual actions to the point where it underestimates the capacity of structures to constrain individual agency and potentially resist change. Archer (2010) argues that Giddens's theory "over-socializes" actors by implying they are completely embedded within and shaped by social structures, neglecting their ability to shape those structures actively. She argued that while structures and agency are interwoven or even interdependent, they should be analytically separated; otherwise, the constraining features of structure over agency fall flat (and vice versa: the potential for change is not there).

Following the macro-level engagement in the financial system, Archer (1995) established that social morphogenesis proffers a fresh perspective for understanding society, program evaluation, and international relations through the morphostatic/morphogenetic framework and analytic framework of structure, agency, and culture—SAC (Van Belle et al., 2023). These frameworks provided relevant resources for critiquing post-structuralist and postmodernist thoughts, offering the potential for a new approach to social investigations to understand the nature and relationships between structure, agency, and culture. Archer explained that the morphostatic/morphogenetic framework "is an explanatory framework, which complements the realist philosophy of science and furnishes specialized practitioners with guidelines for explaining the problems they have in hand" (Archer & Morgan, 2020, p. 183). This chapter explores the potential contribution of social morphogenesis to explain how global decolonization can be achieved.

In the first part of this chapter, I describe the morphostatic/morphogenetic framework of social morphogenesis and its role in understanding the nature and relationships between structure, agency, and culture. In the second part of the chapter, I apply Archer's structure, agency, and culture explanatory framework and framework to unpack the social process of colonization and a potential concrete utopia toward decolonizing global health. Specifically, I focus on Archer's four modes of reflexivity: communicative reflexives, which seek consensus; autonomous reflexives, which prioritize outcomes; meta-reflexives, which emphasize values; and fractured reflexives, which are non- or dis-oriented. I argue that the decolonization of global health can be achieved through subjective powers of reflexivity, which can mediate the colonial matrix of power, invigorating the colonization of global health. To ground my argument of moving from a colonized global health to a decolonized one, I focused on the inter-relational reflexivity.

Morphogenetic Principles and Postcolonial Critical Realism

Archer (1995, 2020) drew inspiration from the biological concept of morphogenesis, describing the transformation and differentiation of cells into tissues and organs with distinct structures and functions to formulate what she described as "Social Morphogenesis." According to Archer (2013), it is only possible to theorize about (radical) social transformation, such as achieving equity and justice in global health, by examining how humans constitute society and the social formation of human agents. On this premise, it is safe to assume that Bhaskar's articulation of what he calls the "transformational model of social action" underpins Archer's (1995) morphogenetic model. Since the concept of social morphogenesis began, its adoption to explain how society and social (sub) systems work has received attention in many fields, such as economics, social work, education, information systems, etc. Archer (2021) used the social morphogenetic approach to explain the current state of our society, including the role of the COVID-19 pandemic. She used the morphogenic framework to explain current societal fragmentation, highlighting how the synergy between globalized capitalism and digital science innovations, starting around 1980, creates divergent pulls on social order. Maccarini (2019) also adopted it to understand the transition to new forms of social order in the global world. Horrocks (2009) also applied the morphogenetic approach to a longitudinal case study of information systems development and organizational change in British local government. The three examples illustrate the morphogenic framework's potential to explain social transformation, thus giving me the impetus to consider it to explore the plausibility of global health decolonization.

There is a shared understanding among critical realists such as Archer (2013), Danermark et al. (2019), and Sayer (2000) that for any process to merit consideration as a generator of social change, it must incorporate structured human relations (context-dependence), human action (activity-dependence), and human ideas—concept-dependence (Archer, 2013; Danermark et al., 2019; Sayer, 2000). According to Archer (2020), these three dimensions make social theorizing non-naturalistic owing to the focus on the interactions between structure, agency, and culture. Social structures and cultural systems are operationalized as entities with causal powers that agents may try to use to change themselves, their situation, and others (Archer, 1995). Social and cultural structures make agency possible and can include material resources, such as money, cultural ideas, patriarchy, and systems like the global healthcare system. Structure also includes roles or positions, practices, recourses, and processes. Structure limits (constraints) and is not deterministic; it is a human interaction influenced by human culture and relationships that instigates change. At a certain point in time, through agential interactions and actions, the structure might be transformed or modified (Danermark et al., 2019). This conceptualization forms the basis of Archer's morphogenetic approach.

Culture and agency are linked to ideas, beliefs (norms), and reasoning. For societal change, "agency" is the property of humans, whether they represent themselves as individuals or as collectives such as organizations or governments (Elder-Vass 2008). While agency represents individual reasons for action or non-action following reflexivity (however influenced by relations), culture reflects collective agreements that may sit at an institutional or wider organizational level (de Souza, 2014). According to Archer (2013), culture and structure have converged in ways that promote morphogenesis. Culture (ideas realm) actively contributes to restructuring social systems. Archer (2013) posits that changes in culture amplify changes in structure and vice versa through a process marked by positive feedback—one does not precede the other. They are mutually constitutive. This phenomenon highlights a new dialectic and synergy between structure and culture. Therefore, from a bird's eye perspective, agency must make gains in structure (and culture) for social transformation to occur.

Political systems and their operations are important for (de)colonizing global health. Political systems and their capitalistic nature with imperialist agendas constituted the social structures that governed how those in the colonized countries acted (agency) and influenced how they reorganized themselves (culture). While capitalism is considered the stronger motive for political colonization, Nkrumah (1965), the former president of Ghana, suggested that imperialism was the greatest driver of neo-colonialism—establishing and heightening the operation of coloniality. According to Nkrumah (1965), the colonizers' political policy and economic systems influenced the colonized nations' socio-economic practices. Galtung's (1967) definition of political colonialism helps us understand the structural role of political systems in perpetuating colonialism in all its forms. Galtung defined political colonialism as a process whereby the center of gravity of a nation is no longer in that nation itself but in some other nation, the colonizer.

Edward Said's *Orientalism* (1977) and *Culture and Imperialism* (1993) illustrate the roles of orientalism, culture, and imperialism in perpetuating colonialism. He argued that culture and imperialism are intertwined and mutually reinforcing. Said argues that Western scholarship and cultural productions, often termed "Orientalism," are not merely objective accounts of the East but rather are deeply rooted in and serve to legitimize imperialist power relations (Said, 1977). He also argues that culture is not a neutral space but is shaped by and, in turn, shapes political and economic contexts. Said expands this analysis, arguing that culture, including literature, art, and popular representations, actively participates in the project of imperialism (Said, 1993).

He examines how cultural productions can be used to justify, perpetuate, or even resist imperial rule.

Using the gravitational metaphor, characterizing political and cultural systems means that the external political system influences what happens and the events in the colonized countries. This metaphor represents the nature of global health practices today, especially on research agendas concerning the provenance of funding opportunities, which is the social structure/institutionalization of the knowledge ecosystem. The system of funding research is institutionalized in the Global North and is now considered a cultural practice. As I and other authors have discussed, because most funding for global health research and practice comes from the Global North and organizations such as the Centers for Disease Control and Prevention and philanthropical structures such as the Bill & Melinda Gates Foundation, there is a propensity for these systems to dictate research and global health agendas and activities in the Global South. Through the cultural practice of research grants, these nations determine the research project's focus, what methodologies should be applied, what philosophical and theoretical frameworks should guide the research, etc. In this way, the conditions under which the grant was obtained become the cultural system guiding how the research is conducted in the Global South without much input from the local scientists.

The Morphogenetic Cycle and Decolonizing Global Health

Following the understanding that social change such as (de)colonization occurs because of the interaction between structure, culture, and agency, Archer further developed this interaction through time, thus introducing the notion of temporality. She explained that structure, culture, and agency operate diachronically over different periods and that structure (and culture) necessarily must predate or precede the action(s) that transform it. The existing structure also exerts systematic causal effects on subsequent action (Archer, 1995). On a larger scale, the structures change because of the activities and choices of the historically situated individuals. Regarding our understanding of decolonization, my starting point will be the colonized status of global health. The colonized status of global health must predate any goals and actions to decolonize global health, and the decolonization of global health can occur after the actions of the relevant stakeholders are taken to decolonize global health. There is some fluidity between the two, as decolonizing global health will be a long-term process.

Archer argued that while temporality is a flow to time and a historicity to reality, it also provides analytical value, so she decided to break up temporality into three temporal sequences of phases: T1 to T4 (Figure 7.1). She ascribed the terms existent conditioning, interaction, and elaboration to the three phases chronologically. T1 represents the situation (colonized state of global health). Archer's phase T1 relates to Bhaskar's prime moment (1M) in his MELD approach to transformative negation. In Bhaskar's 1M, the focus is on

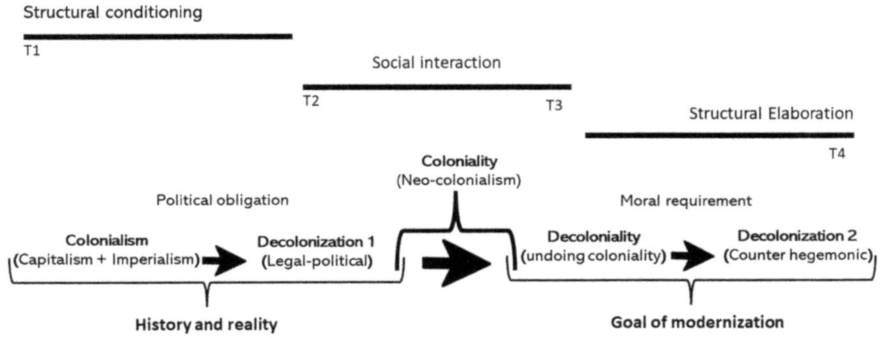

Figure 7.1 The basic morphogenetic diagram juxtaposed on decolonizing global health.

describing the situation (usually oppression, injustice, and inequity) that must be changed (negated). T1–T2 represents the prior structural context that conditioned social interaction. The T2–T3 period represents the thoughts, interactions, and actions of different actors or interest holders in the transformation of the existent social conditioning (colonized global health). This phase answers questions of who did what, with or against whom. T4 is thus the morphostatic or morphogenic state, which enables social interaction and thus becomes the new T1 of the next morphostatic/morphogenetic cycle. Archer and Morgan (2020) explained that at T4, something radical happens to structure and agency. This assertion suggests that there will be a radical disjuncture. Baumgartner and Jones (1991) explained that policies go through long periods of stability and short periods of dramatic reversals. However, it might also be the case that change follows an incremental path. Lindblom (1959) argued that "muddling through" is a more practical approach in complex policy environments where complete information and perfect solutions are often unattainable.

Morphogenesis directs us to think systematically about what occurs in time (Archer, 1995, 2020). Significance is therefore given to the timeframe in which structure, agency, and culture emerge, interact, and redefine each other, constituting the foundation of the explanatory format used to account for any significant change in the social structure (Archer, 2020; Archer & Morgan, 2020). Temporality in the morphogenic cycle is represented in the following chronological sequence of phases: structural conditioning → social interaction → structural elaboration, demarked by time frames illustrated as T1 to T4 (Archer & Morgan, 2020). The idea that structures are adapted and changed by individuals and collectives (social movements) actively interacting and operating within these structures (and processes imbued within them) corresponds to her "social interaction" and "structural elaboration" phases of morphogenesis.

The concept of socio-spatiality, which Bhaskar considered central to social transformation, is critical to understanding how morphogenesis unfolds. Jessop et al. (2008) acknowledged socio-spatiality's polymorphic nature—the organization of socio-spatial relations in various forms. In their socio-spatial theory, they propose that territories (T), places (P), scales (S), and networks (N) should be understood as mutually constitutive and interrelated dimensions of socio-spatial relations. Socio-spatiality, therefore, relates to how the environment (physical and otherwise) interacts with social structures, people, and societies (agency). Likewise, the built environment and existing social structures also impact how processes develop and social transformation occurs. The constructed environment is influenced by the social, cultural, economic, and political processes of the people who utilize it. In the context of colonialism, socio-spatiality relates to the interactions in time and space between colonizers and the colonized. In concrete terms, socio-spatiality relates to how long the colonial relationship existed and the nature of the colonial relationship. Space and the political organization of space are an expression of social relationships (Soja, 1980). Having the colonization rhetoric as a guiding discourse, socio-spatiality in the global health decolonization argument must be considered by viewing the world as a nation–states and ordering them along epidemiological, geographical, and development lines—the Global North and Global South divide. With this conceptualization in mind, socio-spatiality in global health addresses the long-standing power imbalances established during the colonial era, which continue to underpin global health practice and research across institutions through Global North-South cooperations. Socio-spatiality in the global health decolonization discourse thus speaks to engaging with the social, cultural, economic, and political processes that contribute to sustaining health equity and injustice in global health and how these structures and processes can be dismantled to achieve better and equitable global health outcomes.

Archer said the following conditions are necessary for understanding the application of socio-temporality: (i) there are internal and necessary relations within and between social structures; (ii) causal influences are exerted by social structure(s) on social interaction; (iii) there are causal relationships between groups and individuals at the level of social interaction; (iv) social interaction elaborates upon the composition of social structure(s) (Archer, 1995, p. 168). The implications of these underlying principles to the decolonization of global health based on the social morphogenic theory are as follows:

1) The decolonization project must be systematic, that is, the process of dismantling colonial power structures and ideologies needs to be comprehensive and address all aspects of the system, including political, economic, social, and cultural elements, rather than just focusing on isolated changes or superficial actions; it requires a deliberate and coordinated approach to uprooting deeply ingrained colonial legacies across all levels of society.
2) Global health structures can dictate how interest holders act or perceive their roles. For example, funding bodies can control how global health research from the Global North engages and collaborates with the Global

South through the grant guidelines. Like most US National Institute of Health, grant guidelines typically limit the funding allocated towards building construction in the Global South, with a standard percentage often falling around 8% or less, depending on the specific project and research institute involved.

3) The interactions and engagement between the different actors can be harnessed to inform the process of global health decolonization, as these different agents have the agency to change or modify the nature of existing global health structures.
4) Global health decolonization can be achieved through collaborations between different global health organizational structures. For instance, global health departments have been advocating for granting bodies such as the National Institute of Health to change grant conditions that seem to enforce colonial practices. Decolonization should occur not only in global health as it is practiced but also in how the actors and interest holders think and act within the space.

While the importance of temporality may appear obvious, failure to properly incorporate it is a significant issue in social theory and applications. Considering the proper representation of temporality to understand social change, I juxtapose Archer's temporality for social morphogenesis with my conceptualization of how decolonization can be achieved as the desired social change (Figure 7.2).

The morphostatic/morphogenetic temporality model suggests that a structure needs to exist first since a human cannot change or maintain something that does not exist (Danermark et al., 2019). Figure 7.2 illustrates structural conditioning as a state of coloniality where individuals as part of institutions (agency), as well as the institutions themselves (structure), produce, reproduce, maintain, and benefit from intersectional systems of oppression within a colonial framework is necessary for decolonization to be realized. Power is fundamental to colonialism, neo-colonialism, and coloniality. Social interactions

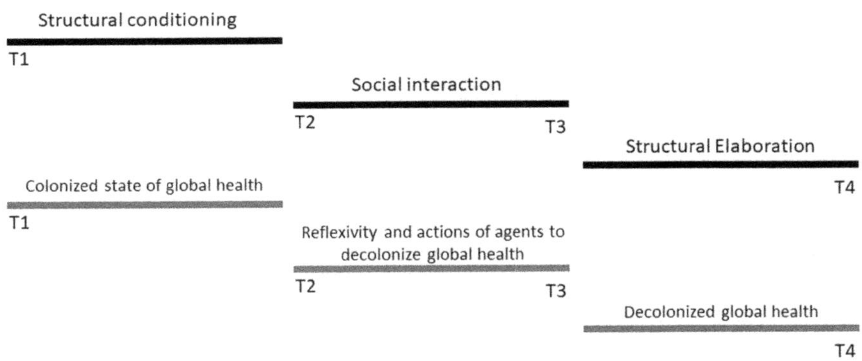

Figure 7.2 The M/M temporality model and the decolonization of global health.

(relations amongst the relevant population) in light of decolonizing global health, therefore, relate to how the Global North should engage in divesting from power-hoarding and ceding power and privilege to allow Indigenous and the Global South to thrive. Power shifting would require a fundamental existential shift in consciousness, imagination, decision-making, and politics that sets the Global North free from its addiction to power and the systems established to preserve the position of power in the global health epistemic hierarchy. Such social interactions must strive to reverse or neutralize the power structures that formulated, perpetuated, and maintained coloniality. Therefore, social interactions geared towards decoloniality must involve adopting counter-hegemonic and equity-based praxis to challenge the colonial matrix of power. According to Opara (2021), social interactions toward decolonization must be intersectional, engaging interdependent systems of oppression and violence in global health's structural, interpersonal, and internalized dynamics.

To put the morphostatic/morphogenetic theoretical framework in the perspective of decolonizing global health, let us consider the inequity in global health research between the Global North and the Global South. The Commission on Health Research and Development identified and reported on what they called the 10–90 disequilibrium, meaning that only 10% of funding is allocated to researching health problems that affect 90% of the world's people who predominantly live in the Global South (Bryant et al., 1996). I present three structural conditions contributing to the observed inequity in global health research. Owing to political colonization, a structured distribution of resources favored the former colonizers. To this end, the Global North is well equipped with better research facilities, institutions, resources, and well-trained researchers to research the diseases affecting their populations, although they have well-established health systems and policies enforcing disease treatment and prevention. The Global North also gained a competitive advantage over nations of the Global South as colonialism allowed them to exploit the colonized nations' local populations as research subjects (this has been discussed in greater detail in Chapter 1 on the historical foundation of global health).

Conversely, with poorly developed and weak health systems, the Global South has fewer disease prevention programs, so these regions' disease burdens tend to be higher. In this way, their disease burden is higher, but they are also ill-equipped to research and generate knowledge and evidence to address the high burdens of disease affecting their populations. Secondly, the suboptimal interest of the Global North in conducting research that addresses the problems of the majority living in low- and middle-income countries is driven by capitalism and ideologies like racism and imperialist agendas. For instance, Big pharma typically invests in diseases they know require a cure, such as cancers, which yield substantial economic benefits. This assertion is supported by all the top ten oncology drugs selling well, recording over $1 billion in sales yearly.

Consequently, pharma is gearing up to usher in the next generation of cancer treatments that are smarter, more targeted, and potentially more curative than ever before, which also means more lucrative. Another reason why the Global North is likely to focus research efforts and resources on a particular disease is that there is a potential that they are likely to be affected if disease incidence is not curbed. For instance, Laxminarayan (2024) noted that each year, the Global Fund to Fight AIDS, Tuberculosis, and Malaria allocates nearly US$5 billion to provide access to treatment for these diseases in the Global South. Together, these three diseases account for approximately 2.8 million deaths annually, a figure that is less than half the number of deaths caused by bacterial infections other than tuberculosis in the Global South. This status of inequity in global health research and associated structures represents T1 on Archer's morphogenic framework (structural condition). More of the structural condition in global health is unpacked in Chapter 2.

Based on the morphogenetic framework, phase T2–T3 is focused on the period when different actors or stakeholders take action to address inequities in global health research. The goal of actors and stakeholders operating in phases T2–T3 will be to address the global health research inequities. Previous attempts to address this inequity aimed to promote need-based funding in research failed because of underfunding (Weisz, 2020). An alternative approach that has been proposed by Pandey and Adhikari (2023) is to create a global health research fund for under-researched diseases that primarily affect the Global South but are often unbound by borders. They contend that this kind of fund, like the COVID-19 pandemic fund, can motivate other countries, especially from the Global North, to commit more research resources. Pandey and Adhikari (2023) proposed that a technical advisory group can be appointed to guide a governing board in the equitable distribution of research resources. Some factors to consider for equitable research funds distribution include the burden of disease, future need, health security, resilience, value for money, and potential for scientific yield, amongst others (Labonte & Spiegel, 2003).

An important consideration in the phase of social interactions is that the stakeholders and actors involved in transforming the inequitable state of global health research operate within different structures (or institutions) with different agendas. These structures or institutions guide their actions as they are meant to represent the interests of these institutions. Therefore, for the idea of a global health research fund to succeed, all the organizations and institutions that represent it must first agree that there is inequity in global health research, and secondly, they should be willing to work towards addressing it. If these two conditions are fulfilled, policies and programs can be designed and implemented to contribute to the global health research fund.

The last phase of the morphostatic/morphogenetic framework, structural elaboration, represents the change from the inequitable state of global health research to one where research agendas are considered equitably. The fund is anticipated to strengthen research capacity in the Global South by supporting local researchers and establishing a more sustainable research infrastructure (Pandey & Adhikari, 2023). This approach would generate contextually relevant evidence, reduce dependence on foreign research ecosystems, and promote epistemic agency within the Global South. Figure 7.3 represents the application of the morphostatic/morphogenetic framework to capture the process of changing the state of global health inequity characterized by the equitable distribution of research funds based on global health and epistemic justice.

Critical realists who regard critical realism as a form of neo-Marxism argue that agents' beliefs are caused by colonial structures (embedded in coloniality) and that this, in turn, causes agents' behavior to be conformist, leading to the sustainment of colonialism (Cruickshank, 2010). This point of view suggests a relationship of functional necessity between colonial structures and agents' misconceptions of colonialism, thus leading to its sustainment. Archer argues that structures are activity-dependent, meaning that structures were created by the activities and actions of agents in the past. According to Archer (1995), agents in the past organized and constructed the various structures—social, economic, cultural, and political systems—that make up our modern society. This understanding is undoubtedly true for colonialism. The colonization of most African nations, also known as the scramble for Africa, was a concerted effort by leaders of Europe between the 1880s and 1914. During this time, European countries used diplomatic pressure, aggressive economic enticement, religious propaganda, and military invasions to gain control of Africa. These structures have shaped global health practice in our modern society, causing health inequities and injustice through unseen causal entities.

The structures that emerged from the activities of agents now possess emergent properties with causal powers. This means that transformation from a colonial state of global health practice can be achieved through the reflections, activities, and actions of global health actors, which occurs at the level of social interaction on the morphogenic cycle. The actions of these global health actors can lead to the emergence of other structures that cause the equitable practice of global health. In the following section, I will focus on the social interactions phase of social morphogenesis as it is critical to transforming structures.

Reflexivity and Morphogenesis

A morphogenic approach to decolonizing global health entails viewing global health as a dynamic system that evolves through the interplay between different forces, shaped by a social context driven by equity and justice, not coloniality. My focus will thus be on global health engagements and practices underscored by how social structures and agencies interact at the level of social interaction. My adoption of the morphogenetic approach will focus on understanding how global health practices change and adapt within the international landscape, considering the influence of broader structural factors on

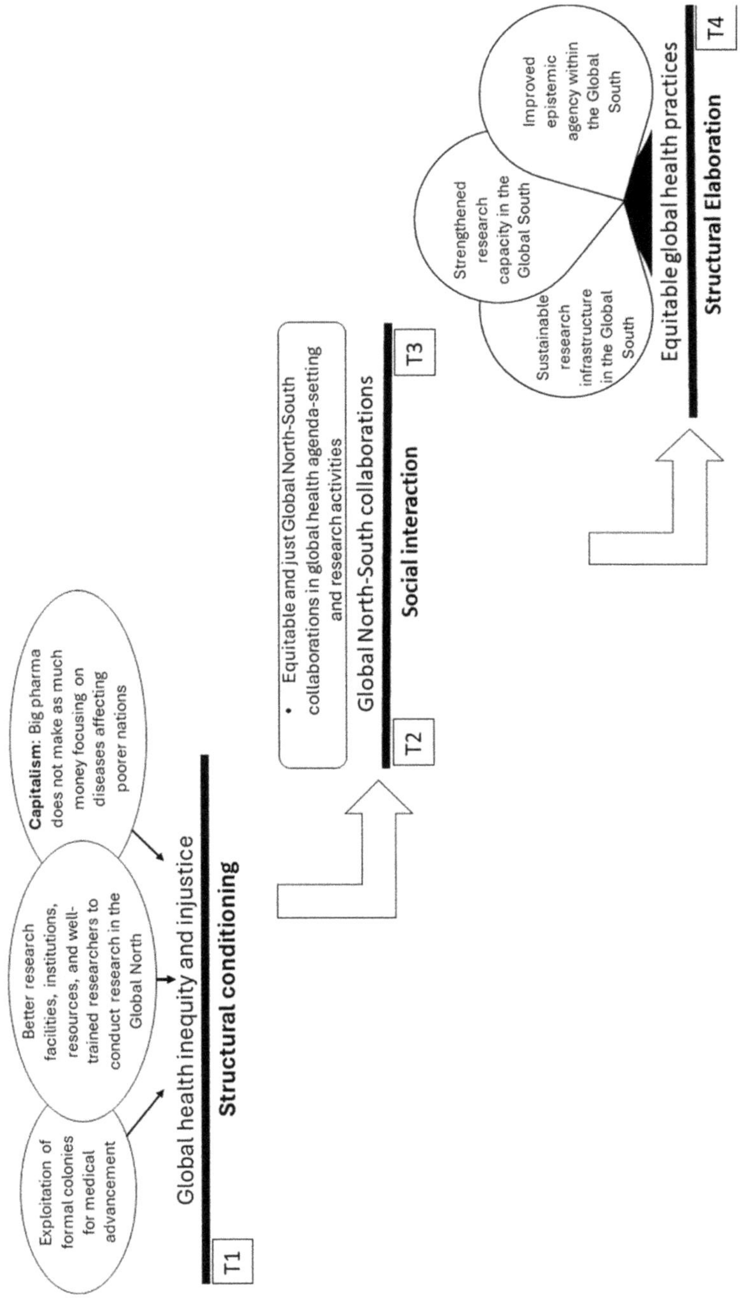

Figure 7.3 A morphogenic representation of global health research inequity.

individual and group actions and the potential for individuals and groups to modify those structures reflexively through their global health practices. Therefore, reflexivity is at the heart of the agency's role in the morphogenic apparatus. Central, therefore, to decolonizing or transforming global health is the reflexivity (exchange of ideas and cultural frames) of the actors involved in global health practice. Consequently, reflexivity—individual and collective reflexivity—as a recursive loop is a vital mediatory and fundamental aspect of the morphogenic approach.

Reflexivity is a term widely used in the social and behavioral sciences.[1] Its use in the field has been categorized into four themes: (1) reflexivity as a general feature of interaction and subjectivity; (2) as a methodological praxis; (3) as a property of discursive and non-discursive systems; and (4) as a key feature of late modernity (Zienkowski, 2017). The application of reflexivity in social morphogenesis relates to its consideration in late modernity or the postcolonial era. The conditions that foster a morphogenic society instigate an agent (an individual or collective agent/actor) to become more self-directed and, in turn, more reflexive. A key aspect of agency within the morphogenic framework is that individuals or the collective can critically reflect on their social situation and make choices that may influence the existing social structures. Before the political decolonization, global health practices were largely informed by imperialist agenda and other colonial-informed structural frameworks, resulting in morphostasis or social maintenance—maintenance of colonial systems, ideologies, mindsets, and practices even after the end of political colonialism. Colonial morphostasis was achieved through coloniality and thus was described as "neo-colonialism" (Nkrumah, 1965).

Archer (2012) argues that, unlike previous historical periods (colonial and neo-colonial periods in this case), we currently exist in a context where structure and culture have synergy, offering an unpredictable environment with morphogenetic consequences. The experience of two global pandemics (COVID-19 and mpox) have also destabilized global health. These pandemics also ushered livelihoods, education, social protection, and economic stability disruptions. Changes in communication technologies and structures characterize the unpredictable nature of modern society, increasing global flows of images, ideas, and finance and cultural exchanges that increase one's awareness of the contingency of one's identities and convictions (Zienkowski, 2017). Most recently, following the announcement by President Donald Trump of the United States of America about their withdrawal from the World Health Organization, there has been much anticipation of structural changes. In this climate, the calls for decolonizing global health are becoming loud, prompting individuals (and groups), especially from the Global South, to become more reflexive. Sennett (1980) suggested that agents adopt a proactive stance to see change in increasingly unpredictable environments, such as the global political turbulence we are currently experiencing. As such, to achieve equity and justice in global health practice, especially in the current climate, there must be reflexivity and actions on the part of the different global health actors to undo the colonial structure and culture that continues to guide global health practice, including research. Reflexivity, therefore, should be used to mediate the colonial matrix of power, underpinning global health practice.

Bhaskar considered individuals or agents and collective action pivotal in his transformational model of social action. He relates the transformative ability to having power, which Sayers conceptualizes as a causal entity (Sayer, 2012). As elaborated in Chapter 6, Bhaskar (2020) describes $Power_1$ as the power held by the oppressors who seek to maintain the status quo (homogenesis), while $Power_1$ is the implicit potentialities of the oppressed, which they can use for their emancipation (freedom). Reflexivity and voice are considered components of $Power_1$ or $Power_2$, which can be used to seek unity through diversity and reestablish transformative action, thus seeking changes in the existing structures and obtaining social morphogenesis. In this way, reflexivity is predominantly conceptualized in social transformation from the perspective of the oppressed, the individuals, groups, or institutions advocating for social morphogenesis. Nevertheless, in situations where the oppressors (the elites) are also interested in contributing to the transformative change, both groups should practice reflexivity (More of this when discussing inter-relational reflexive below). That said, the nature of reflexivity of each of these groups will be different. The reflexivity of the oppressing group should focus on relinquishing some of their authority and control to the oppressed group, while the oppressed group should reflect on empowerment and self-determination. Whatever angle it is considered from, reflexivity examines one's or the group's feelings, reactions, and motives for acting in the way they do within the underlying value systems.

Archer conceptualizes reflexivity as "creative self-mastery that enables individuals to evaluate their social situation and act purposively within it" (Rybczynska-Bunt et al., 2024, p. 1). In social theory, reflexive processes are increasingly considered at the heart of social transformation. Reflexivity speaks to knowledge (and self-knowledge) embedded in the structures of global systems, and its influence is extended to peoples' daily experiences (Caetano, 2014). Although many sociologists recognize the role of reflexivity in social transformation, they lack the theoretical and operational grounds necessary to account for the different dimensions of reflexivity (Caetano, 2014). She argued that most sociologists who have discussed the concept of reflexivity in the context of social transformation tend to simplify the past, undermine the link between reflexivity and social change, and undermine the importance given to structure and the dynamic roles of agency. Archer (2012) addresses these shortcomings in the morphogenic approach to social transformation by identifying and conceptualizing four types of reflexivity and their role in social transformation or morphogenesis: communicative reflexives, autonomous reflexives, meta-reflexives, and fractured reflexives.

- *Communicative reflexives* are characterized by internal conversations that invite completion and confirmation by others before they lead to courses of action. Communicative reflexives have two central tenets: (1) the individual or group have internal conversations and, after having these internal conversations, (2) seek confirmation and approval from others before they act. In communicative reflexives, there is first a deliberation about one's circumstances, and, in the light of these deliberations, we determine our courses of action in society. These internal discussions, however, are not completed internally. Although raised intra-personally, they are resolved through interpersonal engagements.
- *Autonomous reflexives* sustain self-contained internal conversations, leading directly to action. Autonomous reflexives refer to individuals who primarily rely on their internal dialogues and reflections for decision-making. These *reflexives* are predominantly self-directed and less inclined to seek external validation before acting. Essentially, they exhibit high independence in their thought processes and decision-making, relying significantly on their internal contemplation.
- *Meta-reflexives* are critical and reflexive about their internal conversations and the prospects of effective societal action. Meta-reflexivity is the practice of critically re-evaluating one's reflexivity, which involves examining and reflecting on one's inner thoughts and social environment. It is the insertion of an extra reflection loop into an interior dialogue one has.
- *Fractured reflexives* are those whose internal conversations intensify distress and disorientation rather than leading to purposeful courses of action. In fractured reflexives, the individual discovers that their internal conversations create dissonance and distress rather than guide them toward purposeful actions that would benefit them.

While Archer does not specifically engage with the political landscape in her morphogenesis conceptualization, medical practice and public and global health practice must engage with politics as their politics constitute social structures that govern their operations. For instance, in President Donald Trump's political agenda of America First, he stopped all global health funding to America's contributions to the World Health Organization. I contend, therefore, that meaningful global health decolonization cannot be achieved without political engagement. To this end, in my conceptualization of morphogenesis, individuals or agents are considered to lead micro-political lives having the desire to be emancipated or be freed from whatever bondage they find themselves in, and the politics of these individuals contribute to the "macroscopic" structuring and restructuring of society—morphogenesis. Communicative reflexives are considered the foundation of society and its transformation. Restricting my discussion to global health, I can refer to the works of contemporary advocates for equity and epistemic justice in global health, such as Abimbola (2020, 2024), Pai (2021, 2022), Kyobutungi et al. (2021, 2025), and many others who have consistently communicated their reflections on the decolonization of global health through scholarly writings. The autonomous reflexives combine to foster social development by injecting dynamism into the new positions they occupy. They are the source of productivity in its multifarious aspects.

Collectively, the meta-reflexives function as the well-spring of society's social criticism. Through meta-discursive acts, interlocutors can engage with the meanings that fix who and what they are in an unequal and power-infused world whose boundaries can only be imagined through interpretive and critical praxis. According to Archer (2012), only meta-reflexivity enables us to respond properly to the ever-changing, morphogenetic society. In global health, decolonization should lead to transformational acts (e.g., no more academic conferences, no more development aid, no more publishing in academic journals where you must pay to be published).

The fractured reflexives are inclined to passive agency: its proponents' deliberations go around in circles and lack conclusions. Communicative reflexives are particularly liable to recruitment to the pool of fractured reflexives (Archer, 2012).

Reflexivity and Major Systems Change

Major system change is a prominent feature of contemporary health reform (Waring et al., 2023), and the decolonization of global health is critical to this reform. In my conceptualization of the morphogenesis of a colonized global health to a decolonized one, social interaction can be effectively achieved through reflexivity. Global health can be accurately described as a product of negotiations between various actors, including different nations, international organizations like the World Health Organization, educational institutions, and non-governmental organizations, as these diverse entities must collaborate and compromise to address global health challenges that transcend national borders and require collective action. Global health is thus a complex political arena defined by disagreements and struggles and considered to be redefined through negotiated order (Thomas, 1984). Negotiated order is a theoretical perspective developed primarily by Anselm Strauss (1917–1996), who argued that virtually all social order, including global health, is negotiated order (Fine, 1984). Through these ongoing negotiations, the various actors create, maintain, transform, and are constrained by social structures. Negotiated order is a sociological concept that suggests all social order is created through ongoing negotiation and interaction between individuals and groups rather than being solely dictated by formal rules or structures (Fine, 1984; Thomas, 1984). Essentially, meaning and order emerge through continuous processes of bargaining and compromise at various levels within a social setting. The negotiated-order perspective of reflexivity provides a framework for understanding the processes involved in morphogenesis and morphostasis and identifying the social structures and conditions that shape those processes. It also allows for linking actors or agents and social structures by specifying how social actors respond to and change social structure, whether they act on their behalf or as organizational representatives (Copp, 2005).

Central to achieving major systems changes such as decolonizing global health is navigating the micro-politics as manifest in the reflexivity of the agents that are involved in global health practice and research, notably the interest holders involved in agenda setting (including dialogue and negotiation), research, policy making, program designing and implementation, and those using or taking up these programs or interventions. In social settings, including global health, the different actors negotiate with one another to accomplish tasks. Through these ongoing negotiations, individuals create, maintain, transform, and are constrained by social structures.

In its role in decolonizing global health, reflexives should focus on undoing the colonial matrix of power. Reflexivity should be aimed at undoing the generative mechanisms of inequitable and unjust global health because, as we have seen earlier, mechanisms are continuously active due to their enduring properties and powers. Indeed, Archer (2012) considers these reflexives as generative mechanisms fostering upward social mobility—emancipation. Opara (2021) argues that reflexives should focus on divesting from an identity rooted in coloniality and whiteness, necessitating a profound shift in consciousness, imagination, and decision-making. The challenge lies in the innovative task of creating an identity that is free from dominance and oppression. To this end, some authors have called for Global South global health practitioners to start by decolonizing their minds as a first step to emancipating their imagination for liberation (See decolonization of the mind in Chapter 5).

Reflexivity to transform global health practice is not only the responsibility of the disenfranchised or formally colonized individuals. It is also the responsibility of those from the Global North who care about addressing inequities and epistemic injustice in global health. For example, Lawrence and Hirsch (2020) explained that The London School of Hygiene and Tropical Medicine, where they work, is engaged in self-reflexivity—exploring how the school's historical links to colonialism can undergo transformation. Others from the Institute of Tropical Medicine in Antwerp, Belgium, are also thinking through and starting the process of decolonization at their institutions (Affun-Adegbulu et al., 2023). To emphasize the need for reflexivity in global health practice from practitioners from the Global North, Daffé et al. (2021) made the call that "all global health practitioners must be deliberate in how they engage in the work, question their practices, and actively work to be anti-racist and to 'decolonize' global health programs, not only as an ideological but also a pragmatic commitment." They further explained that such reflexives could be achieved by proposing three initial questions as part of a continuous practice of self-reflection on how they engage and design global health programs:

1) How do I understand the legacies of racism and colonialism in global health?
2) How do I value different ways of knowing about global health?
3) What are my motivations for global health?

The goal of the first question is to help the practitioner do an introspection on how their practice proliferates narratives surrounding race and ideas needing to control and intervene in communities deemed incapable of resolving their challenges (Daffé et al., 2021). The second question on how one values different ways of knowing should help the global health practitioner think whether they are (in)advertently devaluing the expertise of local collaborators and indigenous populations—their lived experience or other ways of knowing (Daffé et al., 2021). By questioning one's motivations in global health practice, the global health practitioner interrogates their "motivations for global health beyond the ideas of charity, aid, altruism, or wanting to 'do good'—ideas that may be too reductionist, too accepting of the status quo of a 'Global North and Global South' binary, and that normalize the deep economic injustices that have created global power and resource imbalances" (Daffé et al., 2021, p. 558).

Decolonial Reflexivity

Mechanisms orchestrate outcome(s), with the most proximal outcome being an action taken toward enacting social transformation, such as strike action or developing guidelines to inform global health collaborations. If we consider reflexivity or the reflexives as the nature of social interaction, as causal mechanisms, then it must be followed by action(s), which can and should lead to changes in social structure for any transformation to occur. According to Hartwig (2015), in his final reflections, Bhaskar emphasized the importance of self-transformation in social change. Therefore, simply being aware of one's own or our collective biases and societal issues through self-reflection (reflexivity) is not enough to create social change—individuals or groups will need to take steps based on the insights born of the reflexivity to enact change. While self-reflexivity is a crucial first step in recognizing potential areas for change, it only becomes impactful when translated into concrete actions that address institutional and structural power. For significant social change, self-reflexivity must be combined with collective or social actions, where groups work together to implement solutions based on their shared understanding. Social action—collective action that seeks to transform the social conditions—can only be achieved if we move beyond the "self-reflexivity" of the individual stakeholder or institutions to what Gilbert and Sliep (2009) described as "inter-relational reflexivity" or dialogue reflexivity. In conceptualizing inter-relational reflexivity, they explored the nature of reflexivity in the context of social action and community work.

In collaboration with Donati, Archer developed the concept of the "relational subject," which highlights how an individual's identity and agency are intrinsically tied to their relationships with others (Pierpaola & Archer, 2015). Donati (2016) explained that individuals and social subjects are "relationally constituted" and acquire qualities and powers through internal and external social relations. The movement from self-reflexivity to inter-relational reflexivity is synonymous with moving from a critical appraisal of "self" to a critical appraisal of "self" as a responsible member of collective action (Gilbert & Sliep, 2009). Gilbert and Sliep further argue that:

> [R]eflexivity in social action should involve aspects of the critical appraisal by stakeholders of their own and others' intentions and assumptions and the effects of these on self and other. These processes necessitate a reflexivity that moves beyond the solitary individual being reflexive of self to inter-relational reflexivity in which collective reflexivity is generated that promotes a critical understanding of ongoing joint action.
>
> (Gilbert & Sliep, 2009)

I adopt the term "decolonial reflexivity" as a counter-hegemonic discourse to denote a situation where reflexivity, whether self-reflexivity or inter-relational reflexivity, is aimed at decoloniality. Moosavi (2022) first introduced decolonial reflexivity to redefine academic decolonization. In using the term in curriculum designing, he suggested that decolonial reflexivity entailed introspectively interrogating his approach to generating a decolonial curriculum (Moosavi, 2022). Allen and Girei (2023), while applying the decolonial reflexivity in management and organization knowledge, suggest that it entails confronting white identities and critically engaging with whiteness towards decolonization. Their perspective of decolonial reflexivity engages with how white skin, white identities, and whiteness can engage in decolonial discourse without colonizing them (Allen & Girei, 2023). Moosavi (2022) suggested that decolonial reflexivity is about being reflexive about our interventions, which we purport to be decolonial (p. 144). My conceptualization of decolonial reflexivity as a counter-hegemonic discourse entails engaging in reflective exercises and taking action to undo the drivers of coloniality (hegemony, racism, religious paternalism, white supremacy, and white saviorism). This counter-hegemonic discourse should lead to decolonizing the mind, combating colonial amnesia, going beyond traditional mastery (global health expertise), establishing meaningful global health collaborations, valorizing local knowledge, and having a self-reliant mindset (Figure 7.4).

Decolonial reflexivity in the context of decolonizing global health thus means engaging in reflexivity to decolonize global health practice, research, or any aspect of global health. Decolonial reflexivity in global health should be aimed at anticipating and alleviating potentially harmful practices

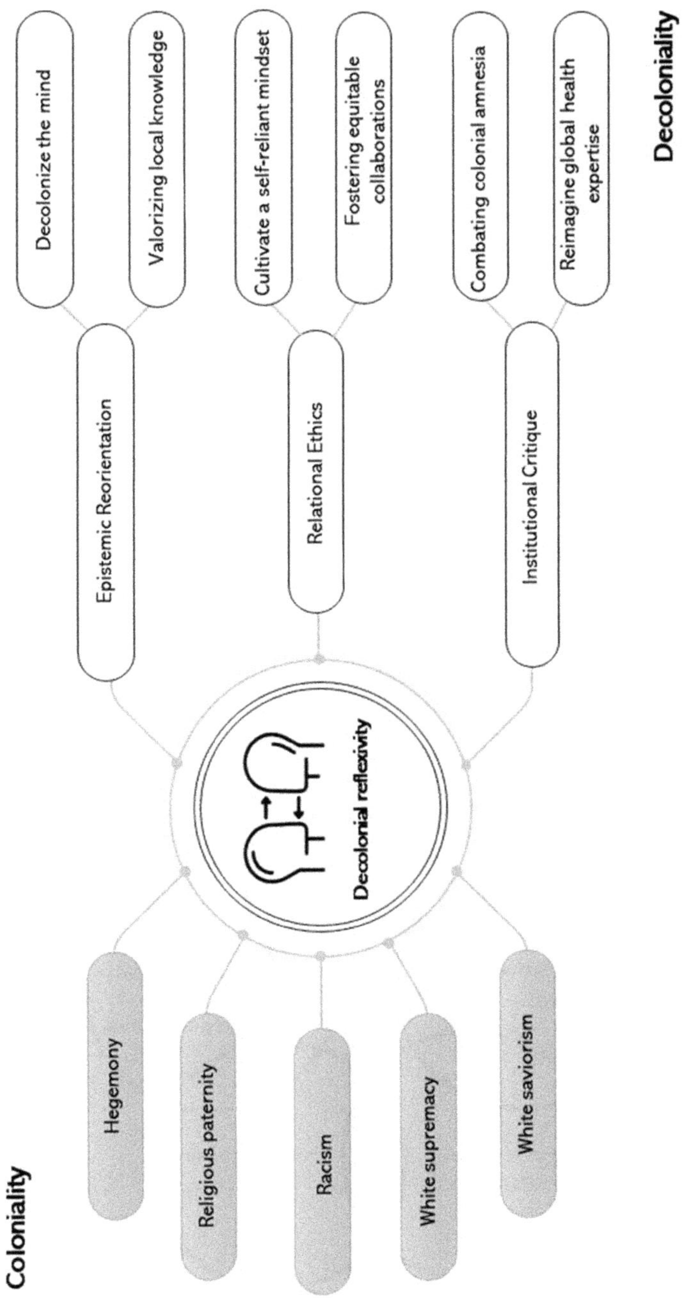

Figure 7.4 Decolonial reflexivity as a counter-hegemonic and equity-based discourse.

inherent in dominant global health practices and research methods (Naidu et al., 2024). The authors argue that decolonial reflexivity in global health practice and research should be ongoing, whereby global health practitioners orient and position themselves toward the formerly colonized and perspectives of the indigenes (Naidu et al., 2024). Following their argument, Gilbert and Sliep (2009) suggested that inter-relational reflexivity involves at least four loops: deconstructing power in the collective, determining moral agency, negotiating accountability and responsibility, and positive "performative" actions. I adapt the inter-relational reflexivity framework in this section to develop a five-loop construct for the decolonial reflexivity approach for global health practice and research (Figure 7.5). In this five-loop construct, I replaced "deconstructing power" in the collective with "deconstructing coloniality," as this term is closer to the decolonial agenda. I also replaced "determining moral agency" with "formulating concrete utopias." Finally, I added the aspect of coalition building as I find it key to the decolonial reflexivity framework.

Coalition Building

Coalition building is focused on harnessing collective power. Coalition building is the strategic process of uniting individuals, groups, or organizations around shared goals despite differing backgrounds, ideologies, or priorities. Following the "America First" mantra, adopted by President Donald Trump

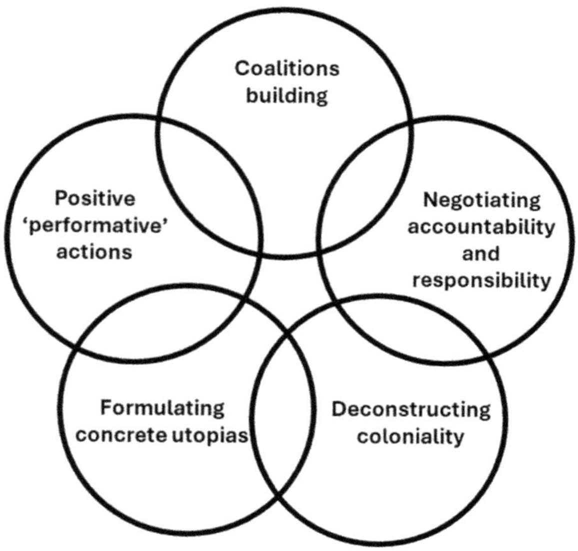

Figure 7.5 Five inter-relational reflexive loops.

during his second presidential term, the global geopolitical climate is defined by polarization and fragmentation. Therefore, the ability to forge alliances across divides has become essential for addressing health inequity and justice in global health. It has been argued that coalitions geared toward decolonizing global health must confront global health inequities and injustices through redistributive justice—shifting resources, authorship, and leadership to Global South actors (Seetah, 2024; Spanaus & De Souza, 2024).

At its core, coalition building relies on "shared goals and objectives" that transcend individual (or a unit's) interests (Beamish & Luebbers, 2009). Coalitions in the decolonization agenda should aim to unite diverse interest holders to challenge systemic oppression and reimagine equitable systems. Successful coalitions, therefore, identify common ground, notably addressing global health inequities and injustices experienced by the Global South in global health research and practice. This diversity strengthened the movement by combining grassroots mobilization, global health expertise, and national advocacy. For example, the Mutual aid networks during COVID-19, like those in Kenya and India, combined local mobilization with global advocacy to challenge vaccine apartheid.

Forming coalitions is critical for the social interaction phase of the morphogenetic framework and occurs at different levels of interaction. While critiques of Global North-driven colonialism, coloniality, and neocolonial power asymmetries remain vital to decolonial discourse, they constitute an incomplete praxis for achieving transformative decolonization in global health. Current paradigms often position the Global South as passive beneficiaries awaiting emancipatory initiatives orchestrated by the Global North—a dynamic that inadvertently reproduces hierarchical dependencies. For decolonization to transcend symbolic gestures, Global South actors must assert an agentive role in this process, critically interrogating their complicities in perpetuating colonial logics through domestic policy inertia, elite capture of resources, and uncritical adoption of externally imposed epistemologies. To this end, coalitions for decolonizing global health should occur at local, national, and international levels to dismantle internalized hierarchies that sustain inequity. Sharma and Sam-Agudu (2023) thus propose that interactions for the decolonization agenda should occur, as illustrated in Figure 7.6.

Global health diplomacy offers an important avenue for these coalitions to take place. Global health diplomacy focuses on health issues that require the cooperation of many countries to address common concerns, but health diplomacy can also play a central role at the regional, bilateral, and national levels. Global health diplomatic commitments from interest holders and actors from the global south would go a long way to fostering the goals of decolonization. Therefore, contact should be established between parliamentarians and other decision-makers regarding health equity, health issues in national security, and national legislation to get them interested and involved in committees where health is impacted. Obtaining commitment from countries in the Global South's global health diplomacy can help develop community trust, create and

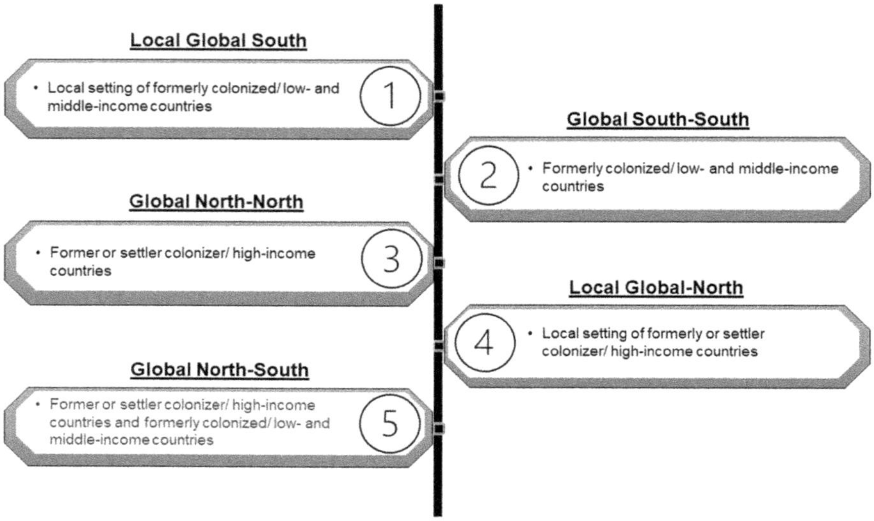

Figure 7.6 Proposed levels of coalition formation for decolonial reflexivity in global health.

coordinate response, improve access, and create an atmosphere for engagement while ensuring harmony with regional cultures (World Health Organization, 2023). According to the World Health Organization (2023), broader engagement between countries would strengthen their ability to evolve common positions. Therefore, engaging countries in the Global South with commitments to work towards their decolonization would strengthen their responses to health issues and other social determinants of health, such as nutrition, food, and access to medicines and technologies. Achieving commitments from countries of the Global South to decolonize global health would also encourage these countries to share best practices and capabilities and to pool technical and other resources and capacities rather than looking to the Global North for rescue, which is costly and can come with other strings attached.

Trust, commitment, and solidarity are equally vital when formulating coalitions (Gawerc, 2021). Coalitions often fracture when members prioritize their agendas over collective goals. Transparent dialogue through self-reflexivity and equitable power-sharing is critical to ensure inclusive participation. Gawerc (2021) identified five coalitional processes and practices empirically found or theorized to be imperative for cultivating solidarity across difference and inequality. These processes include (a) uniting around shared principles while engaging differences, (b) acknowledging and managing inequalities, (c) making space for each other, (d) attention to managing conflicts, and (e) actions that confirm the shared commitments and negotiated identity (Gawerc, 2021). Therefore, coalition building is not merely a tactic but a philosophy of solidarity. It requires humility to listen to marginalized voices, courage to confront power structures, and creativity to reimagine shared futures. As climate activist Vanessa Nakate argues, "No single movement can tackle the climate crisis alone; we need intersectional coalitions." From grassroots organizers to global non-governmental organizations, the future of progress depends on our ability to unite across differences—not despite them, but because of them. In the fight to decolonize global health, coalition building remains a critical component of decolonial reflexivity. Coalitions can transform fragmented efforts into concrete utopias by learning from past struggles, embracing flexibility, and centering justice.

Deconstructing Coloniality

Deconstructing coloniality speaks to undoing power in the context of inter-relational reflexivity (inherently political and predicated on winning allies), which entails critically examining differences in status and authority in the relationships of interest holders. Deconstructing power in global health involves critically examining and dismantling the unequal power dynamics present in the global health system by highlighting and acknowledging how institutions, researchers, and funding in the Global North exert substantial control over health initiatives in the Global South. Such control leads to imbalances in knowledge production, decision-making, and resource allocation, ultimately affecting the effectiveness and equity of global health interventions. Additionally, this reflexivity focuses on historical colonial legacies that continue to influence these power dynamics. Key aspects of deconstructing power in global health include:

1) Examining how research agendas often focus on priorities that may not align with the needs of regions of the Global South.
2) Critiquing the tendency to prioritize Western research methodologies and perspectives over local knowledge systems may lead to neglecting important cultural contexts and community needs.
3) Analyzing the significant influence that international organizations, global health funders, and Western-based research institutions have on global health agendas as they shape policies and priorities. This component can offer ideas on how to reshape or restructure—structural elaboration.
4) Identifying situations where interventions are created and executed without meaningful involvement from local communities perpetuates a power imbalance between "experts" and "beneficiaries."
5) Recognizing that historical colonial power dynamics continue to shape current global health relationships, including the perception of "savior" narratives that portray Western nations as the sole solution to health issues in the Global South (Chaudhuri et al., 2021).

This last activity also involves taking concrete steps to abolish institutional amnesia—an organization's inability to recall and use historical knowledge for present-day purposes (Stark, 2019). To facilitate the reflexivity process and combat institutional amnesia, some global health institutions, such as the University of Washington, through bi-weekly reflexivity meetings, have created a Colonial Power Structure Assessment Framework to achieve equitable collaborations, center projects around local priorities, diversify leadership and promote respectful, collaborative interactions and language/tone in all communications (International Clinical Research Center, 2021).

Actively dismantling the coloniality within the global health system requires a dedicated and sustained effort from individuals, institutions, and governments, involving a shift in power dynamics, knowledge production, and practices to prioritize equity and local needs over a historically dominant Western perspective. Deconstructing coloniality requires those in power ($Power_2$) to be willing to relinquish power and privileges to the previously dominated. As Wiyeh and Mukumbang (2025) argue, deconstructing coloniality to achieve equity and justice in global health is a fundamental paradox in our quest for decolonization. This is because the expectation is that those who have historically benefited from unjust power dynamics support the empowerment of those marginalized. There is also the perspective of the marginalized to trust that those who historically benefited from unjust power dynamics will cede their power to achieve equity in global health practice. Trust is vital in any collaborative endeavor, and deconstructing power in inter-relational reflexivity is no different. Trust becomes an important generative mechanism for deconstructing power as part of inter-relational reflexivity. As an ongoing dynamic process, reflexivity is essential for revealing power, tracking its movement, and identifying the effects of past practices and new methods, along with their accompanying discourses. This process is iterative and continuous; as actions evolve and contexts shift, the reflexive cycle consistently fosters a critical understanding of ongoing activities and transformations.

Formulating Concrete Utopias

Determining moral agency speaks to the question, "What should the nature of the new social relations be?" (Gilbert & Sliep, 2009, p. 473), which relates to the notion of formulating concrete utopias (Wright, 2010). The deconstruction of the colonial matrix of power should facilitate the question of how it is possible to construct the way forward. Deconstructing power in global health should (i) promote greater participation and leadership from researchers, communities, and policymakers in the Global South to shape health agendas, (ii) encourage research methodologies that are culturally sensitive, community-driven, and address local priorities, (iii) advocate for greater accountability and equitable distribution of global health funding, and (iv) encourage researchers and practitioners to critically examine their positions within the global health systems and actively work to dismantle power imbalances (McCoy et al., 2024; Tuhebwe et al., 2023).

Working on redefining the nature of global health practices with various stakeholders from the global North and South entails setting practical utopias to serve the local community. This process might require investing in capacity building in areas where such capacities are needed to address the local community's health needs. For instance, rather than having "global health experts" working in the communities where there is a need, local experts can be trained and empowered to do what needs to be done. Capacity building in the business, politics, and economics of global health is essential for professionals in the Global South. Decolonization in global health demands more than just technical (subject matter) expertise in public health; it requires empowered leaders who can skillfully navigate the complex political and economic landscapes that influence global health funding and policy. These leaders must work to protect their autonomy and promote the health interests of their populations. However, existing Global North or South training programs do not adequately prepare these leaders to tackle global health governance's intricate (multi-scalar) realities. As a result, despite possessing technical skills, many leaders from the Global South find themselves unprepared to engage with the entrenched power structures that control critical resources.

Negotiating Accountability and Responsibility

Negotiating accountability and responsibility is about the coming together of the different parties involved—individuals and groups—in inter-relational reflexivity, understanding existing intentions and assumptions of self and others, and formulating preferred outcomes (Gilbert & Sliep, 2009). Negotiating accountability stems from the relationship shared between the relevant actors and agents, which follows ongoing negotiation and interaction between the individuals and groups as conceptualized through the negotiated order theory. Negotiations are required when the actors involved encounter ambiguity or uncertainty in the reflexivity process, have differing decolonization goals, have different approaches to decoloniality, or create exceptions or loopholes based on coloniality. Common types of negotiation associated with the negotiation order and inter-relational reflexivity include distributive, integrative, and multiparty negotiations. Distributive negotiation often involves making demands and counter-demands, focusing on a "fixed pie" where only a certain number of resources are available and can be likened to a zero-sum game. Integrative negotiation involves exploring interests, brainstorming solutions, and building relationships to find creative solutions that meet the needs of everyone involved. Multiparty negotiation is more about common values and thus requires skills in coalition building, managing multiple perspectives, and finding consensus.

The outcome of these negotiations should be a platform for new social relations between global health practitioners and institutions of the Global North and the Global South. Taking the agenda of ensuring greater accountability and equitable distribution of global health funds, the African Academy of Sciences and the African Union, with financial support from the European Commission, created the African Research Initiative for Scientific Excellence program—a five-year initiative (2022–2026). Following the loop of determining moral agency, the ARISE program seeks to (a) strengthen the capacities of the emerging African research leaders committed to a research and teaching career in Africa, (b) strengthen institutional research management and support systems for research to thrive and, (c) support the generation of cutting-edge research that will contribute towards transforming lives in Africa (Mutua & Nakidde, 2024). At the level of negotiating accountability and responsibility, the Global North and Global South partners use the Good Financial Grant Practice Standards, an innovative tool for enhancing institutional finance and grant management capacity. The African Academy of Sciences developed the Good Financial Grant Practice Standards in partnership with the African Organisation for Standardisation. The Good Financial Grant Practice Standards are designed for institutional teams to self-assess against set criteria and identify and address capacity gaps to inform their financial management actions. According to Gilbert and Sliep (2009), accountability and responsibility negotiations consider the culture of each participant. As we can see in the case of the African Research Initiative for Scientific Excellence program, the African-based institutions were responsible for designing the Good Financial Grant Practice Standards to align with the University and Tertiary university standards and culture in Africa. Because the Good Financial Grant Practice allows grantees and grantors to share best practices in financial and grant management, it permits funding partners to request prospective grantees to comply with the Standard as part of pre-award due diligence (Mutua & Nakidde, 2024). This accountability and responsibility negotiations process creates a cultural space that is co-constructed by everyone involved, allowing for ongoing critical reflection.

As I have argued in the previous chapter, the inequitable representation of Global South researchers as authors in published articles represents inequitable partnerships and collaboration in global health research. To this end, tools have been developed to guide the research team through their reflexivity during publication to enhance equity in global health publications (McIntosh et al., 2023; Morton et al., 2022). The equitable partnership declaration tool contains questions about the research partnerships in the studies, exploring how the research affects and is shaped by researchers, communities, and environments in the study settings (McIntosh et al., 2023). The authors suggested that the equitable partnership declaration should guide reflexivity and publication practices for all studies conducted in the Global South where at least one of the collaborators is from the Global North. These authors are also encouraged to submit their reflexivity statements and manuscripts, and global health-related journals are encouraged to request this reflexivity statement (Morton et al., 2022).

While commitment is integral to decolonizing global health through fostering collaborations where all partners have equal agency and decision-making power rather than a hierarchical structure, it is particularly important when negotiating accountability and responsibility as part of the reflexivity process. This could be achieved by investing more in training and development opportunities for healthcare professionals in the Global South to build local capacity and leadership in global health initiatives.

Positive Performative Actions (Structural Elaboration)

The first order to achieve structural elaboration is bargaining for power, as power negotiations are at the heart of achieving social change. As I have argued above, decolonial reflexivity requires inter-relational reflexivity, which, in a way, requires acting as corporate agents to enact social change. According to Archer (1995), such interaction is resource-dependent, which then lends itself to resource distribution. She argues that within such interaction, the distribution of resources restricts (1) The nature and number of people admitted to transactions, (2) The initial bargaining positions of the agents, and (3) the nature of the demands or change that is required. Based on these three criteria, the Global North would enter the negotiating process from a stronger bargaining position. I have also argued that those possessing $Power_2$ will not be willing to cede their power and privilege and would bring that influence to any negotiation table. Pai et al. (2024) proposed that to reimagine (decolonize) global health, there must be advocacy for leadership by the Global South and allyship by the Global North.

Nevertheless, according to Archer (1995), the initial bargaining position is important in determining what level of social change could be achieved, insisting that agents with low access to resources (in this case, financial capabilities) will have a weaker bargaining position. Pai et al. (2024) proposal entails "shifting power to the Global South." Nevertheless, the pausing and stopping of two key federal grants, which made tremendous contributions to global health, has two implications: (1) the Global North is still whiling the negotiation power, and (2) this is an opportunity for the Global South to become self-reliant and in another way, obtain the resources required to get to the negotiating table on a stronger position. Katumba (2025) pointed out that the Global South has enormous collective bargaining power, particularly concerning its growing population.

The key resources in global health are finances and qualified personnel. It has been argued that the Global South can achieve financial sufficiency by the following means:

1) Enhance its ability to develop domestic funding mechanisms for healthcare infrastructure and minimizing dependence on international assistance.
2) Explore alternative financial mechanisms, including national taxation systems, targeted levies, and collaborations with private sectors to broaden funding streams (strengthened by a strong health system) and secure long-term healthcare funding.
3) Strengthen public health budget oversight through transparent and accountable frameworks that maximize the impact of allocated funds.

4) Utilize digital tools and analytics-backed insights to direct healthcare investments, prioritizing evidence-based decision-making for optimal resource distribution. Having financial resources offers them the ability to have better initial engagements as it increases their potential bargaining power.

Performing decolonial reflexivity requires that actors examine how they narrate and perform with others in the context of global health collaborations and practices. According to Gilbert and Sliep (2009), performing inter-relational reflexivity requires that the different actors involved be transparent about what informs their positions and make commitments to alter their positioning and actions to better serve the social action they have committed. For instance, some global health experts from the Global North strongly advocate for achieving equity and justice in global health practice. Collaborations between these individuals, groups, and institutions, whose reflexivity led to congruent goals and ambitions, notably to decolonize global health, can lead to sharing ideas and engagement in joint reflections. Diplomacy in global health can offer an avenue for reflexivity among global health practitioners in the Global South and those of the Global North for negotiating priorities among international organizations, states, and non-state actors for decolonized global health. While its primary focus is global, it also intersects with domestic policies on complex issues such as climate change, crisis preparedness and response, and health financing.

Conclusion

Approximately 75 of the poorest countries, predominantly in the Global South, contributed less than 4% to the global expenditure. Many of these countries face restrictions on increasing their healthcare spending because they owe significant debts to wealthier nations. Their lending agreements stipulate that repaying these debts must precede public expenditures. This international financial architecture is based on colonial ideologies and remains a structure strongly influencing health promotion and curative services development and delivery. I argue, following the morphogenetic framework, that our reflexivity and the social action that emanate from them must be able to dismantle or, at the very least, reform such laws for countries in the Global South and beyond to attempt to lead global health endeavors and for true allyship to be achieved.

Would the mechanisms of trust, commitment, and motivation generated through inter-relational reflexivity dismantle structures such as the current international financial system, which places intolerable burdens on the countries that can afford it the least? For the meaningful transformation of global health practice, the reflexivity of regulators should lead them to consider what is happening, not only at the level of institutions but also at the level of the entire system, such as the financial system. They should be able to create structures that promote capacity building in the business, politics, and economics of Global Health for Global South professionals. As McCoy et al. (2024) argue, we must create political and economic anticolonialism and social decolonization structures to ensure greater national, racial, cultural, and knowledge diversity within global health structures. The decolonizing global health endeavor is thus multi-scalar, at the level of global health organizations and regional and global interactions, not losing sight of the opportunities posed by global uncertainty.

Note

1 When Archer conceptualized reflexivity in the context of morphogenesis, she focused on self-reflexivity. From the position of the individual demanding change, self-reflexivity refers to a reflection of their current situation and how a situation of emancipation would look like. From the position of an individual in position of power who is supportive of the individual in a vulnerable position, self-reflexivity would mean understanding the way they position themselves and the way their positions and actions reflect dominant discourses and practices. My use of the reflexivity means a combination of both forms of reflexivity. Self-reflexivity according to Archer is always in relation to other people (relational).

References

Abimbola, S. (2020). Beyond positive a priori bias: reframing community engagement in LMICs. *Health Promotion International*, 35(3), 598–609. https://doi.org/10.1093/HEAPRO/DAZ023

Abimbola, S. (2024). *The foreign gaze: Essays on global health*. IRD.

Affun-Adegbulu, C., Cosaert, T., Meudec, M., Michielsen, J., Van De Pas, R., Van Belle, S., Van De Put, W., Soors, W., Robertson, F., & Ddungu, C. (2023). Decolonisation initiatives at the Institute of Tropical Medicine, Antwerp, Belgium: ready for change? *BMJ Global Health*, 8(5), e011748. https://doi.org/10.1136/BMJGH-2023-011748

Allen, S., & Girei, E. (2023). Developing decolonial reflexivity: Decolonizing management education by confronting white skin, white identities, and whiteness. *Academy of Management Learning & Education*, 23(2), 246–264. https://doi.org/10.5465/AMLE.2022.0387

Archer, M. (1995). *Realist social theory: The morphogenetic approach*. Cambridge University Press.

Archer, M. S. (2010). Morphogenesis versus structuration: On combining structure and action. *British Journal of Sociology*, 61(Suppl. 1), 225–252. https://doi.org/10.1111/j.1468-4446.2009.01245.x

Archer, M. S. (2012). *The reflexive imperative in late modernity*. Cambridge University Press.

Archer, M. S. (2013). *Social morphogenesis*. Springer.

Archer, M. S. (2020). The morphogenetic approach: Critical realism's explanatory framework approach. *Virtues and Economics*, 5, 137–150. https://doi.org/10.1007/978-3-030-26114-6_9

Archer, M. S. (2021). The mess we are in: how the morphogenetic approach helps to explain it. *Journal of Critical Realism*, 20(4), 330–348. https://doi.org/10.1080/14767430.2022.1984698

Archer, M. S., & Morgan, J. (2020). Contributions to realist social theory: an interview with Margaret S. Archer. *Journal of Critical Realism*, 19(2), 179–200. https://doi.org/10.1080/14767430.2020.1732760

Baumgartner, F. R., & Jones, B. D. (1991). Agenda dynamics and policy subsystems. *Journal of Politics*, 53(4), 1044–1074. https://doi.org/10.2307/2131866

Beamish, T. D., & Luebbers, A. J. (2009). Alliance building across social movements: Bridging difference in a peace and justice coalition. *Social Problems*, 56(4), 647–676. https://doi.org/10.1525/SP.2009.56.4.647

Bhaskar, R. (2008). *Dialectic: The pulse of freedom*. Routledge.

Bhaskar, R. (2020). Critical realism and the ontology of persons. *Journal of Critical Realism*, 19(2), 113–120. https://doi.org/10.1080/14767430.2020.1734736

Bryant, J. H., et al. (1996). Health research: Essential link to equity in development. www.ncbi.nlm.nih.gov/books/NBK209096.

Caetano, A. (2014). Reflexivity and social change: A critical discussion of reflexive modernization and individualization theses. *Portuguese Journal of Social Science*, 13(1), 93–109. https://doi.org/10.1386/pjss.13.1.93_1

Chaudhuri, M. M., Mkumba, L., Raveendran, Y., & Smith, R. D. (2021). Decolonising global health: beyond "reformative" roadmaps and towards decolonial thought. *BMJ Global Health*, 6(7), e006371. https://doi.org/10.1136/BMJGH-2021-006371

Copp, M. (2005). Negotiated order. In *Encyclopedia of social theory* (pp. 526–529). Sage Publications. https://doi.org/10.4135/9781412952552

Cruickshank, J. (2010). Knowing social reality: A critique of Bhaskar and Archer's attempt to derive a social ontology from lay knowledge. *Philosophy of the Social Sciences*, 40(4), 579–602. https://doi.org/10.1177/0048393109340664

Daffé, Z. N., Guillaume, Y., & Ivers, L. C. (2021). Anti-racism and anticolonialism praxis in global health—reflection and action for practitioners in US academic medical centers. In American *Journal of Tropical Medicine and Hygiene*, 105(3), 557–560. https://doi.org/10.4269/ajtmh.21-0187

Danermark, B., Ekström, M., & Karlsson, J. C. (2019). *Explaining society: Critical realism in the social sciences*. Routledge. https://doi.org/10.4324/9781351017831

de Souza, D., (2014). Culture, context and society: The underexplored potential of critical realism as a philosophical framework for theory and practice. *Asian Journal of Social Psychology*, 17(2), 141–151. https://doi.org/10.1111/ajsp.12052

Donati, P. (2016). The "relational subject" according to a critical realist relational sociology. *Journal of Critical Realism*, 15(4), 352–375. https://doi.org/10.1080/14767430.2016.1166728

Elder-Vass, D. (2008). Searching for realism, structure and agency in actor network theory. *The British Journal of Sociology*, 59(3), 455–473. https://doi.org/10.1111/J.1468-4446.2008.00203.X

Fine, G. A. (1984). Negotiated orders and organizational cultures. *Annual Review of Sociology*, 10, 239–262. https://about.jstor.org/terms

Galtung, J. (1967). Scientific colonialism. *Transition*, 30, 10–15.

Gawerc, M. I. (2021). Coalition-building and the forging of solidarity across difference and inequality. *Sociology Compass*, 15(3), e12858. https://doi.org/10.1111/SOC4.12858

Giddens, A. (1979). *Central problems in social theory: Action, structure, and contradiction in social analysis*. University of California Press.

Gilbert, A., & Sliep, Y. (2009). Reflexivity in the practice of social action: From self-to inter-relational reflexivity. *South African Journal of Psychology*, 39(4), 468–479. https://doi.org/10.1177/008124630903900408

Hartwig, M. (2015). From the anatomy of the global crisis to the ontology of human flourishing. *Journal of Critical Realism*, 14(3), 227–237. https://doi.org/10.1179/1476743015Z.00000000069

Horrocks, I. (2009). Applying the morphogenetic approach. *Journal of Critical Realism*, 8(1), 35–62. https://doi.org/10.1558/JOCR.V8I1.35

International Clinical Research Center. (2021). *Decolonizing global health toolkit*. University of Washington.
Jessop, B., Brenner, N., & Jones, M. S. (2008). Theorizing sociospatial relations. *Environment and Planning D: Society and Space*, 26(3), 389–401. https://doi.org/10.1068/D9107
Katumba, A. (2025, March 21). Beyond dependency: Rethinking Africa's relationship with foreign aid health. https://speakingofmedicine.plos.org/2025/03/21/beyond-dependency-rethinking-africas-relationship-with-foreign-aid/
Kyobutungi, C., Okereke, E., & Abimbola, S. (2025). After USAID: What now for aid and Africa? *BMJ*, r479. https://doi.org/10.1136/bmj.r479
Kyobutungi, C., Robinson, J., & Pai, M. (2021). Charting a new path towards equity, diversity, and inclusion in global health. *PLOS Global Public Health*, 1(10), e0000038. https://doi.org/10.1371/journal.pgph.0000038
Labonte, R., & Spiegel, J. (2003). Setting global health research priorities. *BMJ*, 326(7392), 722–723. https://doi.org/10.1136/BMJ.326.7392.722
Lawrence, D. S., & Hirsch, L. A. (2020). Decolonising global health: transnational research partnerships under the spotlight. *International Health*, 12(6), 518–523. https://doi.org/10.1093/INTHEALTH/IHAA073
Laxminarayan, R. (2024). Stop delaying action on antimicrobial resistance—it is achievable and affordable. *Nature*, 633, 495. https://doi.org/10.1038/d41586-024-02993-3
Lindblom, C. E. (1959). The science of "muddling through." *Public Administration Review*, 19(2).
Maccarini, A. M. (2019). *Deep change and emergent structures in global society: Explorations in social morphogenesis*. Springer. https://doi.org/10.1007/978-3-030-13624-6
McCoy, D., Kapilashrami, A., Kumar, R., Rhule, E., & Khosla, R. (2024). Developing an agenda for the decolonization of global health. *Bulletin of the World Health Organization*, 102(2), 130–136. https://doi.org/10.2471/BLT.23.289949
McIntosh, K., Messin, L., Jin, P., & Mullan, Z. (2023). Countering helicopter research with equitable partnerships. *The Lancet Global Health*, 11(7), e1007–e1008. https://doi.org/10.1016/S2214-109X(23)00278-4
Moosavi, L. (2022). Turning the decolonial gaze towards ourselves: Decolonising the curriculum and "decolonial reflexivity" in sociology and social theory. *Sociology*, 57(1), 137–156. https://doi.org/10.1177/00380385221096037
Morton, B., Vercueil, A., Masekela, R., Heinz, E., Reimer, L., Saleh, S., Kalinga, C., Seekles, M., Biccard, B., Chakaya, J., Abimbola, S., Obasi, A., & Oriyo, N. (2022). Consensus statement on measures to promote equitable authorship in the publication of research from international partnerships. *Anaesthesia*, 77(3), 264–276. https://doi.org/10.1111/ANAE.15597
Mutua, M. N., & Nakidde, C. (2024). How can a realist evaluation adhere to the indigenous research principles? An evaluation protocol of a health research capacity strengthening programme. *International Journal of Qualitative Methods*, 23.
Naidu, T., Gingell, G., & Zaidi, Z. (2024). Decolonial framework for applying reflexivity and positionality in global health research. *Global Health Promotion*, 31(2), 52–58. https://doi.org/10.1177/17579759241238016
Nkrumah, K. (1965). *Neo-colonialism, the last stage of imperialism*. Thomas Nelson & Sons.
Norrie, A. (2024). Dialectical critical realism, complexity and the psychology of blame. *Journal for the Theory of Social Behaviour*. https://doi.org/10.1111/jtsb.12411
Opara, I. N. (2021). It's time to decolonize the decolonization movement. https://speakingofmedicine.plos.org/2021/07/29/its-time-to-decolonize-the-decolonization-movement/
Pai, M. (2021). Decolonizing global health: A moment to reflect on a movement. www.forbes.com/sites/madhukarpai/2021/07/22/decolonizing-global-health-a-moment-to-reflect-on-a-movement/?sh=5887aaed5386

Pai, M. (2022, February 15). Disrupting global health: From allyship to collective liberation. www.forbes.com/sites/madhukarpai/2022/03/15/disrupting-global-health-from-allyship-to-collective-liberation/?sh=1e1bf0ba4e62

Pai, M., Bandara, S., & Kyobutungi, C. (2024). Shifting power in global health will require leadership by the Global South and allyship by the Global North. *The Lancet*, 0(0). https://doi.org/10.1016/S0140-6736(24)02323-7

Pandey, K. R., & Adhikari, B. (2023). Why we need a global fund for health research. *The Lancet Global Health*, 11(7), e1003–e1004. https://doi.org/10.1016/S2214-109X(23)00254-1

Pierpaola, D., & Archer, M. (2015). *The relational subject*. Cambridge University Press.

Rybczynska-Bunt, S., Byng, R., Spitters, S., Shaw, S. E., Jameson, B., & Greenhalgh, T. (2024). The reflexive imperative in the digital age: Using Archer's "fractured reflexivity" to theorise widening inequities in UK general practice. https://doi.org/10.1111/1467-9566.13811

Said, E. W. (1977). Orientalism. *The Georgia Review*, 31(1), 162–206.

Said, E. W. (1993). *Culture and imperialism*. Vintage Books.

Sayer, A. (2000). *Realism and social science*. Sage Publications. https://doi.org/10.4135/9781446218730

Sayer, A. (2012). Power, causality and normativity: A critical realist critique of Foucault. *Journal of Political Power*, 5(2), 179–194.

Seetah, K. (2024). Colonialism, decolonization, and global health. *Sustainable Development Goals Series*, Part F4029, 3–18.

Sennett, R. (1980). Authority and freedom. *The Kenyon Review*, 2(2), 81–110.

Sharma, D., & Sam-Agudu, N. A. (2023). Decolonising global health in the Global South by the Global South: turning the lens inward. *BMJ Global Health*, 8(9), e013696. https://doi.org/10.1136/BMJGH-2023-013696

Soja, E. W. (1980). The socio-spatial dialectic. *Annals of the Association of American Geographers*, 70(2), 207–225.

Spanaus, E. S., & De Souza, E. L. (2024). Decolonising global health: Clarifying concepts for equitable practice. *Epidemiology & Public Health*, 2(3).

Stark, A. (2019). Institutional amnesia and crisis management analysis. *Oxford Research Encyclopedia of Politics*. https://doi.org/10.1093/ACREFORE/9780190228637.013.1526

Thomas, J. (1984). Some aspects of negotiated order, loose coupling and meso-structure in maximum security prisons. *Symbolic Interaction*, 7(2), 213–231. https://doi.org/10.1525/si.1984.7.2.213

Tuhebwe, D., Brittingham, S., Kanagaratnam, A., Togo, E., Olaolorun, F. M., Wanyenze, R. K., Prata, N., & Maragh-Bass, A. C. (2023). Applying a power analysis to everything we do: A qualitative inquiry to decolonize the global health and development project cycle. *Global Health: Science and Practice*, 5(11), e2300187. https://doi.org/10.9745/GHSP-D-23-00187

Van Belle, S., Abejirinde, I. O., Ssennyonjo, A., Srinivas, P. N., Hebbar, P., & Marchal, B. (2023). How to develop a realist programme theory using Margaret Archer's structure–agency–culture framework: The case of adolescent accountability for sexual and reproductive health in urban resource-constrained settings. *Evaluation*, 29(3), 259–275. https://doi.org/10.1177/13563890231185167

Waring, J., Bishop, S., Black, G., Clarke, J. M., Exworthy, M., Fulop, N. J., Hartley, J., Ramsay, A., & Roe, B. (2023). Navigating the micro-politics of major system change: The implementation of Sustainability Transformation Partnerships in the English health and care system. *Original Research Journal of Health Services Research & Policy*, 28(4), 233–243. https://doi.org/10.1177/13558196221142237

Weisz, G. (2020). What happened to the Global Forum for Health Research? *Global Public Health*, 15(8), 1212–1224. https://doi.org/10.1080/17441692.2020.1752767

Wiyeh, A. B., & Mukumbang, F. C. (2025). Global South leaders should strengthen strategic capacity. *The Lancet*, 405(10475), 297. https://doi.org/10.1016/S0140-6736(24)02637-0

World Health Organization. (2023). Health diplomacy. www.emro.who.int/health-topics/health-diplomacy/index.html

Wright, E. O. (2010). *Envisioning real utopias*. Verso.

Zienkowski, J. (2017). Reflexivity in the transdisciplinary field of critical discourse studies. *Palgrave Communications*, 3(1), 1–12. https://doi.org/10.1057/palcomms.2017.7

8 Decolonial Reflexivity in Global Health

Introduction

The discourse on decolonization is ubiquitous in many fields of study. Nevertheless, how decolonization is envisaged in these fields of study differs from global health. In some fields of study, such as philosophy, because of their nature, decolonization is predominantly epistemic. To this end, the goal is epistemic decolonization (Matolino, 2020; Mitova, 2023; Posholi, 2020; Tobi, 2020). Nevertheless, decolonization in global health can be more challenging as it has both epistemic and practical components. This line of thinking is confirmed by Shahjahan et al. (2022), who uncovered that some fields "were easier to decolonize" than others when they reviewed the potential for decolonizing the curriculum (p.97). They uncovered that decolonizing the curriculum in medicine was more challenging because student's enthusiasm diminished as they became increasingly enmeshed in the culture of medicine (Shahjahan et al., 2022).

Decolonizing global health shares similar challenges with decolonizing medical curricula in that decolonization should be achieved at the epistemic and practice levels. In Chapter 5, I discussed six shifts (in mindset and practice) that must be achieved for global health decolonization to be possible: decolonizing the mind, avoiding colonial amnesia, reimagining global health expertise, establishing meaningful global health collaborations, valorizing local knowledge and having a self-reliant mindset. In Chapter 7, decolonial reflexivity is proposed as a guiding principle to decolonize global health, which has the mandate to enhance our confidence by allowing us to scrutinize our epistemic orientations and practices. In this chapter, I assert that decolonial reflexivity should not be an abstract contemplation that detracts from enacting material change. Rather, I operationalize decolonial reflexivity as a vehicle driving us toward the decolonization of global health.

The 2023 WHO Resolution on Decolonial Practices (WHA76.12) offers a template, but implementation hinges on Northern accountability to Southern-led audits. Owing to the interconnected mindsets (racism, hegemony, paternalism, white supremacy, and white saviorism) driving coloniality, decoloniality thus requires a multifaceted approach. The complexity of the concept, process, and movement of coloniality lends decoloniality to take different forms

DOI: 10.4324/9781032700786-8

depending on the sociopolitical positionality of the actor, their colonial history, and their access to power. To understand how decolonial reflexivity can be instrumental in undoing coloniality in global health, I considered some views and approaches that have been explored to achieve political decolonization. I aim to assess how relevant these approaches could be for decoloniality and draw lessons that could inform the conceptualization of decolonial reflexivity for working towards decoloniality in global health.

Views of decolonization

Before I proceed to present decolonial reflexivity as a potential approach to decoloniality, I thought it would be important to examine some of the prevailing approaches that were considered for achieving political decolonization and self-determination. Exploring other views of decolonization is relevant because, as I have previously conceptualized, the goal of decoloniality in global health is global health decolonization. For this reason, I considered the three approaches or views to decolonization and self-determination conceptualized by Stilz (2015): instrumentalist, democratic, and associative views. I will provide a brief description of each of these views or approaches and explore how they can achieve the decolonization of global health through decoloniality.

The Instrumentalist View

The instrumentalist view of Decolonization_1 emphasized the practical necessity and immediate political action to end colonial rule, focusing on structural injustice rather than moral or developmental prerequisites. It argues that decolonization was required primarily because colonial governance was inherently unjust, exploiting and oppressing subject peoples through coercive systems of control (Stilz, 2015). To this end, pragmatic actions were recommended, prioritizing the direct expulsion of colonial powers over resolving questions of national identity or institutional readiness for self-governance (Sultan, 2020).

The instrumentalist view advocated for using colonial tools such as language and administrative structures pragmatically to achieve liberation, in contrast to the developmental view requiring "preparation" for self-rule. Critics argue that this approach risks overlooking deeper sociocultural legacies of colonialism, focusing narrowly on political sovereignty while leaving economic or epistemic inequalities unresolved.

According to the instrumentalist perspective on colonization, decolonization seems plausible when examining the abuses of colonial rule. The instrumentalist approach focuses only on citizens' interests (as institutional "takers") in benefiting from a reasonably just state's rule. Instrumentalists attribute the citizen and their political community solely from a beneficiary's perspective. However, citizens are also interested in deciding how to order their collective lives together. They are not just the passive "takers" of their institutions; they seek to be active "makers" of them.

Decolonizing global health based on the instrumentalist approach entails prioritizing the victim. It strongly affirms the colonized's agency, represented by their capacity to appropriate and take part ownership of their freedom. Towards this end, the instrumentalist approach lends itself to self-determination. Although decoloniality is conceptually and epistemologically different from political decolonization, with decoloniality based predominantly on morality, many scholars today favor the Global South striving for self-termination. The argument is that the Global South cannot continue to rely on the "goodwill" and "benevolence" of the Global North to address their health-related issues as the Global North implicitly or explicitly dictates global health objectives and activities (Khan et al., 2018; Sun et al., 2025), which creates a dangerous dependence on these organizations (see Chapter 5).

The COVID-19 vaccine hoarding during the COVID-19 era exemplified the danger of relying on the Global North for their health issues. The principles of fairness and utility guided the distribution of COVID-19 vaccines. Fairness was meant to ensure equitable access to vaccines for all population groups, while utility prioritizes resource allocation strategies that yield the greatest public health benefit. De Campos-Rudinsky et al. (2024) argued that not including the principle of subsidiarity in Article 4 of the WHO Pandemic Agreement as a pragmatic strategy was a missed opportunity to decolonize global health governance. This dual approach balances distributive justice with outcome optimization in healthcare systems. Many authors perceived the vaccine hoarding incident as an expression of coloniality. Following the vaccine hoarding incidents during the COVID-19 pandemic, there was advocacy for the Global South to invest in producing and distributing vaccines rather than depend on external donors based in the Global North. Achieving this requires the Global South nations to consider dismantling the ideological and structural imbalances perpetuated by foreign aid and aid dependency. This approach will entail establishing fair domestic funding mechanisms for health, overhauling institutional frameworks, and reimagining governance models. Crucially, achieving health sovereignty demands pragmatic policy efforts to construct systems prioritizing healthcare as a collective public resource—moving beyond symbolic assertions of autonomy toward tangible, sustainable infrastructure (Guleid, 2025).

The Democratic View

The democratic view of decolonization is morally required because the colonized do not have democratic representation in global health structures and agenda setting. The democratic view links self-determination to fair procedures for collective decision-making. According to Stilz (2015), the democratic approach to decolonization entails having equal rights to vote for representatives, associate with political parties, express political views, and compete for office. This understanding would mean that the laws reflect the decisions of self-governing people, and as such, they are worthy of respect. The democratic view of decolonization is predicated on the public equality argument. The moral requirement of decolonization, through the democratic view, follows the argument that disenfranchising people is wrong as it brands the excluded as inferior or fails to treat their interests equally (Stilz, 2015). What gives these people self-determination rights is their claim to be politically enfranchised.

The democratic approach insists on fairness in representation. Unfairness in representation is ubiquitous in global health in the forms of (1) asymmetric distribution of power in collaborative work with the Global South, (2) Global South partners feeling less apt to challenge Global North partners, and (3) underground work done by Global North partners requesting tacit approval from Global South partners. These three areas of unfair representation capture the refusal or resistance of Global North partners to learn from local populations, especially those from the margins of society (Gedela, 2021). Approaches to decolonizing global health, which address fairness in representation, would include people with relevant in-country expertise and lived experience of the leading health issues, contexts, and relevant geographies occupying powerful positions on governing bodies and decision-making panels of Global Health organizations. Decoloniality would empower valuable leaders to push forward necessary global health measures when restricted. In the context of the colonization of global health, contributions and participation in decision-making and agenda-setting in the Global South are suboptimal. Decolonizing the global in this sense following the democratic view entails promoting the central role of the World Health Organization in global health, safeguarded by the United Nations Charter requiring that the institutional powers of significant players in global health do not work against the quest for equity.

The Associative View

Decolonization was morally required because the colonized could not affirm the political institutions their rulers imposed on them. In this view of decolonization, citizens desire an equally important interest in self-rule, in being the authors (or "makers") of the institutions to which they are subject. Here, the citizens are interested in benefiting from their nation's rule, their community's self-determination, and the political cooperation that guides these institutions (Stilz, 2015). This view captures two essential levels of decolonization: (a) the personal freedom of the individuals, as "takers," is guaranteed by the country's political institutions, and (b) as "makers," the individuals participate in these institutions. Their claim to be cooperative partners in a political institution they could reasonably affirm gave the colonized self-determination rights.

The associative view of decolonization accommodates nationalism by better incorporating a "maker" perspective—individuals have equally important interests in their institutions as political agents. Political institutions (structures) are valuable for individuals in part because such individuals created those institutions together with others and see those institutions as reflecting a shared project (Stilz, 2015). A paradigm shift would involve actively acknowledging oppressive forces, a leadership shift to include more women, minorities, and experts from the Global South and a knowledge shift from unidirectional to bidirectional flow between the Global North and Global South.

An example of the associative perspective of Decolonization_1 using the maker's perspective as applies to Decolonization_2 is when Sun et al. (2025) argue for the Global South nations to (1) mobilize national and regional assets and (2) expand the role of non-state actors to enhance their relationship and representation within the traditional multilateral organizations to address their health-related concerns. Attaining this requires Global South leaders to confront and redesign the values and structural distortions that Global North foreign aid has introduced into their health systems. It also entails reducing reliance on expatriate expertise and preferring expertise from the Global South for program management and technical operations to strengthen local ownership and sustainability. Based on the taker's perspective, the countries in the Global South can invest in regional efforts to mobilize resources for regional and country public health commons, such as the Africa Epidemics Fund.

A Decolonial Reflexive Approach

The core of Chapter 7 aimed to develop the decolonial reflexivity concept drawing from global health practice and research. I developed decolonial reflexivity based on Gilbert and Sliep's (2009) concept of inter-relational reflexivity as a way of thinking through addressing inequities and injustices in global health. I presented decolonial reflexivity as a counter-hegemonic and equity-based approach to drive the Global South toward self-actualization in global health research and practice. As a step further, I am proposing a four-step decolonial reflexivity approach to provide (not prescribe) practical steps for working towards decoloniality in global health (Figure 8.1):

1) Develop a responsible critique.
2) Ensure commitments (cultivate sustained engagement).
3) Goal setting (concrete utopias).
4) Action.

I developed the decolonial reflexivity approach based on insights from the overarching postcolonial critical realism metatheory. The postcolonial critical realism metatheory was cogently developed from post-colonial theories, the tenets of basic critical realism, Bhaskar's political-moral theory conceptualized through MELD, and Archer's Social Morphogenesis and reflexivity concepts. Where appropriate, I have indicated the elements I drew from in developing the various steps of the decolonial reflexivity approach.

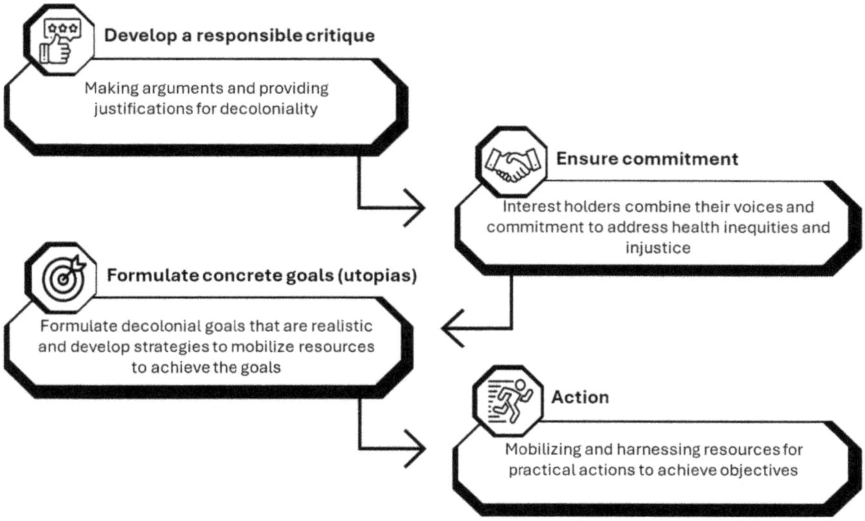

Figure 8.1 A proposed decolonial reflexivity approach to decolonizing global health.

Step 1: Develop a Responsible Critique

Scholarly engagements (philosophical perspectives, empirical inquiries, and narrative discourses) should perform a "critical" function by challenging the socio-political status quo. Although the word "critical" in critical realism was not originally coined to refer to political critique, Roy Bhaskar always intended to support radical politics to illuminate and empower the project of human self-emancipation. Wright (2010) confirmed that diagnosis and critique can be used to explain the systematic ways capitalism harms people. As discussed in Chapter 3, critical realism's "critical" role can be achieved by critiquing the status quo. For instance, a decolonial praxis in global health focuses on subverting the Global North's epistemological dominance, including its institutionalized practices of resource allocation, knowledge production, and policy design that reproduce structural inequities in Global South health systems. Therefore, the "purpose of this critique is to influence political practice by providing reasons and justifications for social change" (Elder-Vass, 2022, p. 540). He used the term "responsible critique" as the kind of critique that can become effective to "recognize when the status quo prevents flourishing and when it creates harm for people, and that requires that we explain the nature of those harms, why we should reject those harms and the things that cause them, and how the status quo contributes to creating them" (p. 540). Chapter 2 describes the colonized nature of global health in detail, which addresses the goal of explaining the nature of the harms of coloniality in global health, and Chapter 4 presents the "things that cause them" (generative mechanisms).

According to Wright (2010), "[to] be a critic of the status quo (existing institutions and social structures) is to identify the harms that are generated by existing arrangements, to formulate alternatives, which mitigate those harms, and to propose transformative strategies for realizing those alternatives" (p. 26). According to Bhaskar, the "concrete" serves to pinpoint the real, but non-actualized possibilities inherent in a situation, thus inspiring grounded hope to inform emancipatory praxis. Formulating critiques to support or empower social change, such as counter-hegemonic discourses to decolonize global health, should be based on the critique that depends on utopianism, ethical commitments, and causal explanation (Elder-Vass, 2022). Zienkowski (2017) states that reflexivity is a precondition for articulating critique (see Chapter 7). This understanding leads to the first step of the decolonial reflexivity approach to addressing inequities and injustices in global health practices and research.

Elder-Vass (2022) identified three characteristics of a responsible critique: it depends on ethics, on causal explanations, and on the development of concrete utopias. Utopianism requires envisioning alternatives to the status quo or possibilities that do not currently exist. In this instance, a decolonized global health will be one without health inequities and (epistemic) injustice, with the status quo being a global health practice underpinned by coloniality. While the argument is that utopias are usually impossible to achieve, it is also argued that formulating them could help us expose the flaws of the status quo (coloniality). Nevertheless, again, unrealistic utopias can be counterproductive, destroying support for change because unrealistic visions can divert the attention of movements away from achievable goals to impossible goals. To this end, Bhaskar advocates for concrete utopias (Archer, 2019), which involves thinking about how a situation or the world could be otherwise, with a change in the use of a given set of resources or with a different way of acting subject to certain constraints (Wright, 2010). The excerpt epistemologically aligns with the counter-hegemonic praxis outlined in Chapter 5 as essential for advancing decoloniality—specifically, the triad of (1) epistemic reorientation (decolonizing the mind and centering Indigenous knowledge systems), (2) institutional critique (confronting historical erasure and redefining expertise hierarchies), and (3) relational ethics (fostering equitable collaboration while cultivating self-reliance and self-determination). This triad operationalizes responsible critique as a grounded methodology and a transformative horizon for global health.

"Useful concrete utopias, though, are not visions of whole alternative ready-made societies but rather partial models that can be built in practice as elements of the larger social world—so that building a better future may involve fitting together a number of concrete utopias that relate to different aspects of social practice" (Elder-Vass, 2022, p. 541). By this statement, Elder-Vass suggests that realistic, useful visions for decolonized global health are not about imagining a perfect, finished society. Abimbola and Pai (2020) have argued that a completely decolonized global health is not feasible. Instead, practical utopias are like building blocks we can create in specific areas and combine over time. In this case, I propose considering the triad of epistemic reorientation, institutional critique, and relational ethics as the components of the Decolonization$_2$ agenda that must be achieved. Think of it like solving a puzzle—each piece (or "concrete utopia") tackles one part of society, and together, they form a bigger picture of progress.

Thinking through better alternatives to the status quo forms the basis of an ethics oriented to change. Elder-Vass (2022) contends that a critique inherently depends on an ethical evaluation of some aspect of the present as a wrong that needs to be addressed through a utopian alternative. Explicit ethical commitments are essential both to the formulation of critique and its expression because to persuade people of why a change is needed, one must be able to unearth the wrong that needs to be addressed (coloniality) and how people could flourish under the utopian alternative (decoloniality). In Chapter 5, I illustrated that ethical/and/or moral considerations drive values and can be informed by facts. Nevertheless, ethical commitments emanate from decolonial reflections through which we must persuade people of our arguments, which entails explicating the ethical commitments and principles on which they are based. Utopian proposals such as decolonizing global health depend on multiple interacting values, requiring continuing ethical discourse. Thus, they commonly believe that good social science should improve the world and our system of moral judgments.

Critical realists believe that social research and theorizing involve value commitments. A responsible critique should first be able to articulate the causal link between the status quo and the lack of human flourishing. In other words, it should provide an assumption that the thing to be changed is causally responsible for repairing the harm. Responsible critique, in essence, requires that to be convinced that coloniality is responsible for the health inequities in the Global South, one must provide a causal link between coloniality and the global distribution of health outcomes to argue for coloniality to be imploded. According to Elder-Vass (2022), while formulating responsible critiques, attention should also be given to the mechanisms involved in the evaluation process and possible outcomes. Formulating such critiques, thus, involves retroducing the mechanisms that generate the adverse effects and outcomes that the status quo perpetuates based on our experience of previous events and structures (see Chapter 4).

Challenging the status quo through responsible critique can be seen as enforcing the "critical" in critical realism. Uncovering how things are is a necessary step to demonstrate the place of human acts in the "reproduction of social structures and relations that stand in the way of emancipation [and human flourishing]" (Wright, 2010, p. 26). Reflections on alternative structures where genuine and equitable (health care) services can be perpetuated (utopia) is a helpful way they strive to contribute to creating structures that overcome inequities and emancipate the disenfranchised (Wilson & Greenhill, 2004). In doing so, one is fulfilling the ethical obligation of addressing unfairness and promoting equity in global health when one examines the abuses associated with coloniality. By considering the concepts of practical utopianism, ethical consideration, and causal explanations, we observe that

"At the philosophical level, critical realism can help us to clarify what is required for productive, responsible critique that can support emancipatory politics" (Elder-Vass, 2022, p. 550).

Mounting a productive and responsible critique to decolonize global health can be achieved through health diplomacy. According to the World Health Organization, health diplomacy refers to "the negotiation processes that shape and manage the policy environment for health." There is an increasing recognition that in the context of health international relationships, health diplomacy can be harnessed to protect populations and health workers and call on donors to support humanitarian action. The main goals of health diplomacy are (1) better health security and population health; (2) improved relations between states and a commitment of a wide range of actors to work together to improve health; and (3) achievement of outcomes that are deemed fair and support the goals of reducing poverty and increasing equity (World Health Organization, 2023).

Developing a responsible critique through decolonial reflexivity to articulate the need for decolonizing global health should lead to understanding the current architecture of global health, its origins, and its impacts. It must highlight how global health architecture reflects historical power asymmetries and competing interests. It must also show how systemic inequities persist while it has driven progress in disease-specific areas. It must argue for reforms to address fragmentation, democratize governance, and prioritize sustainable, equitable health systems.

Step 2: Ensure Commitments (Cultivate Sustained Engagement)

It goes without saying that to achieve a social change, such as decolonizing global health, there must be a commitment from important and relevant interest holders. Ensuring that the parties involved commit to the decolonial project through decolonial reflexivity entails cultivating sustained engagement. To this end, I concur with Sharma and Sam-Agudu (2023) that sustained engagement to decolonize global health should occur at different levels—Global North–Global North, Global North–Global South, and Global South–Global South. I argue that the nature of sustained engagement of the anti-hegemonic praxis should be commensurate to the level of engagement. At the level of the (local) Global South, their decolonial reflexivity should focus on epistemic reorientation (decolonizing the mind and valorizing indigenous knowledge) and relational ethics (cultivating self-reliance and self-efficacy). Epistemic orientation should start with understanding the current architecture of global health, its colonial influence, and how coloniality continues to influence global health research and practice. The Global South should be committed to demanding change, exercising agency, combating elite capture, and fighting for self-determination, self-sufficiency, equity, and justice. The commitment to decolonizing global health required at the (local) Global South should thus focus on a more substantial regional presence in global discussions on health or other issues that potentially impact health, such a representation that we have argued is the symptom of a colonized society. Both health and foreign policy officials from the Global South should be cognizant of the importance of reinforcing their engagement in discussions that are mainly relevant to their region. Equally important is strengthening the interaction and coordination between health, foreign policy, and other governance structures at the regional and domestic levels.

At the Global North–North (former or settler colonizer/high-income country level) engagements, decolonial reflexivity should focus on institutional critique (combating colonial amnesia and redefining global health expertise). Decolonial reflexivity of the Global North should focus on reflecting on and appreciating power, privilege, and positionality. Considering this, they should learn to be authentic allies and co-liberators or part of the decolonization movement. Their commitment should be to shift power and avoid elite capture—the process by which powerful individuals or groups (elites) manipulate systems to divert resources, influence policies, or co-opt initiatives intended for broader public benefit to serve their interests. Commitment to decolonize global health from the Global North–North engagements could focus on:

1) Revising global health programs to center anti-colonial critiques, political economy frameworks, and non-Western epistemologies.
2) Joint commitments to prioritize local leadership in funding decisions, such as the Lacuna Fund (supported by Canada, Germany, and the UK), which directs resources to AI and data science projects led by Global South researchers.
3) Commitments to enforce advocacy for equitable representation in multilateral bodies (e.g., WHO, World Bank) through quota systems or weighted voting to amplify Global South voices.
4) Commitment to collaborative policy efforts to regulate transnational corporations (e.g., pharmaceuticals) headquartered in the Global North.

At the Global North–Global South colonial reflexivity level, the counter-hegemonic praxis should be focused on fostering institutional ethics (equitable collaboration). Decolonial reflexivity and commitments should be toward the collective reimagining of a better version of global health that is genuinely inclusive, diverse, and equitable. The argument here is that the colonized should take the lead and drive the direction of such endeavors, which aligns with Pai's (2022) calls for leadership from the Global South and Allyship from the Global North to decolonize global health. Global North–South commitments could be sought in the following areas:

1) Regarding decolonial co-leadership in governance, commitment should be made for Global North institutions to cede 50%+ decision-making roles in funding bodies (e.g., Global Fund, Gavi) to Global South representatives.

2) Regarding equitable financial mechanisms, commitment should shift from restricted, project-based, or disease-focused aid to unconditional fiscal transfers managed by Global South institutions.
3) Regarding justice in knowledge production, Global North universities should be committed to adopting co-authorship covenants requiring Global South collaborators to lead research design, interpretation, and publications.
4) Commitments to dismantling exploitative labor hierarchies in global health to end "parachute research" by allocating 30%+ of grant budgets to Global South researcher salaries and institutional overheads.

Step 3: Goal Setting (Concrete Utopias)

Of course, the decolonization of global health is an enormous task requiring realistic and achievable goals. As we have seen earlier in this chapter, one of the conditions for constructing a responsible critique is to have plausible concrete utopias—alternatives to the status quo. Archer (2019) illustrated how critical realism aligns with the idea of concrete utopias. According to Bhaskar (2016), formulating concrete utopias is a key feature for thinking about how to effect a transition to a good society and thus "forms an indispensable component in all ethical thinking" (Bhaskar, 2016, p. 16). While formulating a productive and responsible critique is an important step towards understanding why global health must be decolonized, it is equally important to present a picture of how a decolonized global health should look. Imagining the nature of a decolonized global health is known as utopianism. Bhaskar and Hartwig (2010) believe that utopianism is indispensable in postulating a different situation from the actual one, and this different state should convey hope for an alternative future. For example, Hirsch shared her position on decolonizing global health in global health institutions:

> I question whether decolonizing global health institutions is possible. If we want to work towards health justice, the institutions that have been built on and benefited from the racist exploitation of Black, Brown, and Indigenous populations the world over cannot decolonize and keep their epistemic, political, and financial power. If global health institutions are serious about their commitment to working against the legacies of colonialism and fighting racism, then they will need to give up some or all of their power. That means a radical redistribution of funding away from high-income countries, a loss of epistemic and political authority, and a limitation to our power to intervene in low-income and middle-income countries (LMICs). That is unlikely to happen. Systems and institutions protect people, especially white people, all the time.
>
> (Hirsch, 2021, p. 190)

An important question to consider is whether decolonizing global health is a plausible alternative to the current practice of global health. Considering this discussion, would one say decolonizing global health is an unrealistic utopia? I argue that this is how we should envisage decolonizing global health—adopting a process that systematically dismantles coloniality while empowering the Global South. To this end, I considered formulating goals to address the three counter-hegemonic praxis I conceptualized in Chapter 5: epistemic reorientation, institutional critique, and relational ethics. Calls to decolonize global health by formulating concrete utopias are considered under the "reimagining global health" banner.

Real or concrete utopias,[1] for Wright (2010), exist as a subset of the broader enterprise of developing an emancipatory social science, and these utopias should have three criteria: desirability, viability, and achievability. He explained further that not all desirable alternatives are viable and not all viable alternatives are achievable. Desirable alternatives should be based on moral and ethical principles. We have seen that critical realists like Bhaskar, Archer, Lawson, and Elder-Vass agree that the development of alternatives to address harm should be based on ethical and moral principles. I have also argued in Chapter 5 that Decolonization_2 is more an ethical-moral endeavor than a political mandate. Wright (2010) explained that desirable is mainly focused on enjoining abstract principles rather than detailing a plan. For example, the decolonization of global health should be based on the moral and ethical principles of human rights and health for all or the right to health. These have been captured through the politico-moral planar of Bhaskar's dialectical critical realism and Acher's morphogenetic approach to social change. While these principles laid a foundation for providing alternatives to addressing the harms of a global health practice based on coloniality and the relics of colonization, they provide little direction on how to decolonize global health.

Concrete Utopias for Epistemic Reorientation

The goal of decolonizing global health pertains to epistemic reorientation, which involves dismantling colonial-era mental frameworks, including structural racism, and reclaiming cultural, intellectual, and psychological autonomy. Sharma and Sam-Agudu (2023) shared a Four Action framework adapted for the decolonization of global health by the Global South in the Global South, which aligns with the goals of epistemic orientation (decolonizing the mind and valorizing indigenous knowledge). The Four Action Framework had goals that were geared toward (1) eliminating coloniality in individual behavior, (2) reducing systemic inequities, (3) raising neglected areas, and (4) creating (decolonized) new knowledge.

Table 8.1 outlines some practical utopias that can achieve epistemic reorientation. The goals outlined in this segment require the Global South

Table 8.1 Counter-hegemonic praxis for achieving epistemic reorientation

Components of epistemic orientation	*Concrete goals and actions*
Revitalize indigenous languages	• Promote education, media, and official use of marginalized languages to counteract linguistic imperialism (e.g., replacing colonial languages in institutions).
Reform global health educational curricula	• Integrate Indigenous histories, epistemologies, and scientific contributions into mainstream education, challenging Eurocentric narratives.
Integrating anti-racism in education and research	• Reforming curricula to eliminate colonial biases and racist narratives in global health education.
Promote contextually relevant education	• Revise curricula in global health programs to center colonial histories, anti-racism, and indigenous health systems. For instance, schools of tropical medicine—originally tied to colonial projects—should critically reassess their historical roots.
Reclaim cultural narratives	• Support art, literature, and oral traditions rooted in local cosmologies to counteract colonial stereotypes and erasure.
Combat internalized inferiority	• Foster psychological empowerment through community dialogues, mentorship, and platforms celebrating indigenous identities and achievements.
Critique colonial power structures	• Encourage critical analysis of systemic inequities (e.g., racial hierarchies, resource extraction) perpetuated by colonial legacies.
Build intersectional solidarity	• Address overlapping oppressions (gender, class, ethnicity) and collaborate with global movements (e.g., black liberation, indigenous rights).
Amplify grassroots movements	• Support community-led health initiatives and solidarity networks (e.g., African-led malaria control programs) rather than externally imposed solutions. This aligns with the Alma Ata Declaration's emphasis on community empowerment.

communities to empower and uplift their communities, which are grounded in their knowledge systems, beliefs, and practices. For example, Ngũgĩ wa Thiong'o advocates writing in Gĩkũyũ instead of English to reclaim cultural agency. Also, the University of Cape Town has revised curricula to center African philosophies. These actions are relevant for addressing epistemic injustice.

Concrete Utopias for Institutional Critique

Combating colonial amnesia and redefining global health expertise are components of counter-hegemonic practice that require Global North–South

Table 8.2 Counter-hegemonic praxis for addressing colonial amnesia.

Institutional critique	*Concrete goals and actions*
Acknowledge historical and contemporary colonial exploitation	• Explicitly recognize how colonial-era resource extraction, slavery, and racial hierarchies continue to shape health inequities (e.g., Indigenous communities facing higher mortality rates due to historical displacement and underfunded health systems). • Challenge narratives that frame global health as a "neutral" field by exposing its roots in colonial medicine and racialized exploitation.
Reform knowledge production practices	• Prioritize Indigenous and local epistemologies in research design, methodologies (e.g., land-based learning, storytelling), and authorship to counter Western-centric paradigms. Ensure equitable representation of researchers from marginalized communities in journals and editorial boards.
Address historical legacies in health policies	• Explicitly analyze colonial-era practices (e.g., malaria control strategies designed to protect colonizers, not local populations) and their modern implications. Integrate historical critiques into contemporary health interventions.
Decolonize knowledge production	• Shift from Western-centric paradigms to integrating Indigenous and local epistemologies in research, policy design, and training programs.

collaborations. Table 8.2 outlines some counter-hegemonic goals for addressing colonial amnesia.

These goals aim to dismantle colonial power structures in funding, knowledge systems, and governance while centering historically marginalized voices in global health practice. They aim to replace colonial amnesia with historical accountability and structural transformation, ensuring global health systems address root causes of inequity rather than perpetuating coloniality.

Concrete Utopias for Relational Ethics

Relational ethics deals with equitable collaborations and self-reliance. While these may sound oxymoronic, they are not. There should be aspects of global health that the Global South nations should be able to address by themselves, while issues such as epidemics and pandemics would require collaborations to address them. The nature of collaboration refers to Global North–Global South collaborations, while self-reliance speaks to individual countries in the Global South being able to meet the health needs of their populations without the reliance or dependency on aid and grants from the Global North. It also relates to the Global South as a region meeting and being able to collectively provide the requisite health care services required by people from the Global

Table 8.3 Goals for achieving equitable Global North–Global South collaboration

Equitable collaborations	*Concrete goals and actions*
Shift funding and leadership to local institutions	• Redirect research funding and decision-making authority to institutions in the Global South, particularly those historically colonized. For example, address disparities where 99% of malaria research funding flows to institutions in wealthy nations rather than African ones.
Strengthen equitable partnerships	• Adopt mutual-benefit frameworks for Global North–South collaborations, including joint funding mechanisms and technology transfers (e.g., mRNA vaccine production hubs in the Global South). • Reform intellectual property rules to ensure Global South retains sovereignty over health innovations.
Decentralize global health governance	• Challenge power hierarchies in international organizations by transferring leadership roles to experts from the Global South, which includes revising institutions' governance structures like the WHO to reflect equitable geographic and cultural representation.
Combat exploitative research practices	• Link health equity to data ownership by opposing neocolonial practices like helicopter research practices. • Advocate for policies ensuring the Global South retains sovereignty over research data.

South through South–South collaborations. Table 8.3 indicates some goals for achieving establishment.

Indeed, the collaborations (which in reality is reliance) of the Global South with the Global North in this current form have not achieved significant success in addressing the health challenges of the Global South. To this end, authors like Opara (2021) emphasized the need for self-determination, proposing that decolonization should be defined by, led by, and the benefits reaped by the indigenous, formerly colonized, and (neo)colonized, and while doing so, they must reject the external and the internalized white Euro-American gaze and standards and "return to the source." Achieving self-determination in this current dispensation would entail striving to achieve some of the following goals (Table 8.4).

Some global health decolonization proponents advocate for improving the nature of Global North–South collaborations (Lawrence & Hirsch, 2020; Pai et al., 2024). Others, such as Abimbola (2024), see decolonization as addressing the issues of pose and gaze in global health practice and research, while others, like Opara (2021), believe that such collaborations would still lead to dependency, thus insisting on self-determination. While there seems to be a polarity on which relational approach should be adopted to ensure the decolonization of global health, I believe combining both approaches would achieve

Table 8.4 Plurilateral goals toward self-determination

Self-determination	*Goals and actions*
Strengthening domestic resource mobilization	• Redirect research funding and decision-making authority to institutions in the Global South, especially those with a history of colonization. For instance, it is crucial to tackle the disparity in which 99% of malaria research funding is allocated to wealthy nations rather than African institutions.
Expanding and diversifying funding sources	• Expanding and diversifying funding sources is essential for the Global South. • They should pursue grants from regional institutions and non-Western donors while mobilizing diaspora contributions.
Advocating for sustainable funding policies	• Governments should advocate for continent-wide funding policies prioritizing domestic resources and seeking multi-year donor commitments instead of relying on short-term grants.
Investing in local talent and capacity development	• Reducing reliance on expatriate expertise and leveraging local African professionals in program management, fundraising, and technical will enhance local ownership and sustainability.
Scientific autonomy	• Establish conditions that empower Global South scientists to take ownership of their fields through robust research budgets and foster South–South research collaboration.
Technological self-determination	• Increase investment in digital infrastructure and regional innovation to diminish reliance on foreign technology monopolies.
Public health self-reliance	• Achieve self-reliance in public health financing and boost South–South research and human resource training cooperation.
Economic cooperation	• Develop a South–South economic agenda that minimizes dependence on Western products and capital while enhancing trade routes and intercontinental supply chains.
Pharmaceutical innovation	• Adopt a new approach to pharmaceutical innovation and access, which includes regional manufacturing.
Religious freedoms	• Strengthen interfaith initiatives and legal frameworks and ensure they are culturally grounded, ensuring meaningful protections within local contexts while promoting inclusive and pluralistic values.

better results than either of the two positions. In this way, I align with Sharma and Sam-Agudu (2023) that decolonizing globally should be everyone's business, within which we can all play an active role.

Whichever perspective is adopted for decolonization, Wright (2010) proposes forming intermediate reforms to overcome the temptation of setting unrealistic utopias. He suggested that intermediate reforms share two properties: (1) they demonstrate the virtues of the fuller program of transformation, thus contributing to pursuing the alternative as credible and desirable. (2) They enhance people's capacity for action, thus increasing their ability to forge towards transformation. Khan (2022) also agrees that breaking the task down to achievable milestones may be one way to approach the decolonization of the global health agenda. Concrete utopias combine our theoretical understandings of possibilities with an ethical analysis of needs to offer practical schemes for improving human flourishing.

Step 4: Action

Dismantling the historical and contemporary expression of capitalism and imperialism in global health scaffolded by racism, white supremacy, and hegemony requires that the mind decolonization and emancipating our imagination and thinking towards genuine liberation. Decolonizing our minds entails a process of self-recovery to reclaim and restore our indigenous cultures, epistemologies, languages, technologies, art, histories, religions, and science (Opara, 2021). Opara further suggested that:

> We need to be thoroughly purged from centuries of psychosocial conditioning and internalized colonization grounded in European and American myths and lies of who we are, where we come from, our abilities, values, contributions to the world, and how our current state of affairs came to be. These lies were designed for us to internalize their delusion of superiority, even while they depended, and continue to depend, on our wealth, resources, intellect, skills, and labor to survive. We need to engage in individual and collective healing practices to address the cumulative trauma of coloniality, racism, patriarchy, ableism, capitalism, homo-transphobia, and all intersecting systems of oppression that have been transmitted intergenerationally and experienced on the levels of the intrapersonal, interpersonal, institutional, systemic, and structural.
>
> (Opara, 2021)

Opara (2021), in her arguments for Decolonization$_2$, suggests that not only should the Global South purge themselves of the mind control of the Global North, but that they should also strive to move towards emancipating their thinking and imagination to achieve liberation. This argument aligns with Bhaskar's (2009) concept of emancipation, which posits liberation from oppressive structures through emancipation. Through emancipation, he argues that the world becomes meaningful, and values are no longer seen as subjective classifications of the mind but constitute reality. My argument is that the purging of our minds can be achieved through the process of re-education (especially with indigenous knowledge), whereby curriculums are redesigned to uncover our stories of the past, present, future, and in between, integrate an eco-centric liberated ethos, empower us to reject old paradigms of being and create new ones (Opara, 2021).

In a recent lecture at the Open University of Nigeria convocation, the president of the African Development Bank, Dr. Akinwumi Adesina, outlined a visionary path for Africa's economic self-reliance. In his lecture, he said, "The recent dismantling of the official development aid agency in the United States, and similar anti-aid measures in other parts of Europe, means that the old development models that Africa has always relied on will no longer work" (Adesina, 2025). He explained further:

> The era of aid or free money is gone. African countries must now learn to develop via investment discipline. Countries can no longer rely on aid for growth or count it as part of government revenue, as has been the case for decades. Benevolence is not an asset class.
>
> (Adesina, 2025)

The speech by the President of the African Development Bank is a wake-up call for Africa to become self-reliant and seek solutions to the problems plaguing the continent by breaking free from the reliance on foreign aid from the Global North.

Critical realism asserts that knowledge has an emancipatory nature that can free society from the modification of earlier structures of science (Wilson & Greenhill, 2004). According to Bhaskar (2009), emancipation comes with knowledge acquisition, which aims to improve the conditions of the disenfranchised. Emancipation is achieved through essential mechanisms such as consciousness-raising, becoming motivated to act, and finally, acting, a transformative process (Wilson & Greenhill, 2004). The philosophical principles of (postcolonial) critical realism and understanding of value elucidate its contribution to knowledge and the construction of alternatives. Critical realism commits to emancipation and focuses on issues of equality and inequality by questioning the status quo. Critical realism seeks ways of transforming asymmetric relations and calls for action to mobilize research to prevent the degeneration of equity and improve the situation.

Regarding self-reliance, as indicated earlier, members of the decolonizing global health movement advocate for self-reliance as the ultimate indication of decolonization. Tangwa and Munung (2020) explained that during the COVID-19 pandemic, many African countries displayed a sense of self-reliance and self-determination that convincingly demonstrates that African countries can assume responsibility for their health and assert their total decolonization, which means bringing an end to heavy reliance on the Global North for infectious disease control. According to Tangwa and Munung (2020), African leaders held virtual meetings to discuss the continent's response to the epidemic. While the private sector in many African countries donated generously to COVID-19 solidarity funds, the Africa CDC supported the African continent's

COVID-19 response (Tangwa & Munung, 2020). Because the Africa Centres for Disease Control and Prevention receives funding predominantly from external donors like the US CDC, the China CDC, the European Union, and the Gates Foundation, reliance on the Africa CDC does not show self-sufficiency. Therefore, for Africa to show complete self-reliance, Evaborhene et al. (2025) argue that Africa Centres for Disease Control and Prevention must achieve self-sustainability to address the continent's health challenges effectively. Self-dependence, in this sense, would also require African governments to prioritize health security by allocating a larger portion of their national budgets to this area. Additionally, they should explore innovative financing mechanisms, such as public-private partnerships and levies on industries that benefit from health security, including telecommunications and travel (Evaborhene et al., 2025).

Global health diplomacy practiced between Global South nations can be a game-changer for the region and contribute to their global health decolonization. Emphasizing the core issues of social determinants of health, prioritizing the ever-increasing endemics of HIV and Neglected Tropical Diseases, and addressing the challenges of climate change will reap benefits in the immediate and long term. Strengthening the health systems and earmarking specific funds for health from bilateral/multilateral assistance could be done through the successful practice of global health diplomacy in the region. Upgrading health infrastructure and deploying available digital health solutions will improve access and strengthen the fragile health systems to achieve the Universal Health Coverage and related health targets of the Sustainable Development Goals in Africa (Chattu et al., 2021).

Chattu et al. (2021) explained that to address the high burden of disease that disproportionately affects Africa, key Global South actors like the African Union should commit to (i) navigating the politics of global health governance, (ii) developing robust preparedness and disease response strategies to tackle emerging and re-emerging disease epidemics in the region, (iii) address the linkages between health and broader human security issues driven by climate change-induced food, water, and other insecurities and (iv) mobilize resources and capacities to train health officials in the craft of diplomacy (World Health Organization, 2023). The global health diplomats' perspectives, lived experiences, expertise, and knowledge systems should come to the fore and must inform all goal-setting endeavors and language, stance, frameworks, and strategies to achieve the Sustainable Development Goals of the Global South. Funding and infrastructural support must be committed to providing indigenous and (neo)colonized communities the power of their strategies and solutions towards liberation, autonomy, and independence. Global health diplomacy ensures a serious commitment to health-related outcomes by governments, prioritizing context-specific health needs in securing bilateral/multilateral support for addressing the critical macro level and non-medical interventions (outside the national health systems) to achieve the goals of Universal Health Coverage and health-related Sustainable Development Goals.

Regarding Decolonization$_2$ through equitable collaborations with the Global North, the Global South's emancipation can be achieved by developing a particular cadre of global health diplomats that would benefit the region with successful negotiations and policymaking for disease control activities. Therefore, the Global South must significantly strengthen its capacity in global health diplomacy (Wiyeh & Mukumbang, 2025). This endeavor will require pooling financial, technical, and human resources available in the region to address the health issues plaguing the region. One approach in this regard would be to create a capacity-building group that will work with key training and academic institutions in the Global South (both schools of diplomacy and health institutions) to harness experiences in this field and move the health diplomacy agenda forward more quickly. Ministries of foreign affairs need to ensure that global health diplomacy is included in the training and education of diplomats. Joint education and training between health experts and diplomats within the countries in the Global South should also be encouraged.

Discussion

While I was writing this book, a coworker from the Department of Global Health came to my office. He said hello and asked what I was working on. I told him I was writing a book about decolonizing global health. He sighed and replied, "Decolonization is a farce." That got me thinking about decolonization, and the suggestion that decolonizing global health is an unrealistic goal—an unrealistic utopia. Other authors have also questioned how a decolonized global health will look (Abimbola & Pai, 2020). They further insinuate that if we expect a global health that is equitable, inclusive, and diverse without a hint of supremacy, that world "is still elusive." Indeed, Wright (2010) noted that belief in a utopian ideal (such as equitable global health), inclusive and diverse without a hint of supremacy, may be necessary to motivate people, even though the likely actual destination (decolonized global health) may fall short of the utopian ideal. Wright (2010) cautioned that "vague utopian fantasies may lead us astray, encouraging us to embark on trips that have no real destinations at all, or worse still, which lead us toward some unforeseen abyss" (p. 5). For instance, Kwete et al. (2022) proposed that decolonizing global health requires the world's political economy first to be decolonized, which involves removing the underpinning socioeconomic inequity exacerbated by colonization. They argued that the ultimate goal would be "the equitable economic ownership of the global wealth by all human beings" (p. 4). While this utopia helps expose the flaws in the current status quo, it is unrealistic and can divert the attention of decolonization movements away from achievable goals to impossible goals.

Abimbola and Pai (2020) argue, "A future in which global health is decolonized would be one in which there are no longer pervasive supremacist remnants of colonization within global health practice" (p. 1627). Achieving such a future will mean removing all forms of supremacy within all spaces of global health practice, within countries, between countries, and at the global level. Of course, this is an unrealistic goal as every society has some form of supremacy and hegemony orchestrating how things are run, thus dictating human flourishing and freedom outcomes. We see worldwide that whenever there is pushback against a system of oppression, the oppressive regime starts to put structures in place to pacify the situation, in most instances, rather than address the problem. For example, as elaborated in Chapter 1, the fight against political colonialism did not mean to address the problem of colonialism but was converted from direct to indirect colonialism (neo-colonialism). Similarly, as noted by Abimbola and Pai (2020), as the struggle for equity and justice continues in global health, "those in power are likely to fight back—or respond with evasions, token concessions, and changes in appearance but not in substance" (p. 1627).

Does this mean we should give up and not continue to advocate for equity and justice in global health because those in power will continue to fight back? Certainly not! Wright (2010) offered two reasons why we should not despair. His first point suggests that the future has many uncertainties and contingencies, making it impossible to know what is achievable. For example, achieving political decolonization at some point was also seen as an unachievable goal, but today, we are dealing with neo-colonialism. Secondly, Wright (2010) argues that the limits of what is achievable also depend on the beliefs of the people who are working on the goal to achieve it. Wright's framework underscores that decolonizing global health requires transforming beliefs as much as structures. Overcoming colonial amnesia, redistributing power, and centering marginalized epistemologies depend on practitioners and institutions believing in both the necessity and possibility of radical change. Without this shift, efforts risk reproducing coloniality under the guise of reform.

Recent academic work has been geared toward proposing decolonization frameworks. For example, Sharma and Sam-Agudu (2023) proposed a four-action-focused plan for decolonizing global health: (a) eliminate coloniality in individual behavior, (b) reduce systemic inequity, (c) raise neglected areas, and (d) create (decolonize) new knowledge. While I find this attempt commendable, I argue that it lacks a transformation praxis to inform a robust process toward the decolonization of global health. Without a transformation praxis, decolonization risks becoming a metaphor (Tuck & Yang, 2012), a performative gesture divorced from material and epistemic liberation. Even more recently, Tagoe et al. (2025) also shared a four-step transformative approach to decolonizing global health through the following steps: (1) increase consciousness of the extent of colonial legacies, (2) challenge existing health research assumptions and practices, (3) conceptualize a different future, and (4) take the required actions that move us towards that different desired future. While the Decolonization$_2$ approach proposed by Tagoe et al. (2025) mostly aligns with my proposed four-step decolonial reflexivity approach, my approach is grounded in a philosophical paradigm (postcolonial critical realism), which, as I have demonstrated, is commensurable with the decolonization praxis. The four steps of the decolonial reflexivity approach to decolonization are thus informed by philosophical principles and sociological processes offering the foundations for the proposed steps.

A paradigm shift is needed to decolonize global health and its governance structures. Wright (2010) argues that what is needed to achieve change and emancipation is "real utopias," which he defines as having "ideals that are grounded in the real potentials of humanity, utopian destinations that have accessible waystations, utopian designs of institutions that can inform our practical tasks of navigating a world of imperfect conditions for social change" (p. 5). Bhaskar added that real or concrete utopias entail thinking how a situation or the world could be otherwise, with a change in the use of a given set of resources or with a different way of acting subject to certain constraints. In conceptualizing the decolonial reflexivity approach, I envisaged that it should go beyond acknowledging one's bias and positionality in global health research and practice to include actions that address the source of such bias. In my conceptualization of decolonial reflexivity, I envisage a process whereby the colonial influences are acknowledged, identified, and countered through counter-hegemonic and equity-based approaches. For example, the Global South can achieve Decolonization$_2$ by delivering on its health agendas and strengthening its health systems. This way, external resources from the Global North must be fully aligned to support regional (national) health plans, creating a pathway for increased and sustainable (regional) domestic financing.

Unlike Decolonization$_1$, which aims to achieve political and economic self-determination, Táíwò (2022) claims that Decolonization$_2$ has no clear end goal or end date in view. Of course, arguments have been made by various global health scholars that Decolonization$_2$, as it relates to global health research and practice, should aim to achieve equity and justice. Nevertheless, Abimbola and Pai (2020) argue that global health barely achieves diversity and inclusiveness, which are goals that cannot be measured. Abimbola and Pai (2020) argued further that while striving to achieve Decolonization$_2$, we should not only focus on the measurable goals but also on things that matter but are hard to measure, such as meaningful representation of Global South voices on global health agenda-setting with decision-altering contributions. I contend that meaningful representation of the Global South in global health agenda setting can only be achieved through decolonial reflexivity whereby the Global South representatives are considering experts, and their knowledge and epistemic positions are counted as valuable.

According to Wright (2010), while moral and ethical discussions are valuable in providing clarity to normative goals for a desired change, they are limited in informing how to restructure society to achieve these goals. Addressing this limitation would involve considering "the political achievability of the proposed alternative under existing historical conditions, focusing instead on the likely dynamics and unintended consequences of the proposal if it were to be implemented (Wright, 2010, p. 28). He proposes using systematic theoretical models to uncover the social structures, mechanisms, and agents at play and empirical case studies (historical and contemporary) to test the proposed alternatives. Archer's (1995) morphogenetic framework has been explored to unpack the relevant social structures, mechanisms, and agents required to make the alternative plausible and the role of reflexivity in considering the nature of these alternatives. Furthermore, the postcolonial critical realism approach, which underpins this book, provides an ontological framework to explain the structuring relationship between colonial discourses and social change, which was used to understand how the decolonization of global health can be achieved. After establishing the potential viability of the alternative, establishing achievability becomes the next task. Achievability entails making proposals for policies, programs, and interventions. For example, inequitable participation of Global South experts and community representatives in the governance structures and advisory bodies of organizations focusing on improving health in the Global South should have proposals such as ensuring that people from the Global South should hold the most powerful positions in these organizations with the relevant in-country (or regional) experiences and expertise (Khan et al., 2021). The question now remains: would such "narrow" goals have the impact to get to a global health that is free from hegemony, racism, and white supremacy, characterized by justice and equity?

I have established that the challenge with achieving Decolonization$_2$ is that it is based on ethical-moral principles, equity, historical responsibility, and mutual benefit rather than a political mandate. I argue that relying on ethical-moral principles, which the Global North can provide, would not be enough to decolonize global health. Therefore, achieving decolonization in global health will require a political agenda: the drive that self-reliance and self-determination can produce. This line of thinking makes me aligns with Pai et al.'s (2024) proposal of leadership from the Global South and allyship from the Global North. Leadership commands a political mandate and political mandates are more likely to drive social change through resource mobilization to implement counter-hegemonic praxis than rely on ethical-moral principles from the "oppressors" who are unlikely to relinquish their power and privilege.

There are discussions on whether Decolonization$_2$ can be achieved through a "Big Bang" (rapid systemic overhaul) or incrementalism (gradual reform). The debate between a "Big Bang" and incrementalism in decolonizing global health hinges on feasibility, urgency, and sustainability. The "Big Bang" approach advocates urgency in addressing structural inequities through radical decolonial agendas such as Eurocentric research paradigms, exploitative funding models, and Northern-dominated governance (e.g., WHO's donor-driven priorities). A rapid overhaul could immediately dismantle these systems, abolishing "parachute research" policies, redirecting 50% of Global North grants to Global South-led institutions, and transferring intellectual property (e.g., mRNA vaccines) to Global South manufacturers via mandatory tech-sharing agreements. The "Big Bang" approach will also require sudden shifts, signaling an unwavering commitment to justice. For instance, the African CDC's leadership during COVID-19 demonstrated the viability of regional autonomy over pandemic responses, challenging traditional WHO hierarchies.

Conversely, incrementalism focuses on decolonization activities such as capacity building, reducing resistance to decolonization, and evidence-based adaptations. Many Global South health systems lack infrastructure to absorb rapid changes, as observed during the COVID-19 pandemic (Alilio et al., 2022). An incremental approach to decolonizing global health will thus focus on enhancing the structural capacity of the health systems in the Global South to make them more resilient to health system shocks. Gradual steps, like phased local vaccine manufacturing like Rwanda's BioNTech plant, allow skill and institutional development (Sinumvayo et al., 2024). In public policy, incrementalism, which is based on Lindblom's (1959) "muddling through," is a decision-making approach involving small, step-by-step changes rather than large, comprehensive reforms. Lindblom (1959) argued that this method is more realistic and practical than the traditional rational-comprehensive model because it acknowledges the limited information and cognitive capacity of decision-makers. Incrementalism also offers opportunities for evidence-based adaptation of programs and strategies to address colonization-related inequities and injustice. For instance, pilot programs, like decentralized clinical trial networks co-designed with Indigenous communities, requiring iterative learning to minimize unintended harms can be appropriately implemented (Goodson et al., 2022). It is worth noting that incremental reforms risk dilution by entrenched interests. In addition to interest dilution, factors including the polarization of political ideologies and cultural divides generally make reforms a slow and often stagnant process (Baumgartner & Jones, 1991). For example, the COVAX initiative's failure to equitably distribute vaccines underscores how gradualist models often uphold Northern hegemony. To this end, a hybrid approach to decolonization seems appropriate to address the components that require a "Big Bang" or an incremental approach.

Hybridizing strategies to decolonize global health would mean balancing vision and pragmatism. Of course, it will require having targeted "Big Bang" reforms such as the immediate abolition of exploitative practices (ban extractive data-sharing agreements lacking LMIC authorship) and debt cancellation for health-investing nations (e.g., Zambia's 6 billion USD debt relief enabling healthcare expansion). Bump (2025) argues that global health's humanitarian goals (equal rights and entitlements to universal well-being) will not be realized without dramatic changes in the field. He explained that without engaging economic relationships and trade policy, global health limits its attention to downstream consequences of resource inequalities, where its goal of a more egalitarian, healthier world is difficult, if not impossible, to achieve. Concurrent to these "Big Bang" approaches should be phased structural shifts such as five-year transitions to equitable funding models (e.g., Global Fund allocating 50% of grants via Global South-led committees by

2030) and gradual repatriation of health resources, such as relocating WHO's pandemic hub from Geneva to Nairobi. While a "Big Bang" approach addresses the moral urgency of Decolonization$_2$, incrementalism mitigates practical risks. A hybrid model—combining immediate counter-hegemonic and equity-centered mandates (e.g., redistributing power and resources) with phased capacity-building—offers a pragmatic yet transformative path to global health decolonization. Therefore, decolonizing global health requires a multi-dimensional strategy addressing practices, institutions, policies, education, and power dynamics (Spanaus & De Souza, 2024). As Bhaskar (2009) notes, emancipation requires both dismantling oppressive structures and cultivating new, just systems—a dual process achievable through strategic, sustained action. This hybrid approach aligns with Archer's morphogenetic approach, in which she proposes that social change goes through three phases, with the social interaction phase being a critical phase for social change to occur through decolonial reflexivity.

A characteristic feature of morphogenesis is the changes the actors bring to the social structures that govern ("order") them. Reflexivity and its calls for action should lead to changes in social structures. We have seen that emergence proposes that higher-level entities emerge from a collection of lower-level entities. The emergence lens suggests that transformational change, such as the decolonization of global health, might not necessarily be incremental but remain stable for long periods and then rapidly transform. Therefore, while these changes occur at the levels of programs, institutions, and inter-institutional relationships, these "small" changes can lead to bigger changes. For equity and justice (social and epistemic) to be achieved in global health, there is a need for the social, economic, and political structures that govern global health practice to be delinked from their colonial foundations and anchored unto principles of morals and justice.

The role of decolonial reflexivity has not been explored at the level that it is being proposed in this book—Global North–Global North, Global North–Global South, and Global South–Global South. Nevertheless, inferences of the potential effects (of aspects) of decolonial reflexivity can be drawn from its fair application in global health research contexts (Naidu et al., 2024). For example, Russell-Mundine (2012) adopted a decolonial reflexivity approach in an Indigenous tourism development research context and reported that it contributed to the decolonizing and refraining of research. Decolonization, which she operationalized as challenging dominant research paradigms and power structures that may marginalize Indigenous perspectives and knowledge, was achieved by critically examining the researcher's biases and assumptions and the power dynamics inherent in research relationships. The effects of her decolonial reflexivity led to her shifting the research questions, methodologies, and analyses to be more inclusive and respectful of Indigenous knowledge systems (Russell-Mundine, 2012). Nilson (2017) confirmed that decolonial reflexivity was critical to building respect, relationships, and reciprocity between the Global North researcher and the local community in the Global South. This assertion confirms the counter-hegemonic and equity-focused role of decolonial reflexivity in addressing epistemic injustice, unveiling the local research and the community members as the "true" expertise while establishing meaningful global health collaborations. According to Naidu et al. (2024), decolonial reflexivity also allows Global North researchers to access unconscious attitudes underpinned by coloniality in global health practice and research.

While decolonial reflexivity—critical self-examination of colonial power dynamics in knowledge and practice—is essential for equity, it faces several conceptual and practical challenges. Relating to practical challenges, Liwanag and Rhule (2021) explained that the call to be reflexive may run the risk of becoming lip service without clarity on what reflexivity requires. Also, following the application of the colonial reflexivity approach, Russell-Mundine (2012) reported that the approach failed to interrogate the researcher's role in maintaining the dominant Western culture of knowledge creation. She concluded that decolonial reflexivity can only lead to reforming and decolonizing research if it also "addresses deeper issues such as interrogating the systems of the dominant White culture" (p. 1). Concerning its conceptualization, it has been suggested that decolonial reflexivity can become performative (e.g., diversity training or symbolic land acknowledgments) without redistributing power or resources (Liwanag & Rhule, 2021). For example, Universities may add "decolonization" modules to their curricula while maintaining Eurocentric tenure/promotion criteria. Addressing these proposed decolonial reflectivity approaches requires embedding reflexivity in concrete action based on concrete utopias, such as pairing self-critique with redistributive policies (e.g., reparative grants for LMIC researchers). Decolonial reflexivity should be a valuable approach toward answering the urgent political call to challenge the structures that reproduce coloniality within global health.

Conclusion

Decolonizing global health requires more than critiquing the Global North. Countries in the Global South must also confront their role in maintaining outdated systems—like corrupt governance or copying foreign models without adaptation—that hold back equitable progress. True change needs action from within, not just waiting for outsiders to lead. Addressing coloniality-generated health inequities and injustice requires the adoption of a decoloniality framework. In this book, I proposed decolonial reflexivity informed by postcolonial critical realism as an approach toward transformative change and the reimagination of global health research and practice.

Note

1 Real utopias and concrete utopias were used as synonyms. Erik Olin Wright used the term real utopia, while Roy Bhaskar used the term concrete utopia. In *Envisioning Real Utopias*, Wright wanted to provide arguments against the notion of radical social transformation, to which end he proposed "real utopias," which might appear oxymoronic. Wright suggested that real utopias are not fantasies, or not only fantasies. Rather, they are "hard-nosed proposals for pragmatically improving our lives" or utopian ideals grounded in reality.

References

Abimbola, S. (2024). *The foreign gaze: Essays on global health*. IRD.

Abimbola, S., & Pai, M. (2020). Will global health survive its decolonisation? *The Lancet*, 396(10263), 1627–1628. https://doi.org/10.1016/S0140-6736(20)32417-X

Adesina, A. A. (2025). Advancing Africa's positioning within global development and geopolitical dynamics: Lecture delivered by Dr. Akinwumi A. Adesina, CON, CGH president and chairman, boards of directors, African Development Bank Group. www.afdb.org/en/news-and-events/speeches/advancing-africas-positioning-within-global-development-and-geopolitical-dynamics-lecture-delivered-dr-akinwumi-adesina-con-cgh-president-and-chairman-boards-directors-afdb-group-14th-convocation-ceremony-noun-83103

Alilio, M., Hariharan, N., Lugten, E., Garrison, K., Bright, R., Owembabazi, W., Inyang, U., Hassan, S. E. D., & Saldana, K. (2022). Strategies to promote health system strengthening and global health security at the subnational level in a world changed by COVID-19. *Global Health: Science and Practice*, 10(2), e2100478. https://doi.org/10.9745/GHSP-D-21-00478

Archer, M. (1995). *Realist social theory: The morphogenetic approach*. Cambridge University Press.

Archer, M. S. (2019). Critical realism and concrete utopias. *Journal of Critical Realism*, 18(3), 239–257. https://doi.org/10.1080/14767430.2019.1619428

Baumgartner, F. R., & Jones, B. D. (1991). Agenda dynamics and policy subsystems. *Joournal of Politics*, 53(4), 1044–1074. https://doi.org/10.2307/2131866

Bhaskar, R. (2009). *Scientific realism and human emancipation*. Routledge.

Bhaskar, R. (2016). *Enlightened common sense: The philosophy of critical realism*. Routledge.

Bhaskar, R., & Hartwig, M. (2010). *The formation of critical realism: A personal perspective*. Routledge.

Bump, J. B. (2025). Global health and its limitations: An historical perspective. *Health Systems & Reform*, 11(2), 2478681. https://doi.org/10.1080/23288604.2025.2478681

Chattu, V. K., Knight, W. A., Adisesh, A., Yaya, S., Reddy, K. S., Di Ruggiero, E., Aginam, O., Aslanyan, G., Clarke, M., Massoud, M. R., & Jha, A. (2021). Politics of disease control in Africa and the critical role of global health diplomacy: A systematic review. *Health Promotion Perspectives*, 11(1), 20–31. https://doi.org/10.34172/HPP.2021.04

de Campos-Rudinsky, T. C., Bosha, S. L., Wainstock, D., Sekalala, S., Venkatapuram, S., & Atuire, C. A. (2024). Decolonising global health: Why the new Pandemic Agreement should have included the principle of subsidiarity. *The Lancet Global Health*, 12(7), e1200–e1203. https://doi.org/10.1016/S2214-109X(24)00186-4

Elder-Vass, D. (2022). Ethics and emancipation in action: Concrete utopias. *Journal of Critical Realism*, 21(5), 539–551. https://doi.org/10.1080/14767430.2022.2031789

Evaborhene, N. A., Oga, J., & Udokanma, E. (2025). Africa CDC must become financially independent. *Nature*, 640(8059), 602–602. https://doi.org/10.1038/D41586-025-01201-0

Gedela, K. (2021). Undoing supremacy in global health will require more than decolonisation. *The Lancet*, 397(10279), 1058. https://doi.org/10.1016/S0140-6736(21)00383-4

Gilbert, A., & Sliep, Y. (2009). Reflexivity in the practice of social action: From self-to inter-relational reflexivity. *South African Journal of Psychology*, 39(4), 468–479. https://doi.org/10.1177/008124630903900408

Goodson, N., Wicks, P., Morgan, J., Hashem, L., Callinan, S., & Reites, J. (2022). Opportunities and counterintuitive challenges for decentralized clinical trials to broaden participant inclusion. *NPJ Digital Medicine*, 5(1), 58. https://doi.org/10.1038/S41746-022-00603-Y

Guleid, F. (2025, March 28). Why African health systems cannot simply move on. www.internationalhealthpolicies.org/featured-article/why-african-health-systems-cannot-simply-move-on.

Hirsch, L. A. (2021). Is it possible to decolonise global health institutions? *The Lancet*, 397(10270), 189–190. https://doi.org/10.1016/S0140-6736(20)32763-X

Khan, M., Abimbola, S., Aloudat, T., Capobianco, E., Hawkes, S., & Rahman-Shepherd, A. (2021). Decolonising global health in 2021: a roadmap to move from rhetoric to reform. *BMJ Global Health*, 6(3), e005604. https://doi.org/10.1136/BMJGH-2021-005604

Khan, M. S., Meghani, A., Liverani, M., Roychowdhury, I., & Parkhurst, J. (2018). How do external donors influence national health policy processes? Experiences of domestic policy actors in Cambodia and Pakistan. *Health Policy and Planning*, 33(2), 215–223. https://doi.org/10.1093/HEAPOL/CZX145

Khan, S. A. (2022). Decolonising global health by decolonising academic publishing. *BMJ Global Health*, 7(3), e007811. https://doi.org/10.1136/BMJGH-2021-007811

Kwete, X., Tang, K., Chen, L., Ren, R., Chen, Q., Wu, Z., Cai, Y., & Li, H. (2022). Decolonizing global health: What should be the target of this movement and where does it lead us? *Global Health Research and Policy*, 7(1). https://doi.org/10.1186/s41256-022-00237-3

Lawrence, D. S., & Hirsch, L. A. (2020). Decolonising global health: Transnational research partnerships under the spotlight. *International Health*, 12(6), 518. https://doi.org/10.1093/INTHEALTH/IHAA073

Lindblom, C. E. (1959). The science of "muddling through." *Public Administration Review*, 19(2).

Liwanag, H. J., & Rhule, E. (2021). Dialogical reflexivity towards collective action to transform global health. *BMJ Global Health*, 6(8), e006825. https://doi.org/10.1136/BMJGH-2021-006825

Matolino, B. (2020). Whither epistemic decolonization. *Philosophical Papers*, 49(2), 213–231. https://doi.org/10.1080/05568641.2020.1779605

Mitova, V. (2023). Why epistemic decolonisation in Africa? *Social Epistemology*, 37(6), 739–752. https://doi.org/10.1080/02691728.2023.2184218

Naidu, T., Gingell, G., & Zaidi, Z. (2024). Decolonial framework for applying reflexivity and positionality in global health research. *Global Health Promotion*, 31(2), 52–58. https://doi.org/10.1177/17579759241238016

Nilson, C. (2017). A journey toward cultural competence: The role of researcher reflexivity in indigenous research. *Journal of Transcultural Nursing*, 28(2), 119–127. https://doi.org/10.1177/1043659616642825

Opara, I. N. (2021). It's time to decolonize the decolonization movement. https://speakingofmedicine.plos.org/2021/07/29/its-time-to-decolonize-the-decolonization-movement.

Pai, M. (2022, February 15). Disrupting global health: From allyship to collective liberation. www.forbes.com/sites/madhukarpai/2022/03/15/disrupting-global-health-from-allyship-to-collective-liberation/?sh=1e1bf0ba4e62.

Pai, M., Bandara, S., & Kyobutungi, C. (2024). Shifting power in global health will require leadership by the Global South and allyship by the Global North. *The Lancet*, 404(10464), 1711–1713. https://doi.org/10.1016/S0140-6736(24)02323-7

Posholi, L. (2020). Epistemic decolonization as overcoming the hermeneutical injustice of eurocentrism. *Philosophical Papers*, 49(2), 279–304. https://doi.org/10.1080/05568641.2020.1779604
Russell-Mundine, G. (2012). Reflexivity in indigenous research: Reframing and decolonising research? *Journal of Hospitality and Tourism Management*, 19(1), 85–90. https://doi.org/10.1017/jht.2012.8
Shahjahan, R. A., Estera, A. L., Surla, K. L., & Edwards, K. T. (2022). "Decolonizing" curriculum and pedagogy: A comparative review across disciplines and global higher education contexts. *Review of Educational Research*, 92(1), 73–113. https://doi.org/10.3102/00346543211042423
Sharma, D., & Sam-Agudu, N. A. (2023). Decolonising global health in the Global South by the Global South: Turning the lens inward. *BMJ Global Health*, 8(9), e013696. https://doi.org/10.1136/BMJGH-2023-013696
Sinumvayo, J. P., Munezero, P. C., Tope, A. T., Adeyemo, R. O., Bale, M. I., Nyandwi, J. B., Haakuria, V. M., Mutesa, L., & Adedeji, A. A. (2024). Advancing vaccinology capacity: Education and efforts in vaccine development and manufacturing across Africa. *Vaccines*, 12(7), 741.
Spanaus, E. S., & De Souza, E. L. (2024). Decolonising global health: Clarifying concepts for equitable practice. *Epidemiology & Public Health*, 2(3).
Stilz, A. (2015). Decolonization and self-determination. *Social Philosophy and Policy*, 32(1), 1–24. https://doi.org/10.1017/S0265052515000059
Sultan, N. S. (2020). Self-rule and the problem of peoplehood in colonial India. *American Political Science Review*, 114(1), 81–94. https://doi.org/10.1017/S0003055419000601
Sun, L., Selbie, D., Khan, A. S., Karim, S. S. A., Legido-Quigley, H., Ogunsola, F. T., Eamer, G., Matsoso, M. P., Bausch, D. G., & Fisher, D. (2025). Mobilising national and regional assets and non-state actors for pandemic preparedness. *The Lancet*, 405(10487), 1320–1324. https://doi.org/10.1016/S0140-6736(25)00630-0
Tagoe, N., Abimbola, S., Bilardi, D., Kamuya, D., Gilson, L., Muraya, K., Molyneux, S., & Atuire, C. (2025). Creating different global health futures: mapping the health research ecosystem and taking decolonial action. *BMC Health Services Research*, 25(1), 1–10. https://doi.org/10.1186/S12913-025-12566-3
Táíwò, O. (2022). *Against decolonisation: Taking African agency seriously* (1st ed.). Hurst & Company.
Tangwa, G. B., & Munung, N. S. (2020). COVID-19: Africa's relation with epidemics and some imperative ethics considerations of the moment. *Research Ethics*, 16(3–4), 1–11. https://doi.org/10.1177/1747016120937391
Tobi, A. T. (2020). Towards a plausible account of epistemic decolonisation. *Philosophical Papers*, 49(2), 253–278. https://doi.org/10.1080/05568641.2020.1779602
Tuck, E., & Yang, K. W. (2012). Decolonization is not a metaphor. *Decolonization: Indigeneity, Education & Society*, 1(1), 1–40.
Wilson, M., & Greenhill, A. (2004). Theory and action for emancipation: Elements of a critical realist approach. *Information Systems Research*, 143, 667–674. https://doi.org/10.1007/1-4020-8095-6_42
Wiyeh, A. B., & Mukumbang, F. C. (2025). Global South leaders should strengthen strategic capacity. *The Lancet*, 405(10475), 297. https://doi.org/10.1016/S0140-6736(24)02637-0
World Health Organization. (2023). Health diplomacy. www.emro.who.int/health-topics/health-diplomacy/index.html.
Wright, E. O. (2010). *Envisioning real utopias*. Verso.
Zienkowski, J. (2017). Reflexivity in the transdisciplinary field of critical discourse studies. *Palgrave Communications*, 3(1), 1–12. https://doi.org/10.1057/palcomms.2017.7

Index

For Product Safety Concerns and Information please contact our EU
representative GPSR@taylorandfrancis.com
Taylor & Francis Verlag GmbH, Kaufingerstraße 24, 80331 München, Germany

www.ingramcontent.com/pod-product-compliance
Ingram Content Group UK Ltd.
Pitfield, Milton Keynes, MK11 3LW, UK
UKHW020147200926
475702UK00016B/2590
9781032700779